AGEING AND DEMENTIA: A METHODOLOGICAL APPROACH

AGEING AND DEMENTIA: A METHODOLOGICAL APPROACH

Edited by Alistair Burns (MB, ChB, MRCP,
MRCPsych, MPhil, MD, DHMSA)
Professor of Old Age Psychiatry
University of Manchester, UK

Edward Arnold
A member of the Hodder Headline Group
LONDON   BOSTON   MELBOURNE   AUCKLAND

© Edward Arnold

First published in Great Britain 1993

Distributed in the Americas by Little, Brown and Company,
34 Beacon Street, Boston, MA 02108

British Library Cataloguing in Publication Data

Burns, Alistair S.
  Ageing and Dementia:Methodological
  Approach. – (ACIOG Monographs)
  I. Title II. Series
  618.97

  ISBN 0–340–56838–0

Whilst the advice and information in this book is believed to be
true and accurate at the date of going to press, neither the author
nor the publisher can accept any legal responsibility or liability
for any errors or omissions that may be made. In particular (but
without limiting the generality of the preceding disclaimer) every
effort has been made to check drug dosages; however, it is still
possible that errors have been missed. Furthermore, dosage
schedules are constantly being revised and new side effects
recognized. For these reasons the reader is strongly urged to
consult the drug companies' printed instructions before
administering any of the drugs recommended in this book.

Typeset in 10/11 Melior by Wearset, Boldon, Tyne and Wear
Printed in Great Britain for Edward Arnold, a division of Hodder
Headline PLC, Mill Road, Dunton Green, Sevenoaks, Kent TN13
2YA by St Edmundsbury Press Ltd, Bury St Edmunds, Suffolk
and bound by Hartnolls Ltd, Bodmin, Cornwall.

PREFACE

When I was asked to edit this volume, I hesitated slightly but then realized how useful such a book could be and how I would have welcomed the opportunity to read about similar subjects when I started my research career. I have attempted to include reviews on substantive topics in dementia and ageing but have also tried to select some which may not appear elsewhere. Each contributor was asked to summarize their area of interest both drawing on the literature and, where possible, providing some data to help in the discussion of methods.

I hope the individual chapters complement each other. Clinical subjects cover the diagnosis of dementia from a clinician's perspective, treatment, assessment of non-cognitive features, the natural history of dementia (survival and cognitive decline), neurological signs and associated medical disorders. The investigational techniques of neuropathology, epidemiology, neuroradiology, neuropsychology and molecular biology are discussed. Issues of services for demented individuals and problems in carers are included. I hope this gives an overview of what is an exciting and expanding field.

The contributors have all been diligent and have exhibited patience and understanding of my nagging. I am grateful to Edward Arnold Publishers for their hard work on my behalf and to my secretary, Barbara Woodyatt. The omissions and errors (which every reader will find) are all my own work.

Alistair Burns
Manchester, 1993

CONTENTS

NOTES ON CONTRIBUTORS

Alistair Burns, MB, ChB, MRCP, MRCPsych, MPhil, MD, DHMSA, is Professor of Old Age Psychiatry at the Withington Hospital, Manchester, UK. He trained as an old age psychiatrist at the Maudsley Hospital and Institute of Psychiatry in London and has spent the last eight years mainly in research in old age psychiatry, with a particular interest in Alzheimer's disease. His major research interest is biological aspects of Alzheimer's disease. His published work includes papers on single photon emission tomography and computed tomography, noncognitive features of dementia, survival of patients with Alzheimer's disease, the natural history of Alzheimer's disease and validation of clinical criteria for Alzheimer's disease.

Hans Förstl, MD, MADAC, is Head of the Alzheimer's Disease Research Programme at the Central Institute of Mental Health, Mannheim, Germany. He took his MD in neurophysiology at the Ludwig Maximillians University, Munich in 1982. He was trained in neurology at the Bogenhausen Hospital in Munich and completed his specialization in neuropsychiatry at the Central Institute of Mental Health in 1989. From 1990 to 1992 he participated in several research projects at the Section of Old Age Psychiatry, Institute of Psychiatry in London. His major interests are old age and Sumo wrestling.

Emile H. Franssen, MD, is Assistant Research Professor and Senior Clinical Investigator at the Department of Psychiatry, New York University. He is a neurologist–neuropathologist and psychiatrist by training. Since 1984, when he joined the Ageing and Dementia Research Center at New York University, he has been extensively involved in longitudinal dementia research. His main area of research and field of publication is the neurology of Alzheimer's disease. He is co-author of *Alzheimer's Disease, Broken Connections* Parts I and II.

Walter Hewer, MD, is a Consultant at the Central Institute of Mental Health, Mannheim, Germany. He is in charge of the medical–psychiatric intensive care unit and a day care hospital unit for elderly patients. He is currently carrying out research on the neuropsychological sequelae of diabetes mellitus in the elderly. He has published mainly on problems of medical morbidity and mortality of psychiatric patients.

Alan R. Hipkiss, BSc(Tech), PhD, is a Senior Lecturer in Biochemistry (Molecular Biology and Biophysics Group) at King's College, London. His major research interest concerns the fundamental basis of ageing as expressed at the cellular and molecular levels, and the factors which might regulate them.

Specific topics studied are age-related changes in how cells deal with altered proteins, and the control of nonenzymic glycosylation of proteins by dietary agents. He has many publications on the selective catabolism of altered proteins in mammalian and bacterial cells, and more recently on the relative susceptibility of proteins to oxygen free radical-mediated damage. He also teaches extensively on ageing biology and is an organizer of courses in this area for final year undergraduates at King's College, for the Age Concern Institute of Gerontology MSc in Gerontology, and for the Certificate in Gerontology for extramural students at Birkbeck College.

Tony R.A. Hope, BM, BCH, PhD, MRCPsych, is Leader of the Oxford Skills Project and Honorary Consultant in Psychiatry. His two main research interests are the behaviour of people suffering from dementia and medical ethics. After carrying out basic research on the development of the nervous system he became clinically qualified, specializing in psychiatry. For several years he has been engaged in a study, principally funded by the Medical Research Council, investigating the range of behavioural problems which occur in dementia. He is interested particularly in the rôle that specific brain damage might have in causing particular behavioural difficulties. He has been editorial assistant to the *Journal of Medical Ethics* and two years ago became Leader of the Oxford Practice Skills Project which aims to develop and evaluate a teaching programme for clinical medical students in ethics, communication skills and the law. In addition to papers in his two main fields he has written a textbook of general medicine *The Oxford Handbook of Clinical Medicine* (Oxford University Press, 1993).

Carol Jagger, BSc, MSc, PhD, Hon MFPFM, is a Lecturer in Medical Statistics in the Department of Epidemiology and Public Health, University of Leicester. She has special responsibility for the longitudinal studies of the elderly in Melton Mowbray, Leicestershire from which she has published widely on aspects of the physical and mental functioning and mortality of the elderly. Her current research interests also include measurement of dementia-free life expectancy through her membership of the international network REVES.

Michael D. Kopelman, PhD, FBPsS, FRCPsych, is a Senior Lecturer in Neuropsychiatry and Honorary Consultant Psychiatrist in the Division of Psychiatry at the United Medical and Dental Schools of Guy's and St Thomas's Hospitals, London. He is also a Chartered Psychologist. His major research interests are in organic and psychogenic amnesia, dementia, the psychopharmacology of memory, and other aspects of neuropsychology. He has had publications in *Brain, Neuropsychologia, Journal of Neurology, Neurosurgery and Psychiatry, Psychological Medicine* and the *British Journal of Psychiatry*. He is a member of the Memory Disorders Research Society and a Fellow of the British Psychological Society.

Mony, J. de Leon, BA, MA, MEd, EdD, is Associate Professor of Psychiatry and Director of the Neuroimaging Research Laboratory at the New York University School of Medicine. The laboratory was established in 1976 and is dedicated to structural and functional studies of the ageing human brain. Over 100 publications related to normal ageing and Alzheimer's disease have been generated by the laboratory. Dr de Leon also serves as Research Director of the New York University based Alzheimer's Disease Research Center which is supported by the National Institute of Aging. He is on the editorial board of *Psychiatry*

Research: Neuroimaging and reviews research articles for more than 10 other journals. His current research interests include *in vivo* neuroimaging in the study of diagnostic and predictive markers for pathologic brain ageing.

Enid Levin, BA, DASS, Dip Soc Anth, is a Senior Researcher at the National Institute for Social Work Research Unit. She has a long-standing interest in services for people with dementia and their carers, particularly in their effects upon mental health. She is well known in this area of social policy at a national and international level. Her interests have led her to work with the Alzheimer's Disease Society and Mental Health Foundation.

Glyn Lewis, MA, MsC, PhD, MRCPsych, is a Senior Lecturer in Epidemiology and General Practice at the Institute of Psychiatry and Epidemiology Unit, London School of Hygiene and Tropical Medicine. He has trained in both psychiatry and epidemiology and has an interest in applying epidemiological methods to the major public health problems of psychiatry. His main areas of research include the aetiology of schizophrenia and depression, devising standardized measures of psychiatric disorder and the management of neurotic disorder in primary care using computerized assessments.

James Lindesay, MA, DM, MRCPsych, is Professor of Psychiatry for the Elderly at the University of Leicester. His research interests are in the epidemiology of psychiatric disorders in the elderly population, service evaluation, and neurosis in late life. He has contributed publications to journals and books on these topics, and is co-author of *Delirium in the Elderly*. He is also an Honorary Consultant Psychogeriatrician working to develop psychiatric services for the elderly in Leicester.

Adrienne Little, BA, MPhil, PhD, is a Consultant Clinical Psychologist at the Bethlem Royal Hospital and Maudsley Hospital and an Honorary Senior Lecturer in Clinical Psychology at the Institute of Psychology, London. She is responsible for co-ordinating the clinical psychology services for elderly people at the Institute. She has contributed to several research projects with elderly people with dementia, including clinical drug trials and studies evaluating methods of monitoring and predicting change. Her current research interests are monitoring the impact of packages of care for people with dementia and examining the mental health needs of elderly black people.

Philip J. Luthert, BSc, MB BS, is Senior Lecturer in Neuropathology at the Institute of Psychiatry and Honorary Consultant Neuropathologist to the Bethlem Royal Hospital and Maudsley Hospital. He is primarily interested in mechanisms of neuronal death in neurodegenerative disease and AIDS and in the definition of different types of neurodegenerative disorder including diffuse Lewy body disease and corticobasal degeneration. Other interests include morphometry of the nervous system, particularly in relation to pattern, and the pathology of the blood–brain barrier. He has published widely on these topics.

Joanna Moriarty, BA, RMN, is a Researcher at the National institute for Social Work Research Unit. She has spent the last three years working with Enid Levin on a study looking at the effectiveness of respite services. Previously, she worked on a project examining ways of monitoring patients' views in the National Health Service.

Lorna Morris, MSc, is a Clinical Psychologist with Tunbridge Wells Health Authority. She was previously Higher Scientific Officer at the Medical Research Council Social and Community Psychiatry Unit, Institute of Psychiatry, London. She has published on psychosocial aspects of caring for people with dementia. Her current research interests are the treatment of depressed patients who are vulnerable to repeated episodes of depression because of the quality of their relationships and childhood adversity which they experienced. This research is being conducted in conjunction with Professor Julian Leff and Professor Chris Brewin.

Robin G. Morris, MA, PhD, is a Senior Lecturer in Clinical Psychology at the Institute of Psychology, London. He studied for his MA in Psychology and Physiology at the University of Oxford and his PhD at the Medical Research Council Applied Psychology Unit, Cambridge, UK where he conducted research into the neuropsychology of Alzheimer's disease. Subsequently he conducted post-doctoral studies into cognition and ageing at the University of Toronto and is now Head of the Neuropsychology Unit at the Institute of Psychiatry, London. More recently his research interests have been the neuropsychology of Alzheimer's disease and Parkinson's disease and the neural basis of executive and memory functioning.

Chris Q. Mountjoy, MB, BS, FRCPsych, DPM, is a Consultant Psychiatrist in Geriatric Psychiatry at St Andrew's Hospital, Northampton. Under the direction of Sir Martin Roth at Newcastle and Cambridge, he conducted collaborative studies in clinical and neuropathological changes in dementia and in the development of the CAMDEX schedule. He is joint author of a number of papers on neuropathological changes in dementia and their relationship to clinical and post-mortem biochemical observations.

Adrian M. Owen, BSc, PhD, is a research neuropsychologist and has spent the last five years in the Department of Experimental Psychology, University of Cambridge and at the Institute of Psychiatry, London designing and developing computerized tests of cognitive dysfunction. His research interests include the neuropsychological basis of cognitive deficits in Parkinson's disease and the neuropsychology of frontal lobe function. He has published in both fields. He has recently moved to the Neuropsychological Laboratory at the Montreal Neurological Institute, Canada.

Vikram Patel, MBBS, MSc, MRCPsych, is Beit Research Fellow and Honorary Senior Registrar at the Section of Epidemiology of the Institute of Psychiatry, London. His main research interest is studying traditional models of mental illness and the use of traditional healers in developing countries and he will be shortly beginning a two year field project in Zimbabwe. He arrived in the UK on a Rhodes Scholarship from India and his initial research was in studying aggressive behaviour in people suffering from dementia. He has also worked in Australia and done research in methods of suicide in Sydney.

Chris Q. Mountjoy
St Andrew's Hospital
Northampton

1 AGEING AND DEMENTIA: A NOSOLOGICAL AND NEUROPATHOLOGICAL OVERVIEW

INTRODUCTION

Dementia is the name given to a clinical cluster of symptoms which are the common presentation of many different pathological processes.

In the glossary to the ninth revision of the International Classification of Disease (ICD9), (World Health Organization, 1978) dementia is a clinical diagnosis of organic psychotic states of a chronic or progressive nature which, if untreated are usually irreversible and terminal. DSM-IIIR (American Psychiatric Association, 1987) on the other hand depends on certain clinical symptoms being present and carries no connotation concerning prognosis. Both systems include similar core clinical symptoms, namely impairment of memory, comprehension, orientation, learning capacity and judgement.

The presence of dementia may be evident from clinical examination and investigation of the patient and an account of the development of the illness given by an informant. The presence of dementia may also be inferred from 'dementia scales', usually comprising a short battery of items on orientation for time, place and person, memory and general knowledge (Kahn *et al.*, 1960; Lifschitz, 1960; Blessed *et al.*, 1968; Hodkinson, 1972; Folstein *et al.*, 1975; Pfeiffer, 1975; Jacobs *et al.*, 1977; Pattie and Gilleard, 1979; Katzman *et al.*, 1983; Bickel, 1988).

The type of dementia, may be inferred from scales such as the Hachinski (Hachinski *et al.*, 1975) and standardized diagnostic schedules such as the Geriatric Mental Status Schedule (GMS) (Copeland *et al.*, 1976), CARE (Gurland *et al.*, 1977), SHORTCARE (Gurland *et al.*, 1984), the Cambridge examination for mental disorders of the elderly (CAMDEX) (Roth *et al.*, 1986) or the Canberra Interview for the Elderly (CIE) (Social Psychiatric Research Unit, 1992) and from the results of specialized investigations such as magnetic resonance imaging (MRI) scans and position emission tomography (PET).

However, the diagnosis of the commonest type of primary degenerative dementia, senile dementia of the Alzheimer's type, depends on the exclusion of other causes of dementia because there is no definite investigation at present which allows a diagnosis in life except possibly for brain biopsy. This procedure, to diagnose what is at present an untreatable disease, is hard to justify in spite of the fact that in the Manchester series (Neary *et al.*, 1986) there was no evidence of deterioration as a result of the biopsy.

Most pathological studies have shown senile dementia of the Alzheimer type to be the commonest of the diagnoses made in demented patients (Corsellis, 1962; Tomlinson *et al.*, 1970; Ulrich *et al.*, 1986, Joachim *et al.*, 1988). In a study of 50 autopsies of demented people Tomlinson *et al.* (1970) found

Alzheimer changes in 50% of cases compared with vascular dementias which were found in 17% of cases. Fifteen per cent showed a mixture of vascular and Alzheimer changes. Ten per cent of clinically demented patients were not found to have any characteristic pathological change. This of course could be due to the clinician mistaking cases of pseudo-dementia for dementia, but it could also be due to types of dementia not then identified pathologically.

Yet the changes of Alzheimer's disease are found in normal brains and the difference between these and those of Alzheimer's disease are ones of distribution and quantity. There are four main microscopic abnormalities in the brains of patients suffering from Alzheimer type of pathology:

1. Neuronal loss
2. Large numbers of neuritic plaques
3. Neocortical neurofibrillary tangles
4. Deposition of amyloid.

Neurofibrillary tangles, the characteristic change of the dementia described by Alzheimer with the aid of the then new silver stains, are also found in the normal brain in the hippocampus and parahippocampus with increasing age. Similarly, neuritic plaques, found in profusion in most cases of Alzheimer type dementia are also found in the brains of apparently normal individuals although in smaller numbers. Neuronal loss is found both in normal ageing and in dementia but to a greater extent in dementia (Terry *et al.*, 1981; Mountjoy *et al.*, 1983). The differences between normal ageing and Alzheimer's dementia are differences in distribution, for example in the presence of large numbers of neocortical neurofibrillary tangles in SDAT. Plaques are usually more frequent in dementia than in controls but occasionally nondemented subjects may also have large numbers of plaques. There is no clearly defined and widely agreed cut off point between demented subjects and controls. An attempt to provide tentative recommendations has been suggested (Khachaturian, 1985) which give different criteria for different age groups and by a working party of the Medical Research Council (MRC), (Wilcock *et al.*, 1989).

Amyloid deposition occurs in approximately 30% of normal people. The deposition occurs in the superficial cortex, leptomeninges, in blood vessels and in the cores of senile plaques. It is found in approximately 80% of those suffering from Alzheimer's disease (Esiri and Wilcock, 1986) in a similar distribution. The demonstration that the gene for amyloid formation is located on the long arm of chromosome 21 and the finding of the gene associated with familial Alzheimer's disease was located nearby led to speculation that the two were one in the same. Evidence from Tanzi *et al.* (1988) shows that the genetic defect of familial Alzheimer's disease is not tightly linked to the amyloid beta protein gene.

PROBLEMS OF PATHOLOGY

Post-mortem bias
Most investigations into the differences between normal ageing and dementia have depended on consecutive post-mortem cases and these inevitably are affected by a selection bias. Demented patients with behavioural problems which preclude their management at home are more likely to be admitted to hospital. Post-mortem examinations are more likely to be requested for hospital patients than for those who die in the community and are also more likely to be requested for those patients with features which interested the clinicians.

For research purposes the obvious advantage of using hospital subjects is that they are more easily available for psychological testing and observation of behaviour during life compared with subjects in epidemiological studies who often need to be visited at home. Post-mortem consent is more likely to come from the relatives of patients who have died from a dementia because they are concerned to know the type of dementia and the diagnostic implications it carries for them and their children. However, post-mortem consent may be withheld, so a hospital sample, already biased because the majority of demented patients are cared for at home, becomes even less representative.

Similar but greater problems apply to the collection of 'control' brains from those who die without evidence of neurological or psychiatric disorder: it is easier to obtain brains from those who die in geriatric hospitals rather than from subjects in the community. Further, patients are admitted to hospital because of physical illness which can and does effect any psychological testing that may be undertaken during life and, therefore, these subjects are not true 'normals'. The relatives of 'control' 'normal' patients do not have the same positive incentives to give permission for post-mortem examination as do the relatives of demented patients. Furthermore, the cause of death in 'normals' is more varied than the usual cause of death in dementia, i.e. bronchopneumonia (Tomlinson and Corsellis, 1984; Burns et al., 1990g), and some neuropathological and biochemical measures may be affected by the mode of death. In research 'normal' brains have sometimes been obtained at a post-mortem ordered by the Coroner because the subject has died suddenly and the cause of death is uncertain. These people are more likely to have died from vascular causes, such as myocardial infarction, compared with demented subjects, and their mental and cognitive status during life is unlikely to have been adequately assessed.

TECHNICAL PROBLEMS

Because normals and dements differ only in respect of distribution and frequency of lesions, much effort has been directed to quantification as a method of relating structural changes to psychological deficits. Thus early studies in Newcastle (Blessed et al., 1968) showed a correlation between severity of dementia in life and the average count of plaques made from representative areas in each of the four lobes of the neocortex. It was unusual for demented subjects in that study to have less than 18 plaques per microscopic field. The von Braunmühl silver stain was used. The study implied that there was a threshold of plaque counts above which most cases are demented. However, in serial sections different plaque counts are obtained when different stains are used (Tomlinson and Corsellis, 1984), the distribution of plaques is not evenly spread throughout the cortex and there is, for example, a tendency for greater numbers of plaques to be found at the base of a sulcus (Braak and Braak, 1991).

It is therefore difficult for the investigators to decide on the most typical area of cortex in which to make plaque counts and this may lead to observer bias. The investigator also has to resolve the problem of deciding what constitutes an individual plaque when the packing density is high and the many small plaques appear to coalesce into one large atypical mass.

Traditional silver stains for neurofibrillary tangles are also fickle; minor variations in processing may lead to different counts (Yamamoto and Hirano, 1986). The counting of tangles is tedious and therefore estimates of density have frequently been made (Corsellis, 1962; Mountjoy et al., 1983) rather than the recording of absolute counts of tangles in nucleolated neurons. Such estimates do not allow the question of continuity with normal ageing to be addressed.

PATHOLOGICAL DIAGNOSIS

In the past it was considered sufficient in the absence of other pathology for the diagnosis of Alzheimer's disease to be made if neurofibrillary tangles are found in significant numbers in the neocortex (Tomlinson and Corsellis, 1984), but these pathological rules have changed. For example, Terry et al. (1987) described Alzheimer dementia without tangles but with many plaques.

An American task force (Khachaturian, 1985) decided on the pathological criteria for Alzheimer's disease including criteria for the amount of pathological change required in different age groups. The numbers of plaques and tangles present in each age group seem to have been selected on the basis of opinion rather than on empirical neuropathological studies from representative samples. As already stated, the criteria set for counts may well be affected by the stains and techniques used. Khachaturian allows that in the presence of a positive clinical history of AD these criteria should be revised downwards to an extent that needs to be determined by further research. This caveat is often forgotten and investigators may reject true cases of Alzheimer's disease from a study because insufficient numbers of plaques and tangles were found to meet the published criteria.

The pathological diagnosis of pure Alzheimer disorder also depends on how the neuropathologist chooses to deal with vascular lesions. Tomlinson et al. (1970) found a significant number of normal individuals also had some areas of cerebral softening. It may well be that these individuals would have shown abnormality on exhaustive psychological testing but it does imply that there might be a need for the pathologist to use judgement in deciding on how much vascular change is necessary before a case should be assigned to a vascular or mixed Alzheimer vascular diagnosis. Tomlinson demonstrated a normal distribution of the volume of softening with increased diagnostic probability of vascular dementia if the volume was high. Esiri (1991) writes that it is a matter of judgement to decide whether in any individual case the cerebrovascular lesions contributed to clinical dementia. Depending on the neuropathological opinion a case with a small vascular lesion may be assigned to a 'mixed' Alzheimer vascular diagnosis or accepted as a case of pure Alzheimer's disease.

The advent of new histochemical stains has demonstrated a greater pathological heterogeneity within clinical dementia than had previously been recognized. Now instead of vascular dementia and vascular dementia mixed with Alzheimer's disease as the principal problem of differential diagnosis from Alzheimer's dementia, the new disorders of frontal lobe dementia and of Lewy body disease have been added to the list of common causes of dementia. These new categories may amount to as much as 15% of all post-mortems of clinically demented patients (Perry et al., 1989; Lennox et al., 1989, Perry et al., 1990).

Both of the newly described disorders seem to differ from traditional Alzheimer's disease.

Frontal lobe dementia
Frontal lobe dementia differs pathologically from Alzheimer's disease in having no plaques or tangles, and having severe neuronal loss in the frontal lobe.

In 1987 workers in Sweden reported a longitudinal study of 158 patients suffering from dementia (Gustafson et al., 1987). At post mortem approximately 10% of patients were found to have predominately frontal lobe atrophy caused by neuronal degeneration in the absence of the classical changes of Alzheimer or Pick (Brun, 1987; Englund and Brun, 1987). In life this atrophy had corresponded to measurements of reduced frontal cerebral blood flow (Risberg, 1987). The clinical picture of these cases was also different. The onset of the illness was insidious and was associated with early change in personality, lack of insight, disinhibition and later by stereotopy and increased apathy (Gustafson et al., 1987). There was also a progressive dysphasia ending in mutism, though spatial functions and memory were comparatively spared. Evidence for this type of dementia has also been produced independently in the UK (Neary et al., 1988).

According to Tomlinson (1991) it has long been recognized that Pick inclusions are not always detected in cases of Pick's disease, so it is possible that frontal lobe dementia might be examples of Pick's disease that lack Pick cells or Pick bodies rather than a new syndrome. Whether it is a new syndrome or a variant of Pick's disease, frontal lobe dementia may lead to a faulty clinical diagnosis of Alzheimer's disease.

Lewy Body dementia

The characteristic pathological change in Parkinson's disease is loss of neurons from, and the presence of Lewy bodies in, the substantia nigra. Lewy bodies have been found more frequently in dements of the Alzheimer type than in age matched controls (Gibb et al., 1989).

Perry et al. (1989) described a senile dementia of Lewy body type. The patients with Lewy Body disease do not have as many plaques and tangles as one would find in Alzheimer's disease in its purest form but do have neocortical Lewy body inclusions.

Retrospective clinical examination of the notes of patients with pathologically defined Lewy Body Senile Dementia, showed that these cases compared with Alzheimer cases, were more likely to have presented acutely with confusional states, and showed some fluctuation in the subsequent clinical course, often causing clinicians to make an erroneous diagnosis of vascular dementia. They suffered more frequently from visual hallucinations and transient episodes of loss of consciousness. They had a shorter duration of illness than typical Alzheimer cases and often had severe or fatal neuroleptic sensitivity (McKeith et al., 1992). Perry et al. (1990) estimate that Lewy Body dementia may account for as many as 20% of the hospitalized demented population.

It is probable that such patients are over-represented in post-mortem series because of clinical interest aroused by the patients behavioural problems and the rapid progression of the disease will lead to requests for autopsy.

Lennox et al. (1989) in Nottingham had similar findings. They examined fifteen brains using antiubiquitin staining. This stain is far more reliable in demonstrating Lewy bodies than the traditional haematoylin and eosin stains in which the bodies are hard to identify. The use of this stain may explain why the syndrome was not previously described and may account for some of the clinically demented cases for whom no apparent abnormality was noted at post-mortem. They noted that tangles were rarely seen, while plaques were seen in large numbers in the neocortex. They found that the severity of the dementia related to cortical Lewy body density, whilst subcortical abnormalities made a much less significant contribution. Diffuse Lewy body disease was found in 27% of demented subjects from a consecutive series of 216 post-mortems, and was thus the second commonest cause of dementia.

It is clearly desirable that any clinical study should strive to obtain neuropathological examination of as many cases as possible in order to confirm the diagnosis while recognizing the impurities that may exist within the 'gold standard' of neuropathological diagnosis.

CLINICAL STUDIES

Dementia is a clinical diagnosis and a diagnosis of dementia of Alzheimer type is made by a process of exclusion of other causes (McKhann et al., 1984, Wilcock et al., 1989). Although there are some statistically significant differences between some of the symptoms found in Alzheimer's Disease, Frontal Lobe Dementia and Lewy Body dementia the disorders cannot be separated with assurance on clinical examination alone (Hansen, 1990; Byrne, 1992). Indeed there is wide variation of symptomatology within Alzheimer's disease (Burns et al., 1990b; 1990c; 1990d; 1990e; 1990f).

Criteria for clinical diagnosis are formalized in DSM-IIIR and ICD9; both classifications were codified before the newer forms of dementia were recognized. Because DSM-IIIR does not include the progression of the disorder as part of its diagnosis it is likely to misclassify cases of delirium as dementia. The proposed DSM-IV does take progression into account but abolishes the notion of dementia and refers instead to disorders of cognitive deficit. If adopted there will be a welcome congruence between the American system and ICD-10 classification.

Studies which have used contemporary classifications depend for validation on neuropathological confirmation or on evidence of cognitive decline over time.

In general the clinical classification bears up moderately well to pathological scrutiny, most studies producing an agreement in diagnoses in between 60% and 80% of cases (Tierney et al., 1988; Erkinjuntti et al., 1988a; Joachim et al., 1988). The accuracy of the clinical diagnosis is increased when strict research criteria such as NINCDS/ADRDA (McKhann et al., 1984) are applied (Tierney et al., 1988; Burns et al., 1990a). Homer et al. (1988), showed that a number of patients fully investigated in a leading London teaching hospital had different pathological diagnoses at post mortem. The greatest area of discrepancy was in cases of mixed and vascular dementia. This may in part be a reflection of the way in which vascular dementia was defined pathologically. In the study of Homer and colleagues the presence of any vascular lesion in an Alzheimer brain was regarded as evidence for a pathological diagnosis of mixed dementia.

Other studies have shown that the greatest area of misclassification is for the mixed cases of dementia. Clinicians tend to assign any patient with dementia who also has evidence of vascular disease to the vascular dementia group though pathological examination may show the signs of co-existing Alzheimer change. The problem may arise in reverse when undetected vascular disease is found at post-mortem.

Gilleard et al. (1992) attempted to identify factors which impaired overall diagnostic accuracy but age, comprehensiveness of investigation, severity of dementia and length of delay between investigation and autopsy did not influence diagnostic accuracy.

Evidence of progression of dementia over time has been demonstrated by both the GMS (Copeland et al., 1976) and the CAMDEX (Roth et al., 1986). The

GMS which is a modified version of the Present State Examination (Wing *et al.*, 1974) can be administered by trained lay interviewers and a computer algorithm (AGECAT) is used to make diagnoses.

Because the origin of the GMS lies in the PSE it is particularly useful for the diagnosis of affective disorder and schizophrenic disorders of later life. The absence of an informants interview in its early stages of its development probably detracted from its ability to diagnose dementia. This deficiency has been rectified by the introduction of the HAS (Copeland and Dewey, 1991).

Data can then be collected in an efficient, highly reliable fashion on lap top computers which produce a diagnosis. Follow-up studies provide an important check of validity by showing a deterioration in scores of demented patients over time. For example psychiatrists agreed with AGECAT diagnosis of mild and more advanced dementias in 28 out of 31 patients (Copeland *et al.*, 1988). But in a separate report only six of the 12 subjects diagnosed as mild organic cases using the AGECAT system were rated as demented by psychiatrists 1 year later. Two were judged to be depressed, one schizophrenic and three normal (Copeland *et al.*, 1986). Copeland and colleagues suggested that some of the recovered cases may have been suffering from delirium at the initial interview but the psychiatrists deciding diagnosis were aware of respondents medical and psychiatric histories and took this information into account when making their original decisions.

In a further follow-up Copeland *et al.* (1992) showed a deterioration in the performance of the definite demented cases.

The CAMDEX (Roth *et al.*, 1986) was developed as a schedule designed, to differentiate between dementia and depression. It is therefore less useful than the GMS in diagnosing non-depressive functional disorders. It incorporated an informants interview because this was an important aspect of diagnosis which, at the time CAMDEX was developed, was missing from the GMS.

The CAMDEX is a lengthy interview more useful for research purposes than for routine administration. At present it is not computerized to provide for easy scoring of its diagnostic and severity scales. The CAMCOG examination part of the CAMDEX is a useful short cognitive examination which includes various tests including the MMSE, and some questions from the WAIS. It is a schedule which gives a good clinical 'feel' of a patients abilities, can be administered quickly to normals without giving offence but possibly is too long for moderately severely affected subjects. However, it is the larger number of questions which allows greater flexibility and avoids the problem of ceiling effects of the MMSE. It is of interest that many of the items from the CAMCOG were included in the tests recommended by the MRC Alzheimer's Disease Workshop (Wilcox *et al.*, 1989).

Information concerning the progression of disease and the validity of the CAMDEX are provided from the studies of O'Connor *et al.* (1990, 1991). They reviewed 137 elderly subjects who had been diagnosed as demented using CAMDEX, 38 of the surviving 67 mildly demented respondents were rated identically 1 year later; 25 were rated as moderately or severely impaired; two were graded as minimally demented (both were diabetics whose physical health had improved in the interim) and two were classed as normal; in one case for reasons which remain unclear. Clinical validity seems to be satisfactory though diagnosis was confirmed using identical procedures and was not completely independent. Neither of these studies has had adequate neuropathological studies of the deceased.

Whether such lengthy interviews are necessary is questioned by the recent study by Orrell and colleagues 1992 which compared four rating scales including the MRC test items.

A logistical analysis showed that eight items only were necessary to discriminate between depressed patients and dements and only one of the items was not a memory or orientation test.

DISEASE OR CONTINUUM

To the general public ageing is always associated with some degree of intellectual decline and dementia is regarded as an advanced senility. If dementia is an accelerated form in the ageing process the psychological deficits found in dementia should be similar to those found in normal ageing and the biochemical and pathological changes found in the brains' of clinically demented people should be similar to those found in the brains of very elderly normal people. If on the other hand changes in patterns of behaviour, in biochemistry or in pathology are found which are unique to dementia and related to the severity of the dementia the hypothesis that dementia is an extreme form of ageing can be rejected.

Examples of where a continuum thinking seems more appropriate than the categorical model are hypertension, osteoarthritis, atherosclerosis and possibly senile dementia. The point at which dementia is recognized or diagnosed may well depend on the environment which in the individual exists, on the perceptions of his or her family and by the way in which behaviour and personality changes (Blass and Gibson, 1988).

When changes along such a continuum reach the point when an elderly person or his relatives seek the help of a clinician, it may be appropriate to speak of them as diseased. According to the continuous model, changes along the continuum can be described simply in terms of the degree of change along the continuum and the rate of progression of the change. The greater the change the greater the likelihood of disability; in this model there is no discrete point at which people necessarily move from health to disability as the disease model implies. Perhaps the question should not be whether a subject has a syndrome or not but how much does he have (Rose, 1985).

The view that dementia is a disease that can be distinguished from the normal ageing process has been challenged on the grounds that the scores on cognitive and behavioural scales which act as markers for dementia are distributed in a unimodal fashion in community populations (Brayne and Calloway, 1988). Hofman et al. (1988) disputed this finding on the grounds that the scales used were crude and subject to measurement error which might blur a true bimodality.

The very old
Although the incidence of dementia increases with age there does not seem to be an increase in the incidence of senile dementia in centurians (Hauw, 1986). This conclusion is based on very small samples, biased by their selection criteria that need to be confirmed in larger more representative studies. Similarly normative data on the morphology of the brain is needed for those who are not disabled and die at a very late age. The only way in which these doubts and uncertainties can be addressed is by means of longitudinal studies. Epidemiological prospective longitudinal studies are also needed to collect data on potential risk factors.

Neuropsychological aspects of ageing

Studies which correct for cohort effects generally show far more selective effects of chronological age on mental function than cross sectional studies which do not correct for such confounding variables as education, nutrition and intercurrent disease (Katzman and Terry, 1983). Some generalizations can be made about cognitive function in ageing humans. Judgement and retrieval of learned information tends to be preserved in healthy ageing. Vocabulary, information and comprehension tends to show little decline from the age of 25 to 75 years even in cross-sectional studies. The distribution of vocabulary skills in individuals above 75 years of age tends to be bimodal suggesting that impairments may reflect subclinical disease rather than ageing. Speed and central processing slows with ageing whether measured by such techniques as backward masking or simply by the time required to memorize a list of words. A common problem in ageing is the degeneration of the sense organs with the resulting reduction of sensory information (O'Connor et al., 1989). It is statistically normal for older people to complain about their hearing or vision which is often attributable to disorders such as cataracts or macular degeneration. Sharp cognitive decline has proved to be a good predictor of mortality in older people. This preterminal decline can reflect the sensitivity of the ageing brain to systemic illness as well as the effects of dementing syndromes on mortality. Including data from individuals who died shortly after a study is completed can skew the results of neuropsychological tests of the elderly downwards (Blass and Gibson, 1988). Frank depressive illness is not rare in the elderly; depending on the definition it occurs at some time in 30%. Grief over bereavement or other losses are even more common. Failure to correct for emotional and other motivational factors can skew downwards the results of neuropsychological evaluation in older people.

Alzheimer's disease is associated with deficits in a variety of cognitive functions for example, memory, language, visuospatial abilities. A variety of cognitive and neuropsychological tests have been used as tools for assessing dementia. The present tests are quite good at discriminating between healthy ageing and those with disability due to dementia, especially in the more advanced stages. Studies vary however with respect to the magnitude of the cognitive deficit seen in Alzheimer's disease and different conclusions are drawn as to whether there are quantitative or qualitative differences in cognitive functioning in Alzheimer's disease compared with normal ageing.

Early diagnosis

In order to achieve early diagnosis of dementia it is necessary to develop a means of determining the pre-morbid state in order to identify any decline in the individuals memory or personality. Research should explore a variety of methods for measuring the pre-morbid state in addition to the present common practice of relying on an informant. Individual change in physiological and behavioural functions is important because of variability in the normal pre-morbid state. This makes it impossible to decide on a single threshold value of current function which would apply to all persons. There is an assumption that senile dementia follows a progressive downward course from the mild stage to the severe stage and death. There is a need however for more natural history studies to determine if there are plateaus (Storandt et al., 1988).

It is impossible to decide what if any are the earliest signs and symptoms of dementia unless longitudinal studies are carried out in which a wide range of recordings are made and repeated during life and the brain is examined after death. There is a danger that if the phenomenological net is not cast wide enough at the start of the investigation a huge investment of time and money is wasted because large numbers of subjects are needed to provide a representative sample.

Ante-mortem markers

An ideal diagnostic technique according to Murphy and Sunderland (1990) should include, (1) Specificity with no overlap or misidentification of other sources of dementia, (2) Sensitivity to detect disease in its earlier stages, (3) Ability to find a relation for a progression of the disorder, (4) A relatively noninvasive procedure, (5) Technical reliability and simplicity, (6) Low cost. So far no ante-mortem marker has been found which meets these criteria for identifying cases of Alzheimer's dementia.

Until recently investigations of the cerebrospinal fluid (CSF) failed to produce any promising results either in respect of neurotransmitters or neuropeptides. Van Nostrand et al. (1992) have described decreased levels of soluble amyloid β-protein precursor in the CSF of live Alzheimer patients and more recently Farlow et al. (1992) have produced evidence showing a low concentration of soluble amyloid β-protein precursor in hereditary Alzheimer's disease. Six members of a family affected by presenile Alzheimer's disease associated with a point mutation of the precursor gene were studied. One gene carrier with clinical signs of the disorder had a low CSF concentration of the precursor similar to those of three patients with sporadic Alzheimer's disease subsequently confirmed at post-mortem. Two symptom-free gene carriers had levels similar to those of three nondemented controls, although one of the gene carriers who had deficits on neuropsychological testing had a lower value than the other. The authors conclude that the low concentrations of soluble amyloid precursor proteins in the CSF reflect the process that results in amyloid plaque formation and vascular deposition in Alzheimer's disease. If these results are confirmed in a larger series and are proved to be specific there has clearly been a major advance in the diagnosis of SDAT.

A report by Joachim et al. (1989) that β-amyloid deposition occurs in the skin and intestine of Alzheimer patients has not proved useful in practice because some Alzheimer cases are negative and a proportion of normal elderly controls are positive.

Molecular genetic studies have provided evidence that Alzheimer disease is not a single homogenous disorder (St George-Hyslop et al., 1990). Some early onset familial forms of Alzheimer's disease show linkage with chromosome 21 but others do not. This finding indicates both deviation from normal distribution and heterogeneity within Alzheimer's disease. Late onset cases have not shown such a linkage and appear to be sporadic and it is unlikely that screening will provide a specific test. A claim by Harrington and colleagues (Harrington et al., 1990; Harrington et al., 1991; Mukaetova-Ladinska et al., 1991) that paired helical filaments (PHF) preparations using antibodies directed at different regions of tau have shown a twenty-fold increase in levels of PHF activity in grey matter extracts of Alzheimer's brain compared with extracts from age matched controls is encouraging, but the specificity of the test in differentiating Alzheimer cases from other types of dementia which also have neurofibrillary tangles has yet to be determined.

METHOD OF INVESTIGATION

Research into Alzheimer's disease has been hampered by the absence of a suitable animal model. Recently it seemed that a model has been created by inserting a human gene for beta amyloid protein into transgenic mice. Such mice appeared to produce typical lesions of Alzheimer's disease. Unfortunately experiments of two separate investigators have been found to be flawed and it is not yet known whether the mice who develop the pathological lesions of Alzheimer's disease actually suffer from a failing memory (Cherfas, 1992).

Until an animal model or a biological marker is found Alzheimer's dementia research needs to concentrate on epidemiological samples in order to identify risk factors and the prevalence and incidence of dementia.

Epidemiological studies can either be cross sectional or longitudinal. Cross sectional investigations give information about the prevalence of a disorder and may be carried out by a full investigation of all subjects or by screening to identify likely sufferers and then the examination of the likely sufferers in detail. This is thought to be more economic of time and money.

Longitudinal studies provide cross-sectional information at first and, subsequent follow-up surveys but also give information about the incidence of the disease and clues as to likely risk factors. Risk factors themselves are probably better investigated by means of case controls studies in which subjects with a condition of interest are compared with control subjects in which that condition is absent.

Epidemiological studies may be subject to inaccuracy, the potential for which was demonstrated in the Gospel Oak study (Livingston *et al.*, 1990). It was found that a list of pensioners provided by General Practitioners, Social Service and Community Workers was potentially very inaccurate. A 'door knock' survey of the whole of Gospel Oak revealed that 50% of the pensioners on the final list were different from those on the first list.

The identification of cases may be subject to error especially where screening instruments such as the Mini Mental State Examination (MMSE) are used as the preliminary screening test for identification of cases. Performance on this test is partly determined by educational and cultural background and the scoring of it, as of many other tests, although appearing precise has room for variance on the part of the examiner. Highly educated people with early to moderate levels of intellectual decline will probably score sufficiently highly on a screening instrument to be excluded from a study of dementia though it may be evident to their families that their abilities have deteriorated quite considerably.

Performance on the screening test and on the instruments administered at the time of investigation may be influenced by the patients mental and physical state on that day. For example, depression delirium or just a poor nights sleep may interfere with the patient's ability to cooperate and respond appropriately. This doubtless is the reason why in most epidemiological studies where the subjects have been followed up, there is evidence that some of those diagnosed initially as demented appear to have improved. Because of day to day fluctuations in performance it is extremely valuable to have information from an informant about the patient's previous mental state and of any deterioration that has occurred.

The validity of clinical rating scales has not been satisfactorily confirmed by post-mortem series but may be inferred by the decline in rating scores over time. However, in view of potential pathological heterogeneity it may not give evidence of the type of dementia. Most epidemiological studies depend on the definition of the case either by use of DMS IIIR or ICD 9 or its successor ICD 10. The case is therefore defined as a case because the illness is either present or it is not. If one takes into account the possibility of dementia being an extreme of normal ageing then it is possible that some of the diagnostic features of dementia may be present but insufficient to meet the criteria for DMS IIIR or

ICD 9. Here the AGECAT diagnostic system has an advantage in identifying possible cases as well as definite cases. Most longitudinal studies suffer from the failure to obtain post-mortem consent. Such surveys are difficult to organize and coordinate but until pathological evidence has produced in a representative proportion of these epidemiologically identified cases it will be impossible to be sure that the cases identified were truly cases of Alzheimer's disease.

Longitudinal epidemiological studies such as that conducted by Copeland and colleagues (1992) are able to give figures for the prevalence of organic disorders and for their incidence. In the Liverpool study prevalence figures were 3.8% for moderate and severe cases and the incidence rate, clinically confirmed by six year follow-up was 9.2 per 1000 per year (Alzheimer type 6.3, Vascular 1.9, Alcohol related 1). The expense of running such a community based survey is illustrated by the fact that the initial cohort consisting of 1070 people aged over 65 years yielded only 100 cases diagnosed by the AGECAT programme and only 54 cases judged to be cases of dementia by psychiatrists.

The study was important in drawing attention to the greater number of subjects suffering from depression and anxiety compared with the number of dements and by showing the high mortality rate with those diagnosed as having depression.

Of the original 54 organic cases diagnosed at year one, 5 had recovered and were probably acute confusional states at the time of initial diagnosis. One was depressed and one suffered from mental handicap. There was evidence of progression of the disorder in the remaining cases. The follow-up interview was enhanced by the use of an informant interview which had not been available at the time of the original survey. It is to be expected that this important addition to the schedule will contribute to improved diagnostic capabilities with the AGECAT. Conclusions from individual studies can only give limited information.

If comparable studies are identified the data may be reanalysed using meta-analysis.

Meta-analysis refers to the analysis of analyses. This is a statistical analysis of a large number of analysed results from different studies with the purpose of integrating the findings. It connotes a rigorous alternative to the casual, narrative discussions of research studies which typify attempts to make sense of the rapidly expanding research literature (Glass, 1976). The principal source of error in conducting meta-analyses is failure to include the results of unpublished studies. This is especially true for comparison of drug treatments, as non-significant results are rarely published, but is much less likely to be a factor in the evaluation of epidemiological studies because the large investment of time and money makes it essential to publish results. Meta-analysis may be rendered uninterpretable if 'poorly' designed studies are included with the results with 'good' studies. An incorporation of multiple results from the same study may bias or invalidate the meta-analysis and make the results appear more reliable than they are because the results are not independent (Glass *et al.*, 1981).

Participants in the EURODEM group made available data from their prevalence studies conducted between 1980 and 1990. The data from six suitable studies were subjected to a meta-analysis which showed that prevalence of dementia increased with age and that there was a considerable comparability between studies. Rocca *et al.* (1991a) showed that when age and sex were considered there were no major geographic differences in prevalence of Alzheimer's disease across Europe. Overall European prevalence (per 100 population) for the age groups 30–59, 60–69, 70–79 and 80–89 years was respectively 0.02, 0.3, 3.2 and 10.8. Prevalence increased exponentially with advancing age and, in some populations, was consistently higher in women. In some respects the comparability between different centres was a disadvantage in that it made the ability to tease out environmental factors more difficult.

EURODEM also conducted a series of meta-analyses on potential risk factors in dementia. One (van Duijn *et al.*, 1991) showed that the relative risk of developing Alzheimer's disease was increased by a factor to 3.5 for those with at least one first degree relative with dementia. The more relatives affected the greater the risk. The risk decreased with increasing age though still remained significantly greater than for those without affected relatives. The same paper reported an increased relative risk of developing Alzheimer's disease if there was a family history of Downs Syndrome or Parkinson's disease. Mortimer *et al.* (1991) was able to show that there was an increased relative risk of developing dementia for those patients who had suffered head trauma with loss of consciousness and that increased risk was independent of family history of dementia, of level of education and level of alcohol consumption. Maternal age of 40 years and over carried an increased relative risk for the child (Rocca *et al.*, 1991). Breteler *et al.* (1991) showed no association between neurotropic viruses, allergic conditions, general anaesthesia and blood transfusions and Alzheimer's disease. A history of hypothyroidism and epilepsy within 10 years of the onset of dementia carried an increased risk. Jorm *et al.* (1991) were able to show that a previous history of depression sufficiently severe to require admission to hospital increased the relative risk of developing dementia though exposure to antidepressive drugs did not.

The relative risk of developing Alzheimer's disease was not increased by low, medium of high alcohol intake though smoking reduced the risk and the higher the consumption the lower the risk (Graves *et al.*, 1991a). There was no evidence that occupational exposure to solvents or lead increased the risk of developing dementia (Graves *et al.*, 1991b).

CONCLUSION

Major difficulties of research into dementia have been the way in which samples are collected. There has been a tendency to examine people who are admitted to hospitals, or old people's homes rather than to take a proper epidemiological sample. Even where a sample is properly derived there are great problems in deciding what constitutes early or mild dementia. Biochemical and neuropathological studies of brains have not been based on epidemiological samples and so called control brains have usually been obtained from non-demented patients suffering from other physical diseases who had died in hospital.

Research into the dementias suffers from problems relating to circularity in which the clinical syndrome is defined and redefined and then confirmed by a pathological examination using criteria which also change from time to time. Research into the dementias also suffers because it is relatively rare for clinical studies to be followed to post-mortem or for pathological studies to have good clinical evaluation and investigations obtained from subjects while alive.

The redefinition of clinical diagnostic criteria means that the results of previous work are diminished in importance or totally disregarded by new investigators using the new definitions. Advances in pathological techniques have delineated new diseases and therefore earlier work must be viewed with suspicion or discarded for fear that some of the cases included in those studies though regarded as not absolutely typical at the time of investigation might, with the benefit of new techniques, have been diagnosed as belonging to one of the new syndromes. Studies into phenomenology on a purely clinical basis are suspect without pathological confirmation of diagnosis as are the development of scales of severity and diagnosis. Much has been learnt from cross sectional studies of small groups of patients suffering from Alzheimer's disease. Results to date have not been sufficiencly precise to resolve the question of whether or not Alzheimer type dementia is the end part of a continuum of normal ageing and therefore represents an accelerating form of ageing. The question of whether dementia of Alzheimer's type represents a continuum or a category will be resolved either by the discovery of a specific marker or by evidence of discontinuity in results found in longitudinal studies of aged people who develop dementia. Genetic evidence showing that at least some types of Alzheimer's disease have an hereditary basis with known genetic location, suggests that at least some cases of Alzheimer's disease are distinct from the process of normal ageing.

REFERENCES

American Psychiatric Association (1987). *Diagnostic and Statistical Manual of Mental Disorder*, 3rd edition, revised. American Psychiatric Association, Washington DC.

Bickel, H. (1988). Psychogeriatrisches Screening im Allgemeinkrankenhaus. *Zeitschrift fur Gerontopsychologie und-psychiatrie*, **4**, 259–75.

Blass, J.P. and Gibson, G.E. (1988). Aging and the brain. In *Etiology of Dementia of Alzheimer's Type*. Henderson, A.S., Henderson, J.H. (Eds), pp. 5–17. John Wiley and Sons, Chichester.

Blessed, G., Tomlinson, B.E. and Roth, M. (1968). Association between quantitative measures of dementing and senile change in cerebral grey matter of elderly subjects. *British Journal Psychiatry*, **114**, 797–811.

Braak, H. and Braak, E. (1991). Neuropathological stageing of Alzheimer-related changes. *Acta Neuropathologica*, **82**, 239–59.

Brayne, C. and Calloway, P. (1988). Normal ageing, impaired cognitive function, and senile dementia of the Alzheimer's type: a continuum? *Lancet*, 1265–6.

Breteler, M.M., van Diujn, C.M., Chandra, V. *et al.* (1991). Medical history and the risk of Alzheimer's disease: a collaborative re-analysis of case-control studies, *International Journal of Epidemiology*, **20**, 36–42.

Brun, A. (1987). Frontal lobe degeneration of non-Alzheimer type. I: Neuropathology. *Archives of Gerontology and Geriatrics*, **6**, 193–208.

Burns, A., Luthert, P. and Levy, R. (1990a). Accuracy of clinical diagnosis of Alzheimer's disease. *British Medical Journal*, **301**, 1026.

Burns, A., Jacoby, R. and Levy, R. (1990b). Psychiatric phenomena in Alzheimer's disease. I: Disorders of perception. *British Journal of Psychiatry*, **157**, 72–6.

Burns, A., Jacoby, R. and Levy, R. (1990c). Psychiatric phenomena in Alzheimer's disease. II: Disorders of perception. *British Journal of Psychiatry*, **157**, 76–81.

Burns, A., Jacoby, R. and Levy, R. (1990d). Psychiatric phenomena in Alzheimer's disease. III: Disorders of mood. *British Journal of Psychiatry*, **157**, 81–6.

Burns, A., Jacoby, R. and Levy, R. (1990e). Psychiatric phenomena in Alzheimer's disease. IV: Disorders of behaviour. *British Journal of Psychiatry*, **157**, 86–94.

Burns, A., Jacoby, R. and Levy, R. (1990f). Neurological signs in Alzheimer's disease. *Age and Ageing*, **20**, 45–51.

Burns, A., Jacoby, R., Luthert, P. and Levy, R. (1990g). Cause of death in Alzheimer's disease. *Age and Ageing*, **19**, 341–4.

Byrne, E.J. (1992). Diffuse Lewy body disease. *Recent Advances in Psychogeriatrics*, **4**, 33–43.

Cherfas, J. (1992). Mice found not to have Alzheimer's disease. *British Medical Journal*, **304**, 734–5.

Copeland, J.R.M., Kelleher, M.J., Kellett, J.M. *et al.* (1976). A semi-structured clinical interview for the assessment of diagnosis and mental state in the elderly: the Geriatric Mental Status Schedule. 1: development and reliability. *Psychological Medicine*, **6**, 439–49.

Copeland, J.R.M., McWilliam, C., Dewey, M.E. *et al.* (1986). The early recognition of dementia in the elderly: a preliminary communication about a longitudinal study using the GMS-AGECAT package (community version). *International Journal of Geriatric Psychiatry*, **1**, 63–70.

Copeland, J.R.M., Dewey, M.E., Henderson, A.S. *et al.* (1988). The Geriatric Mental State (GMS): replication studies of the computerised diagnosis AGECAT. *Psychological Medicine*, **18**, 219–23.

Copeland, J.R.M. and Dewey, M.E. (1991). Neuropsychological diagnosis (GMS-HAS-AGECAT package). *International Psychogeriatrics*, **3** (suppl.), 43–9.

Copeland, J.R.M., Davidson, I.A., Dewey, M.E. *et al.* (1992). Alzheimer's Disease, Other Dementias, Depression and Pseudodementia: Prevalence, Incidence and Three-Year Outcome in Liverpool. *British Journal of Psychiatry*, **161**, 230–9.

Corsellis, J.A.N. (1962). Mental illness and the ageing brain. *Oxford University Press*, Oxford.

Englund, E. and Brun, A. (1987). Frontal lobe degeneration of non-Alzheimer type. IV. White matter changes. *Archives of Gerontology Geriatrics*, **6**, 235–43.

Erkinjuntti, T., Haltia, M., Palo, J. *et al.* (1988). Accuracy of the clinical diagnosis of vascular dementia: A prospective clinical and post-mortem neuropathological study. *Journal of Neurology, Neurosurgery and Psychiatry*, **51**, 1027–44.

Esiri, M.M. (1991). Neuropathology. In *Psychiatry in the Elderly*, Jacoby, R. and Oppenheimer, C. (Eds), pp. 113–47. Oxford University Press, Oxford.

Esiri, M.M. and Wilcock, G.K. (1986). Cerebral amyloid angiopathy in dementia and old age. *Journal of Neurology, Neurosurgery and Psychiatry*, **49**, 1221–6.

Farlow, M., Ghetti, B., Benson, M.D. *et al.* (1992). Low cerebrospinal-fluid concentrations of soluble amyloid β-protein precursor in hereditary Alzheimer's disease. *Lancet*, **340**, 453–4.

Folstein, M.F., Folstein, S.E. and McHugh, P.R. (1975). Mini-mental state: a practical method of grading the cognitive state of patients for the clinician. *Journal of Psychiatric Research*, **12**, 189–98.

Gibb, W.R.G., Mountjoy, C.Q., Mann, D.M.A. and Lees, A.J. (1989). A pathological study of the association between Lewy body disease and Alzheimer's disease. *Journal of Neurology, Neurosurgery and Psychiatry*, **52**, 701–8.

Gilleard, C.J., Kellett, J.M., Coles, J.A. *et al.* (1992). The St. George's dementia bed investigation study: a comparison of clinical and pathological diagnosis. *Acta Psychiatrica Scandinavica*, **85**, 264–9.

Glass, G. (1976). Primary, secondary, and meta-analysis of research. *Educational Researcher*, **5**, 3–8.

Glass, G., McGaw, B. and Smith, M.L. (1981). *Meta-Analysis in Social Research*, Sage Publications, Beverly Hills.

Graves, A.B., van Duijn, C.M., Chandra, V. *et al.* (1991a). Alcohol and tobacco consumption as risk factors for Alzheimer's disease: a collaborative re-analysis of case-control studies. EURODEM Risk Factors Research Group *International Journal of Epidemiology*, **20** (Suppl. 2), 48–57.

Graves, A.B., van Duijn, C.M., Chandra, V. *et al.* (1991b). Occupational exposures to solvents and lead as risk factors for Alzheimer's disease: a collaborative re-analysis of case-control studies. EURODEM Risk Factors Research Group *International Journal of Epidemiology*, **20** (Suppl. 2), 58–61.

Gurland, B.J., Kuriansky, J.B., Sharpe, L. *et al.* (1977). The Comprehensive Assessment and Referral Evaluation (CARE)—rationale, development and reliability. *International Journal of Ageing and Human Development*, **8**, 9–42.

Gurland, B.J., Golden, R.R., Teresi, J.A. and Challop, J. (1984). The SHORT-CARE: an efficient instrument for the assessment of depression, dementia and disability. *Journal of Gerontology*, **6**, 209–23.

Gustafson, L. (1987). Frontal lobe degeneration of non-Alzheimer type. II: Clinical picture and differential diagnosis. *Archives of Gerontology and Geriatrics*, **6**, 209–23.

Hachinski, V.C., Iliff, L.D., Zilkha, E. *et al.* (1975). Cerebral blood flow in dementia. *Archives of Neurology*, **32**, 632–7.

Hansen, L., Salmon, D., Galasko, D. *et al.* (1990). The Lewy body variant of Alzheimer's disease a clinical and pathologic entity. *Neurology*, **40**, 1–8.

Harrington, C.R., Edwards, P.C. and Wischik, C.M. (1990). Competitive ELISA for the measurement of tau protein in Alzheimer's disease. *Journal of Immunological Methods*, **134**, 261–71.

Harrington, C.R., Mukaetova-Ladinska, E.B., Hills, R. *et al.* (1991). Measurement of distinct immunochemical presentations of tau protein in Alzheimer's disease. *National Academy of Science U.S.A.*, **88**, 5842–6.

Hauw, J.J., Vignolo, P. Duyckaerts, C. *et al.* (1986). Etude Neuropathologique de 12 centenaires: La fréquence de la démence sénile de type Alzheimer n'est pas particulièrement élevée dans ce groupe de personnes très agées. *Revue Neurologique (Paris)*, **142** (2), 105–15.

Hodkinson, H.M. (1972). Evaluation of a mental test score for assessments of mental impairment in the elderly. *Age and Ageing*, **1**, 233–8.

Hofman, A., van Duijn, C.M. and Rocca, W.A. (1988). Is Alzheimer's disease distinct from normal ageing. *Lancet*, **2**, 226–7.

Homer, A.C., Honovar, M., Lantos, P.L. *et al.* (1988). Diagnosing dementia: Do we get it right? *British Medical Journal*, **296**, 894–6.

Jacobs, J.W., Bernhard, M.R., Delgardo, A. and Strain, J.J. (1977). Screening for organic mental syndromes in the medically ill. *Annals of Internal Medicine*, **86**, 40–6.

Joachim, C.L., Morris, J.H. and Selkoe, D.J. (1988). Clinically Diagnosed Alzheimer's Disease: Autopsy Results in 150 Cases. *Annals of Neurology*, **24**, 50–6.

Joachim, C.L., Morris, J.H. and Selkoe, D.J. (1989). Amyloid-protein deposition in tissues other than brain in Alzheimer's diseases. *Nature*, **341**, 226–30.

Jorm, A.F., van Duijn, C.M., Chandra, V. *et al.* (1991). Psychiatric history and related exposures as risk factors for Alzheimer's disease: a collaborative re-analysis of case-control studies. EURODEM Risk Factors Research Group. *International Journal of Epidemiology*, **20** (Suppl. 2), 43–7.

Kahn, R.L., Goldfarb, A.I., Pollack, M. and Peck, A. (1960). Brief objective measures of the determination of mental status in the elderly. *American Journal of Psychiatry*, **117**, 326–8.

Katzman, R., Brown, T., Fuld, P. *et al.* (1983). Validation of a short orientation-memory-concentration test of cognitive impairment. *American Journal of Psychiatry*, **140**, 734–9.

Katzman, R. and Terry, R. (1983). *The Neurology of Aging*. F.A. Davis Co., Philadelphia.

Khachaturian, Z.S. (1985). Diagnosis of Alzheimer's disease. *Archives of Neurology*, **42**, 1097–105.

Lennox, G., Lowe, J., Landon, M. *et al.* (1989). Diffuse Lewy body disease: correlative neuropathology using anti-ubiquitin immunocytochemistry. *Journal of Neurology, Neurosurgery and Psychiatry*, **52**, 1236–47.

Livingston, G., Hawkins, A., Graham, N. *et al.* (1990). The Gospel Oak Study: prevalence rates of dementia, depression and activity limitation among elderly residents in inner London. *Psychological Medicine*, **20**, 137–46.

Lifschitz, K. (1960). Problems in the quantitative evaluation of patients with psychoses of the senium. *Journal of Psychiatry*, **49**, 295–303.

McKeith, I., Fairbairn, A., Perry, R. *et al.* (1992). Neuroleptic sensitivity in patients with senile dementia of Lewy body type. *British Medical Journal*, **305**, 673–8.

McKhann, G., Drachman, D., Folstein, M. *et al.* (1984). Clinical diagnosis of Alzheimer's disease: Report of the NINCDS-ADRDA Work Group under the auspices of Department of Health and Human Services Task Force on Alzheimer's Disease. *Neurology*, **34**, 939–41.

Mortimer, J.A., van Duijn, C.M., Chandra, V. *et al.* (1991). Head trauma as a risk factor for Alzheimer's disease: a collaborative re-analysis of case-control studies. EURODEM Risk Factors Research Group. *International Journal of Epidemiology*, **20** (Suppl. 2), 28–35.

Mountjoy, C.Q., Roth, M., Evans, N.J.R. and Evans, H.M. (1983). Cortical neuronal counts in normal elderly controls and demented patients. *Neurobiology of Ageing*, **4**, 1–11.

Mukaetova-Ladinska, E.B., Harrington, C.R., Hills, R. *et al.* (1991). Regional Distribution of Paired Helical Filaments and Normal Tau Proteins in Aging and in Alzheimer's Disease with and without Occipital Lobe involvement. *Dementia*, **101**, 1–14.

Murphy, D.L., Sunderland, T. (1990). The need for early markers in Alzheimer's disease. *Dostert, R, Riederer, P, Strolin Benedetti M, Ronucci R (eds). Early markers in Parkinson's and Alzheimer's diseases*, Springer-Verlag, Wien, pp. 137–46.

Neary, D., Snowden, J.S., Bowen, D.M. *et al.* (1986). Cerebral biopsy in the investigation of presenile dementia due to cerebral atrophy. *Journal of Neurology, Neurosurgery and Psychiatry*, **49**, 157–62.

Neary, D., Snowden, J.S., Northen, B. and Goulding, P. (1988). Dementia of frontal lobe type. *Journal of Neurology, Neurosurgery and Psychiatry*, **51**, 353–61.

O'Connor, D.W., Pollitt, P.A., Brook, C.P.B. and Reiss, B.B. (1989). A community survey of mental and physical infirmity in nonagenarians. *Age & Ageing*, **18**, 411–14.

O'Connor, D.W., Pollitt, P.A., Hyde, J.B. *et al.* (1990). A follow-up study of dementia diagnosed in the community using the Cambridge Mental Disorders of the Elderly Examination. *Acta Psychiatrica Scandinavica*, **81**, 78–82.

O'Connor, D.W., Pollitt, P.A., Hyde, J.B. *et al.* (1991). The progression of mild idiopathic dementia in a community population. *Journal of the American Geriatrics Society*, **39**, 246–51.

Orrell, M., Howard, R., Payne, A. *et al.* (1992). Differentiation between organic and functional psychiatric illness in the elderly: An evaluation of four cognitive tests. *International Journal of Geriatric Psychiatry*, **7**, 263–75.

Pattie, A.H. and Gilliard, C.J. (1979). *Manual of the Clifton Assessment procedures for the elderly*. Hodder and Stoughton, London.

Perry, R.H., Irving, D., Blessed, G. *et al.* (1989). Clinically and Neuropathologically distinct forms of dementia in the elderly. *Lancet*, **i**, 166.

Perry, R.H., Irving, D., Blessed, G. *et al.* (1990). Senile dementia of Lewy body type. A clinically and neuropathologically distinct form of Lewy body dementia in the elderly. *Journal of the Neurological Sciences*, **95**, 119–39.

Pfeiffer, E. (1975). A short portable mental status questionnaire for the assessment of organic brain deficit in elderly patients. *Journal of the American Geriatrics Society*, **23**, 433–41.

Risberg, J. (1987). Frontal lobe degeneration of non-Alzheimer type III. Regional cerebral blood flow. *Archives of Gerontology and Geriatrics*, **6**, 225–33.

Rocca, W.A., Hofman, A., Brayne, C. *et al.* (1991a). The prevalence of vascular dementia in Europe: facts and fragments from 1980–1990 studies. EURODEM Prevalence Research Group. *Annals of Neurology*, **30** (6), 817–24.

Rocca, W.A., van Duijn, C.M., Clayton, D. *et al.* (1991). Maternal age and Alzheimer's disease: a collaborative re-analysis of case-control studies. EURODEM Risk Factors Research Group. *International Journal of Epidemiology*, **20** (Suppl. 2), 21–7.

Rose, G. (1985). Sick individuals and sick populations. *International Journal of Epidermiology*, **14**, 32–9.

Roth, M., Tym, E., Mountjoy, C.Q. *et al.* (1986). CAMDEX: A standardized instrument for the diagnosis of mental disorder in the elderly, with special reference to the early detection of dementia. *British Journal of Psychiatry*, **149**, 698–709.

Social Psychiatry Research Unit, National Health and Medical Research Council, Australian National University (1992). The Canberra Interview for the Elderly: a new field instrument for the diagnosis of dementia and depression by ICD-10 and DSM-III-R, *Acta Psychiatrica Scandinavica*, **85**, 105–13.

St George-Hyslop, P.H., Haines, J.L. Farrer, L.A. *et al.* (1990). Genetic linkage studies suggest that Alzheimer's disease is not a single homogeneous disorder. *Nature*, **347**, 194–7.

Storandt, M., Aufdembrinke, B. *et al.* (1988). Group report relationship of normal aging and dementing diseases in later life. In *Etiology of Dementia of Alzheimer's Type*, Henderson, A.S. and Henderson, J.H. (Eds), pp. 231–9. John Wiley and Sons, Chichester.

Tanzi, R.E., McClatchey, A.I., Lamberti, E.D. *et al.* (1988). Protease inhibitor domain encoded by an amyloid protein precursor MRNA associated with Alzheimer's disease. *Nature*, **331**, 528–30.

Terry, R.D., Peck, A., DeTeresa, R. and Schechter, R. (1981). Some morphometric aspects of the brain in senile dementia of the Alzheimer type, *Annals of Neurology*, **10**, 184–92.

Terry, R.D., Lawrence, M.D., Hansen, A. *et al.* (1987). Senile dementia of the Alzheimer type without neocortical neurofibrillary tangles. *Journal of Neuropathology and Experimental Neurology*, **46**, 262–8.

Tierney, M.C., Fisher, R.H., Lewis, A.J. *et al.* (1988). The NINCDS-ADRDA A work group criteria for the clinical diagnosis of probable Alzheimer's disease: A clinicopathological study of 57 cases. *Neurology*, **38**, 359–64.

Tomlinson, B.E., Blessed, G., Roth, M. (1970). Observations on the Brains of Demented Old People. *Journal of the Neurological Sciences*, **11**, 205–42.

Tomlinson, B.E., Corsellis, J.A.N. (1984). Ageing and the dementias. In *Greenfield's Neuropathology* (4th Edition). Hume-Adams, J., Corsellis, J.A.N. and Duchen L.W. (Eds). Edward Arnold, London.

Tomlinson, B.E. (1991). Ageing and the dementias. In *Greenfield's Neuropathology* (5th Edition). Hume-Adams, J. and Duchen, L.W. (Eds). Edward Arnold, London. 1284–410.

Ulrich, J., Probst, A., Wüest, M. (1986). The brain diseases causing senile dementia. A morphological study on 54 consecutive autopsy cases. *Journal of Neurology*, **233**, 118–22.

van Duijn, C.M., Clayton, D., Chandra, V. *et al.* (1991). Familial aggregation of Alzheimer's disease and related disorders: a collaborative re-analysis of case-control studies. EURODEM Risk Factors Research Group. *International Journal of Epidemiology*, **20** (Suppl. 2), 13–20.

van Nostrand, W.E., Wagner, S.L., Shankel, W.R. *et al.* (1992). Decreased levels of soluble amyloid B-protein precursor in cerebral spinal fluid of live Alzheimer disease patients. *Proceedings of the National Academy of Science USA*, **89**, 2251 5.

Wilcock, G.K., Hope, R.A., Brooks, D.N. *et al.* (1989). Recommended minimum data to be collected in research studies on Alzheimer's disease. *Journal of Neurology, Neurosurgery and Psychiatry*, **52**, 693–700.

Wing, J.K., Cooper, J.E. and Sartorius, N. (1974). *The measurement and classification of psychiatric symptoms*. Cambridge University Press, Cambridge.

World Health Organization (1978). *Mental disorders: glossary and guide to their classification in accordance with the ninth revision of the International Classification of Diseases*. World Health Organization, Geneva.

Yamamoto, T. and Hirano, A. (1986). A comparative study of modified Bielschowsky, Bodian and thioflavin S stains on Alzheimer's neurofibrillary tangles. *Neuropathology and Applied Neurobiology*, **12**, 3–9.

Alan R. Hipkiss

Division of Biomedical Sciences
King's College London

2 MOLECULAR GERONTOLOGY: UNDERSTANDING THE MECHANISMS OF AGEING

INTRODUCTION

The phenomenon of ageing is almost universal, occurring in all higher animals, some plants and even some microorganisms. Ageing is manifested as deleterious changes with respect to time which ultimately result in death of the organism. When the physiology of ageing animals is examined a decline in functional efficiency in virtually all areas is observed. For example, changes in the muscular, skeletal, endocrine, reproductive, immune and neurological systems are found from mice to humans. The timing of these events is particularly interesting. In each species the initiation of the decline in the various physiological functions appears to be more or less coincident; for example, in humans this appears to be in the fourth decade of life whereas in rodents the decline starts in less than one year. It is possible to see some physiological rationale behind these timings, which appears to be the time required for progeny to be independently capable of breeding and raising young. One is then led to the questions: (a) what are the processes which prevent the decline in physiological efficiency prior to the age-related onset? and (b) what factors are responsible for the thirty-fold delay in age-related physiological decline when humans and mice are compared? This is effectively a restatement of Leonard Hayflick's (1987) observations on the approach to obtaining an understanding of ageing: ' "Why do we age?" may be the wrong question. The right question may be "Why do we live as long as we do?" '. In this account of the possible bases of ageing it is proposed that living is dangerous even at the molecular level; sooner or later, depending on the species, changes occur that affect the structure and function of cellular macromolecules that in turn compromise physiological activity and are ultimately responsible for the finitude of the individual.

The cause of ageing is still debated. Fundamentally most arguments about ageing centre on whether it is a deterministic or nondeterministic process. It has been proposed that ageing is specifically determined genetically. This implies the existence of specific genes, whose activities are expressed only at the latter part of the animal's life, to induce the onset of senescence and death. Genes which specify cell death have been clearly detected in model systems, and mutations in them can delay or prevent degeneration of the appropriate cells (Driscoll and Chalfie; Raff, 1992). However, developmentally associated cell death (apoptosis) is different from the necrosis-type death which usually accompanies ageing. There are strong evolutionary arguments against the idea of specific ageing-inducing genes. In the wild most animals live for only about one-third of the life-span observed in captivity, with death occurring from predation, starvation and disease. Therefore, because the vast majority of animals do not survive in the wild to remotely close to their maximum life-span, it is difficult to envisage the selection of a gene or genes to induce specific ageing events which are only expressed when the organism is old. However, to suggest that the existence of specific ageing genes is unlikely is not to deny a genetic component to ageing. Clearly the maximum life-span of an organism is genetically determined, and the onset of age-related changes in physiology is genetically controlled, as shown specifically by the progeroid syndromes. It is more likely that the roles of such genes would be to delay the onset of ageing rather than provoke it, and mutations in them result in early or premature senescence. It is the author's opinion that ageing is more likely the result of the deleterious effects of a number of processes, endogenous and exogenous in origin, which ultimately compromise the systems which maintain cellular and molecular integrity. Genes which affect the timing of onset of ageing and senescence might be called longevity assurance genes whose functions may control directly or indirectly the cellular ability to resist insults. The effects of such genes are seen when humans and mice are compared; both show similar age-related changes such as atherosclerotic conditions, tumour incidence and cataracts, but these phenomena are delayed for at least thirty times longer in humans than in mice. Identification of longevity assurance genes and their regulation may be fundamental to our understanding of ageing in general and possibly to the control of the onset of specific age-related pathologies.

Maintenance of molecular integrity (i.e. molecular homeostasis) is important for effective and efficient cell function, and processes which compromise homeostatic function contribute significantly to the ageing 'process' (better stated as 'processes'). In this review some of the agents or events which contribute to molecular instability, together with the genes and enzymes thought to control them, will be discussed. It will be argued that a major function of the proposed longevity assurance genes is associated with maintenance of molecular integrity.

SOURCES OF MOLECULAR INSTABILITY

The processes of ageing are multifactorial in origin. Changes to the genetic material and the major structural and catalytic elements in the cell derive from endogenous and exogenous events. Neither DNA nor proteins are chemically stable even in the absence of exogenous factors. In addition there are the hazardous effects of environmental agents such as toxins, mutagens, and ultraviolet (UV) and ionizing radiations, as well as the deleterious actions of normal cellular metabolites (oxygen, glucose and other sugars).

Spontaneous changes in DNA
The ends of chromosomal DNA usually consist of tandem telomeric repeats, TTAGGG, which protect the DNA ends from recombination and allow the chromosomal length to be maintained. The telomere repeats are attached by the enzyme telomerase. In human somatic cells telomeric repeats are lost at a rate of 10–80 base-pairs per year during *in vivo* ageing (Harley, 1991). Cultured human fibroblasts lose telomeres at rates between 50 and 200 base-pairs per cell doubling. The chromosomes from premature ageing syndromes such as progeria possess shorter telomeres. The mechanism by which the telomeres are lost and the processes which regulate telomerase are not understood. However, the gradual shortening of average chromosomal DNA length could conceivably

increase the probability of dysfunction, especially of any DNA coding for regulatory genes present towards the end of the DNA molecules.

Mammalian DNA is enzymically methylated at about 5% of its cytosine residues. It is thought that such modifications are important for gene regulation in that methylation of specific CG sequences inhibits gene expression. Both *in vivo* and *in vitro* studies suggest that there is a decline in the percentage of methylated cytosines with age (Vincent *et al.*, 1987). In cultured fibroblasts the loss of methyl groups from DNA is associated with cell division rather than elapsed time, and decreases between 10 and 19% have been detected in heart and intestine. Whilst the mechanisms by which the losses occur are unknown, this partial or complete failure of epigenetic control may explain the examples of inappropriate gene expression seen in ageing cells.

The glycosidic bond which links purines to deoxyribose in DNA is somewhat unstable leading to the spontaneous generation of apurinic sites in DNA (Lindahl and Nyberg, 1972; Setlow, 1987). Loss of pyrimidines, though not unknown, is less frequent because of the greater stability of the pyrimidine–deoxyribose bond. The products, apurinic and apyrimidinic sites (collectivelly called AP sites) create noncoding changes in DNA and the potential for cross-linking between the aldehyde function of the sugar and an adjacent amino group deriving from either DNA or protein. Such cross-links are deleterious to chromosomal function.

The bases containing amino groups (cytosine, adenine and guanine) can spontaneously deaminate to uracil, hypoxanthine and xanthine, respectively (Lindahl and Nyberg, 1972; Setlow, 1987). The presence of latter bases is recognized by specific glycosylases which cleave them out to generate AP sites. Another spontaneous alteration to a DNA base is the formation of O^6-methylguanine following its reaction with S-adenosylmethionine. Again a specific glycosylase is thought to cleave out the modified base to yield an AP site. Single strand breaks in the DNA are also formed but their origin is unclear, although they could be related to the presence of AP sites (above) in the DNA and the lability of the phosphodiester bond to cleavage by a β-elimination process following loss of the base from deoxyribose. Estimates of the occurrence of such processes suggest that each cell has to content with 580 depurinations, eight cytosine deaminations, 130 O^6-methylguanines and 2300 single strand breaks per hour at 37°C (Saul *et al.*, 1987).

DNA damage induced by endogenous and exogenous agents
Not only is DNA intrinsically unstable (above) but it is also subject to attack by a variety of insults. Agents which damage DNA include environmentally derived toxins and mutagens, the byproducts of oxygen metabolism and deleterious interaction with normal constituents of the cell (e.g. reducing sugars).

A major source of DNA damage results from the effects of oxygen free radicals. Such radical species are formed from the incomplete reduction of oxygen to produce a number of species including superoxide and hydroxyl radicals, the latter being particularly reactive. Over 50 different products of oxygen free-radical damage to DNA have been detected (Halliwell and Aruoma, 1991), including cytosine and thymine glycols, 5-hydroxymethyluracil, 8-hydroxyadenine and 8-hydroxyguanine. Ring cleavage can also occur resulting in the generation of 4,6-diamino-5-formamido-pyrimidine and 2,6-diamino-4-hydroxy-5-formamidopyrimidine from adenine and guanine, respectively. The deoxyribose is also subject to oxygen free-radical damage. Many of these products have also been isolated from human urine and, assuming that they are not of dietary origin, calculations show that there are at least 1000 oxygen free-radical-mediated DNA-damaging events per cell per day (Saul *et al.*, 1987). Excretion of thymine glycol corresponds to oxygen consumption rates in animal studies. It should be noted that much of the DNA damage caused by UV and ionizing irradiation involves formation of oxygen free radicals. The most frequently investigated products of UV-mediated DNA damage are thymine dimers; thymine–cytosine and cytosine dimers can also be formed. Formation of such photoproducts may play a role in ageing of tissues normally exposed to UV irradiation as shown by the increased tumour incidence in xeroderma pigmentosum patients who are genetically deficient for an enzyme involved in excision repair of the damaged DNA. However, such patients do not show premature ageing of internal tissues.

Another form of DNA damage induced by oxygen free radical attack is the formation of DNA–protein cross-links (Nackerdien *et al.*, 1991). Model studies show that exposure of chromatin to hydrogen peroxide and copper or iron ions promotes the production cross-links between thymine and tyrosine residues. Interestingly the presence of ascorbic acid (vitamin C) increases the yield of the cross-linked material probably by reducing the divalent copper ions back to the monovalent form to maintain production of hydroxyl radicals. Thymine–lysine cross-links have also been identified. Ascorbic acid may also promote cleavage of phosphodiester bonds in DNA, illustrating that many anti-oxidants can also behave as pro-oxidants.

The subcellular location of the DNA is important when considering oxygen free-radical-mediated damage. DNA is found in mitochondria as well as the nucleus. Mitochondria are the organelles intimately associated with oxygen metabolism, that is, its step-wise reduction to water, and are therefore a likely source of free radicals because about 1% of the electron flux along the electron transport chain are thought to generate incompletely reduced oxygen molecules. Studies show that the frequency of 8-hydroxyguanosine, a product of free-radical-mediated damage, is sixteen times greater in mitochondrial DNA than nuclear DNA (1/8000 compared to 1/130 000) (Richter *et al.*, 1988). This implies either a great hit frequency or a lower repair function, or both, in the mitochondrial DNA compared to that in the nucleus. In the ageing rat mitochondrial 8-hydroxyguanosine increases a further three-fold in liver, kidney and intestine, but not in the brain or testes. The explanation for the tissue differences is not understood.

Another form of DNA damage found in mitochondrial DNA are specific mutations and/or deletions which usually accompany rare neuromuscular diseases such as myoclonic epilepsy and ragged red fibre syndrome and Parkinson's disease. Using polymerase chain reaction (PCR) technology as an amplification process, it has recently been shown that certain specified deletions accumulate with age in nondividing tissues but not in dividing tissues (Yen *et al.* 1991; Bittles, 1992). Brain and heart, which have high and absolute oxygen demands, accumulated the deletion to the greatest extent. The incidence ranges from 0.1 to 0.5% in old human brain, but the deletion is not found in foetal tissue. The presence of the deletion also varies in different parts of the brain, most being present in the basal ganglia. It has been suggested that other deletions may also be present such that the brain may possess a mosaic of mitochondrial DNAs. However, the biological significance of these studies remain in doubt because, as yet, less than 1% of the mitochondria have been shown to possess DNA with deletions. This implies that the remaining 99% of the mitochondria contain complete copies of the DNA and therefore any general effects on cellular adenosine triphosphate (ATP) synthesis are unlikely, especially as there are in excess of 1000 mitochondria per cell.

Control of DNA damage

Many of the events which deleteriously modify DNA are mediated by the action of oxygen free radicals, frequently thought to be hydroxyl radicals. It appears that two strategies have evolved as defence mechanisms: anti-oxidant agents and enzymes which remove the damaging species prior to interaction with polynucleotides, and the specific repair of the damaged DNA. A number of general anti-oxidants have been identified such as vitamins A, C and E, uric acid and carnosine, all of which have been claimed to decrease oxygen free-radical-mediated damage. However, it should be remembered that many anti-oxidants are also pro-oxidants in appropriate circumstances and could be another causative factor of, or contributory to, some types of radical-mediated damage. For example, ascorbic acid can increase the rate of hydroxyl radical damage to DNA (see above). The major anti-oxidant enzymes are superoxide dismutase (SOD), peroxidase and catalase; SOD converts the superoxide radical to hydrogen peroxide while the other enzymes convert hydrogen peroxide to water and oxygen. It appears important that such enzymes are present at appropriate activities as hydrogen peroxide is potentially more destructive than superoxide. The presence of copper or iron ions can provoke formation of highly reactive hydroxyl radicals from hydrogen peroxide via Fenton chemistry. Thus microorganisms genetically engineered to synthesize high levels of superoxide dismutase show increased mutation frequencies (Scott *et al.*, 1987; Yarom *et al.* 1988).

The second line of defence is to eliminate the affected region from the DNA should any of the changes outlined above occur. Should a base become modified, a base excision repair will first remove the changed base and then excise the section of the polynucleotide strand. There are a number of specific glycosylases which recognize the presence of damaged or modified bases in DNA. For example, there is a specific enzyme which detects the presence of uracil arising as a result of deamination of cytosine. This and other glycosylases cleave the glycosidic bond between the damaged base and deoxyribose to leave an apurinic or apyrimidinic (AP) site. Cleavage of the phosphodiester bonds either side of the AP then occurs somewhat analogous to excision repair in response to formation of thymine dimers following UV irradiation, i.e. eight nucleotides from the 5' side of the damaged site and four nucleotides from the 3' side to release a 13 nucleotide fragment. A replacement segment of DNA is then synthesized complementary to the opposite strand. Although the enzymes for excision repair of thymine dimers have been characterized, specific enzymes in repair of AP sites have yet to be identified.

Generally the enzymology of DNA repair in mammalian cells is not well advanced. In fact the best characterized eukaryotic DNA repair system is found in yeast, and homologous enzymes have been identified in mammalian and human cells. For example, the yeast RAD 14 protein is thought to be analogous to enzyme which is responsible for the defect in excision repair in xeroderma pigmentosum group A patients, while the yeast RAD 4 protein appears to be analogous to the absent activity in xeroderma pigmentosum group C (Bankmann *et al.*, 1992; Barnes, 1992; Legerski and Peterson, 1992). Other human genes thought to be important in DNA repair called Excision Repair Cross Complementary (ERCC) genes have yeast equivalents. It is in the lower eukaryote where the details of the repair processes will be elucidated, especially given the availability of repair mutants and recombinant DNA technology to restore effective function. That DNA repair may be important in ageing is suggested by the example of the ERCC-3 gene product. This protein, which has a yeast homologue, is thought to be defective in Cockayne's syndrome where there is a defect in repair of damaged DNA in active genes. Cockayne's syndrome is regarded as a form of premature ageing, and gives rise to neurodegeneration.

There has been much discussion as to whether DNA repair activity is affected by ageing and whether clear species (life-span) differences can be detected. Essentially the jury is still to report on the verdict as claims for and against such propositions have been reported. The reader is directed to Warner *et al.* (1987), pp. 183–98 for a clear discussion. See also Kirkwood (1989).

Poly(ADP-ribose)

Intracellular production of poly(ADP-ribose) from nicotinamide adenine dinucleotide (NAD^+) is induced by agents that generate strand interruptions in DNA. Poly-ADP ribosylation of proteins is restricted to the nucleus and is thought to be required for DNA repair, perhaps by way of a nick-protection mechanism to prevent formation of chromosomal aberrations or initiation of DNA synthesis before repair (Satoh and Lindahl, 1992). The capacity to synthesize poly(ADP-ribose) appears to decrease with animal age in rats and the poly(ADP-ribose) transferase activity is linearly related to animal maximum life-span (Dell'Orco and Anderson, 1991).

LIPIDS AND AGEING

Lipids present in cell membranes are thought to be potential sites of oxygen free-radical-mediated damage. Polyunsaturated fatty acids (those containing double bonds) are especially prone to attack leading to the formation of lipid peroxides and propagation of chain reactions promoting oxidation and cross-linking to other molecules (Harman, 1984). Should these events occur in cell membranes changes in function would result leading to cell lysis and death. Paradoxically, however, it is thought that saturated lipids, though less likely to be targets for free-radical attack, promote formation of atheroma and consequent atherosclerosis, a major age-related disease.

Lipofuscin, the so-called age pigment which accumulates with age in muscle and nerve cells, is thought to derive, at least in part, from oxidatively damaged cellular lipids cross-linked to proteins (Poot, 1991). Despite the fact that lipofuscin was identified many decades ago, relatively little is known about its molecular origin or whether it is deleterious to cell function.

Mitochondria are intimately associated with oxygen, possess considerable amounts of lipid and have therefore been thought to play a major or causal role in cellular ageing. Model studies in mitochondria have shown that hyperoxides (e.g. tertiary-butyl hydroperoxide) cause changes in calcium flux, electron transport and membrane polarization, and initiate mitochondrial lipid peroxidation. It is also thought that efficient anti-oxidant systems would protect cells against free-radical-induced lipid damage (Harman, 1984; Poot, 1991). However, much of the recent studies by the proponents of the free-radical theory of ageing have tended to neglect lipid damage concentrating instead on effects on DNA and proteins.

PROTEINS AND AGEING

As mentioned in the introduction to this chapter, proteins, the major structural components of cells as well as catalytic agents, also undergo changes with time. Like those occurring in DNA the sources of such change are the results of exogenous insults and endogenous instability. It is essential that the sources and consequences of alteration of protein structure be considered because the most common feature of ageing cells and tissues is the accumulation of altered proteins (Adelman and Dekker, 1985; Rosenberger, 1991).

Spontaneous changes in proteins

Denaturation

The function of a protein, whether structural or catalytic, is determined by its shape. Therefore, any process which alters the shape of a protein may affect its function; frequently the extent to which a protein's action is changed is a reflection of the degree to which its structure is perturbed. Some mutant proteins appear to produce no deleterious effects whereas others can be fatal to the organism. However, mutation is not the major source of alteration in protein structure as mutation rates are surprisingly low (about 1 in 10^9) which is testament to the efficacy of the DNA repair mechanisms. Most of alterations to proteins, many of which accumulate with age, are the results of changes at the postsynthetic level. Protein denaturation involves a change in the macro-molecule's shape through the action of physical (e.g. temperature or pH changes) or chemical (e.g. detergents, heavy metals) agents such that it becomes biologically nonfunctional. It should be remembered that a protein's structure is not fixed but subject to changes due to the probability of making or breaking certain bonds (e.g. salt bridges and hydrogen bonds) which promote the association of one part of the polypeptide chain with another. Hence there is at least a theoretical likelihood that some polypeptide chains of a particular protein species (varying between 10 and 200 000 000 in total per cell) will adopt conformations at any instant in time different from that required for biological function. That is to say the complexity of protein structures in themselves must be considered as a potential source of altered proteins.

In addition to the denaturation events mentioned above which do not involve a change to the composition of the protein there are a number of processes where alteration to the amino acid residues does occur.

Deamidation and generation of isopeptides

Both asparagine and glutamine residues are somewhat unstable and therefore undergo deamidation to aspartic acid and glutamic acid residues, respectively. Both result in the addition of an extra negative charge to the protein molecule which could affect proper biological function. Other potentially deleterious effects are associated with deamidation especially of asparagine residues. The mechanism by which the asparagine residue spontaneously deamidates in-volves the formation of a cyclic succinimide intermediate with the imino group of the peptide bond (Stephenson and Clarke, 1989). This intermediate cleaves at either of two positions to produce an aspartate or isoaspartate residue, the latter involving an additional methylene group in the polypeptide backbone. Not only could the isopeptide bond compromise the protein's proper function but it also impairs its susceptibility to proteolysis as isopeptide bonds appear to be somewhat refractile to attack by proteases responsible for protein turnover (to be considered later) and have been detected in urine.

Racemization

The biosynthesis of proteins by ribosomes employs only the L-isoforms of the 19 amino acids which bear an asymmetric alpha carbon atom. Both L-serine and L-aspartic acid residues are particularly prone to spontaneous racemization to their respective D-isomers which results in their side chains being in an incorrect position, i.e. on the opposite side of the polypeptide backbone (Adelman and Dekker, 1985). Again such a change will perturb the shape of the protein molecule. Although such racemizations are somewhat slow occurring at between 0.1 and 0.3% of the aspartate and serine residues per year, such changes can be detected in proteins which show little or no turnover such as the crystallins in the core of the eye lens and enamel of teeth. In fact the precipitated crystallins which constitute the opacity in senile cataracts are enriched in D-aspartic acid residues; presumably the changes in macromolecular conformation which racemization induces contribute to the alteration in protein solubility to result in crystallin precipitation. Whether changes induced by racemization are sufficient in themselves to create the cataractogenic state is unlikely because its rate is species independent but cataract onset varies considerably between species of differing maximum life-span. Calculations show that in humans by the age of 50 years on average each crystallin molecule in the eye lens core will contain at least one D-aspartic acid residue. Other agents which provoke changes in protein conformation at a more rapid rate should therefore be considered (see below).

Induced protein damage

Amongst the processes which could contribute to the age accumulation of altered proteins are errors during their synthesis. Crude estimates of error rates at translation (the most error-prone step in protein biosynthesis) are put at 3 in 10^4 codons, although this figure is thought to vary considerably depending on codons and context. The error catastrophe theory of ageing (Poot, 1991), proposes that the error rate increases with age, but there has been little unambiguous experimental observation in support of this and some which suggests that the mistranslation rates remain unchanged in ageing cells. However, it should be pointed out that the error frequency of bacterial (70S) ribosomes is at least five times that of the larger eukaryotic (80S) cytoplasmic ribosomes. Hence one would predict that those mitochondrial proteins synthesized within that organelle could provide a source of error proteins, although most mitochondrial proteins are of cytoplasmic origin. Whether erroneous mitochondrial proteins contribute to the age-related decline in mitochondrial structure and function is uncertain. However, but in a different context, the differences in error rates between 70S and 80S ribosomes should be given due consideration by biotechnology companies which use bacteria for synthesis of human proteins for therapeutic application (e.g. recombinant insulin).

The action of oxygen free radicals on proteins is now regarded as a major source of altered proteins in ageing in general and in causation and/or progression of certain disease states (emphysema, atherosclerosis, arthritis and cataractogenesis) (Harman, 1984). As in the effects on DNA oxygen free radicals can produce a range of modifications to the target molecule. Much current opinion regards the hydroxyl radical as the most dangerous species; it can modify amino acid side chains (e.g. histidine, tyrosine, tryptophan, glutamic acid, methioinine) to alter the chemistry of the protein to change its structure and function (Stadtman, 1992). Free radicals can also induce covalent cross-linking between protein molecules and to DNA.

Hydroxyl radicals can also cleave peptide bonds to create protein fragments.

There is a considerable body of evidence to show that protein fragments, especially those derived from hydrophobic regions of the molecule, can interact indiscriminately and deleteriously with other cellular macromolecules probably to compromise proper cell function. It cannot be insignificant that during normal protein turnover the initial cleavage of the polypeptide chain is the rate-limiting step, the resultant fragments do not accumulate being catabolized to very small peptides or amino acids almost as soon as they are produced. A fuller discussion of proteolysis, ageing and the generation of altered proteins is given below. It may be significant that Down's syndrome patients possess an extra copy of chromosome 21 which bears not only the gene for the amyloid precursor protein, a fragment of which accumulates in an aggregated form as amyloid plaque (see elsewhere in this volume), but also is the location of the superoxide dismutase gene. It is unknown whether the extra gene dosage of superoxide dismutase without an additional catalase gene plays a role in the decreased life-span of Down's patients. However, one can envisage a situation where there is increased conversion rate of the relatively innocuous superoxide radical by extra superoxide dismutase to hydrogen peroxide without a compensating increase in catalase activity. Such a condition could increase the potential for transition metal-mediated conversion of the peroxide to the far more reactive hydroxyl radical by Fenton chemistry (Minc-Golomb et al., 1991). As noted above extra copies of the superoxide dismutase gene increases mutagenesis in bacteria (Scott et al., 1987; Yarom et al., 1988).

Not all proteins are equally susceptible to free-radical-mediated damage. For example, bovine crystallins prepared from the lens, and nonlenticular proteins such as serum albumin, haemoglobin and lactate dehydrogenase were treated with hydroxyl radicals generated from a mixture of hydrogen peroxide and copper ions (i.e. Fenton chemistry). It was found that the lenticular proteins were far more resistant than the nonlenticular proteins as judged by their fragmentation (Carmichael and Hipkiss, 1991). While the mechanism responsible for this difference is not known, such a differential susceptibility would be anticipated given that many lenticular proteins are required to last the life time of the animal because those in the lens core are not replaced. Interestingly, the amino acid sequence of some crystallins is very similar, and even identical in some cases, to that of the small stress proteins whose synthesis can be induced following exposure of cells to agents which provoke the formation of altered proteins (see later).

Protection from oxygen free-radical-mediated damage to proteins is afforded by the anti-oxidant apparatus outlined above which includes vitamins A, C and E as well as superoxide dismutase, peroxidase and catalase. A number of other potential anti-oxidants have also been proposed such as uric acid and carnosine. In some tissues an age-related decline in certain possible anti-oxidants has been observed, and the total anti-oxidant level is thought to be higher in longer lived species (Barja de Quiroga et al., 1990). However, as yet feeding extra anti-oxidant vitamins does not result in any increase in longevity in experimental animals.

In addition to the interception of the reactive oxygen radical prior to its (deleterious) interaction with a cellular macromolecule, there is also a process whereby the altered proteins which are the products of oxygen free-radical attack are removed by proteolysis (Doherty and Mayer, 1992). In recent years it has been clearly demonstrated that altered proteins in general are selectively catabolized intracellularly. Details of this important homeostatic process will be discussed later.

Effects of glucose and other sugars

Oxygen is not the only commonly occurring agent which can bring about damage to cellular macromolecules. In mammals glucose is a major energy transport molecule and nervous tissues, for example, show an essential requirement for it except under conditions of extreme starvation. However, many years ago it was recognized that sugars such as glucose and others which possess aldehyde or ketogroups (i.e. reducing sugars) can react, nonenzymically, with amino groups on, for example, proteins eventually to produce high molecular weight cross-linked material and finally to advanced glycosylation end-products (AGE-products) (Baynes and Monnier, 1989). This process, called the Maillard reaction, is usually thought to be very slow at mammalian body temperature and has been neglected by biological gerontologists until comparatively recently, but is understood by food chemists in terms of the ability of the process to create brown products. It appears that glucose is the slowest reacting sugar in terms of the Maillard reaction because the active species is the linear or straight chain form of the molecule; the cyclic form does not participate as it does not contain an available aldehyde or keto group, and only 0.002% of glucose is in the linear form at any instant in time. Other common sugars such as galactose, fructose, ribose and deoxyribose are up to 200 times more reactive. Even intermediates in the glycolytic pathway such as glyceraldehyde-3-phosphate and dihydroxyacetone phosphate (and their unphosphorylated forms) react readily with amino groups including those present in proteins. Hence there may be considerable potential for this process called nonenzymic glycosylation or glycation, although the extent to which the protein glycation contributes to intracellular ageing phenomena is as yet unknown. However, it has been found that superoxide dismutase from erythrocytes from Werner's syndrome patients show increased glycation (Taniguchi et al. 1989), and the enzymic activity is severely impaired.

In addition to the 'classic' Maillard reaction leading to AGE-products, glucose can itself promote the formation of hydroxyl radicals via an auto-oxidative reaction involving transition metals and the production of ketoaldehyde intermediates whose effects are similar to those which result from oxygen free-radical-mediated protein damage (Hunt et al., 1988). In the latter case protein fragmentation can also result.

It is clear that protein glycation is an important age-associated process especially when proteins with long half-lives are considered. The proteins present in basement membranes, blood vessel walls, connective tissue and the eye lens become increasingly glycated during normal ageing and could therefore provide a partial explanation for some age-related declines in physiological function. In addition the resultant new structures may be immunologically different from the original proteins and may therefore be recognized as nonself by the immune system and could provide a basis for some autoimmune conditions whose incidence increase with age (Wiztum and Koschinsky, 1989). Similarly protein glycation on or in the long-lived memory T-cells could also affect immunological efficiency.

In uncontrolled diabetes the potential for glycation is increased and the process is increasingly thought to play a causative role in the initiation or progression of many of the diabetes-associated conditions such as atheroma, kidney damage, retinopathy and cataractogenesis. Interestingly, fibroblast cultures obtained from diabetics show a decreased proliferative potential compared to age-matched controls.

The metabolic effects of glycation have been investigated to a limited extent. For example, the Maillard products of lysine and glucose incubations can inhibit aminopeptidase N and carboxypeptidase A, and feeding experiments with glucose/amino acid reaction products have been shown to decrease pancreatic amylase activity in rats (Shibamato, 1989; Wiztum and Koschinsky, 1989). There have been a number of reports showing that Maillard products of glucose–amino acid incubations are genotoxic and mutagenic (Shibamato, 1989). Therefore, should the Maillard reaction occur *in vivo* to any extent, the products could increase the mutagenic load on the cells and inhibit some of the enzymes responsible for the degradation of proteins and polypeptide fragments.

Nucleic acids too are also potentially glycatable as some of the bases possess amino groups (Lee and Cerami, 1989). Additionally it should be remembered that depurination of DNA is a common event (see above) which then exposes the ^1C of the deoxyribose which bears the reactive aldehyde group. This then provides the potential for reaction with an amino group either in a base or deriving from a lysine residue present in any closely associated nucleoprotein. Although it is known that DNA–protein cross-links do increase with age, the extent to which glycation events contribute to their formation is as yet unknown.

Control of protein damage

Continuous turnover of proteins
The majority of cellular proteins are subject to continuous synthesis and degradation, collectively called turnover. Protein half-lives vary from minutes to months according to their structure and intracellular location, the degradation being carried out by a combination of cytoplasmic and lysosomal proteolytic enzymes. Some of the factors which apparently determine the rates of protein breakdown include amino acid sequences specific for lysosomal-mediated catabolism (Dice, 1990), the PEST hypothesis which indicates that regions of polypeptide rich in proline, aspartate, serine and threonine residues (or P, E, S, T according to their single letter abbreviations) are targets for attack by intracellular proteases (Rogers *et al.*, 1986), and the N-end rule which proposes that proteins with the basic amino acids lysine or arginine at the amino terminus have short half-lives (Varshavsky *et al.*, 1988). As indicated above, the eye lens core is an exception as protein turnover does not occur because the cells lose their nuclei during an early stage in development. Similarly, in erythrocytes protein turnover is absent, although the cells are removed from circulation after 120 days in humans.

As proteins are generally turned over and are also subject to the postsynthetic changes and insults outlined above, it follows that the degradation rate of a particular protein can have a major role in controlling the accumulation of altered polypeptide forms. Thus, proteins with short half-lives are unlikely to show the effects of the somewhat slow events such as deamidation, racemization and glycation, whereas such postsynthetic changes are readily observed in the proteins in eye lens core where turnover is absent.

Selective catabolism of aberrant proteins
During the last 20 years much evidence has been accumulated to suggest that proteins whose structures differ from that of the normal gene products are selectively and rapidly degraded. This property appears to be present in all cells capable of protein biosynthesis. The types of proteins degraded include polypeptide fragments, those modified by free-radical attack and heat denaturation. Many mutant gene products containing amino acid substitutions are also

rapidly degraded. However, it is clear that not all mutant proteins are rapidly catabolized especially when the tertiary structure is not significantly perturbed, a finding which has evolutionary implications by allowing the persistence of some altered proteins. Thus, the absence of absolute stringency for the removal of all altered proteins, thereby permitting evolutionary changes in polypeptide forms, may also play a causative role in the eventual accumulation of aberrant proteins leading ultimately to senescence and death.

The mechanisms by which altered proteins are degraded bear examination not only for reasons of curiosity but also because of possible pathological implications. Most mammalian cells contain a small protein called ubiquitin (Rechsteiner, 1988; Jentsch et al., 1991; Mayer et al., 1991). This protein has a molecular weight of around 8500 and its primary structure is the most highly conserved sequence in evolution. One of the functions of ubiquitin is to flag or signal aberrant proteins for rapid proteolysis. It appears that abnormal proteins are targeted for destruction by the attachment of a ubiquitin by way of an isopeptide bond via ubiquitin's terminal carboxyl group and a side chain amino group belonging to a lysine residue in the aberrant molecule. Then another ubiquitin forms another isopeptide linkage to the single lysine of the conjugated ubiquitin; the process repeating such that between 10 and 47 ubiquitins become attached branch-like to the target polypeptide via a single lysine residue. Such multi-ubiquitinated proteins are then degraded either by the lysosomes or by the high molecular weight multicatalytic protease (also called a proteosome). The enzymology of this process of rapid intracellular proteolysis is complex and certainly different from the simply protein digestion as seen in the gut. Furthermore, except for the catabolism of small protein fragments (McKay and Hipkiss, 1982), the selective intracellular catabolism of aberrant proteins is energy-requiring (for the attachment of ubiquitin and proteolysis), an observation thermodynamically inconsistent with the fact that protein synthesis consumes energy. As the evolving life forms have apparently found it necessary to possess such a complex mechanism for the selective catabolism of aberrant polypeptides, demanding resources in terms of energy and information, one presumes that the process is crucial and the presence of the substrates must be deleterious to the cell. Therefore, the observation that altered proteins accumulate in ageing cells and tissues may point to a causative role for such aberrant structures in the aetiology of ageing and associated disease states. A system which may be responsible for the removal of glycated proteins has also been described (Vlassara et al., 1985).

Not only do most cells possess constitutive activities which are responsible for the removal of altered proteins but under certain circumstances additional inducible proteins are synthesized. This phenomenon was originally called the heat-shock response because it was first described following the exposure of cells to hyperthermic conditions and the proteins induced termed 'heat-shock' proteins (Parry et al., 1987). However, it was subsequently found that many processes which bring about the formation of proteins with altered structures elicit the de novo synthesis of heat-shock or 'stress' proteins. It appears that processes which promote the stress response, which include synthesis of mutant proteins, polypeptides containing amino acid analogues, oxygen free-radical attack as well as thermal denaturation all result in the formation of altered proteins, the induction resulting presumably because the constitutive proteolytic system becomes saturated with aberrant proteins. Up to 17 different stress proteins have been characterized including the 'chaperone' proteins which are also involved in protein folding and transportation to intracellular organelles such as mitochondria (Ellis and Van der Vies, 1991). Ubiquitin is both a stress protein as well as being synthesized constitutively. This is because there are separate genes for ubiquitin, a polyubiquitin gene under stress response control as well as ubiquitin which is synthesized coordinately with certain ribosomal proteins. Thus when protein synthesis is greatest in cells containing large numbers of ribosomes ubiquitin will be present in sufficient amounts to cope with the normal level of mistranslation. In stress conditions synthesis of extra copies of ubiquitin is promoted. Ubiquitin appears to play a role in Alzheimer's disease as aggregates of ubiquitinated aberrant proteins accumulate in the brain (Matsumoto and Fujiwara, 1991), inferring possible dysfunction in some aspect of protein degradation. Similarly in motor neuron disease aggregates of ubiquitinated neuronal proteins accumulate. Details of the molecular pathology of Alzheimer's disease will be discussed elsewhere in this volume.

Ubiquitin may have an additional role in molecular homeostasis because an enzyme responsible for one of the activation steps for ubiquitin attachment to the target polypeptide also is the RAD6 gene product a protein involved in DNA repair (Reichsteiner, 1988; Jentsch et al., 1991; Mayer et al., 1991). The full implications of this observation have yet to be revealed but it may not be coincidence that aberrant forms of DNA and proteins accumulate with age.

Changes in protein turnover during ageing
In most tissues the rate of protein synthesis decreases with age as part of the control of the eventual size of the animal. The molecular mechanisms might involve changes in ribosome numbers or decreases in the amounts of labile elongation factors (Rattan, 1991), brought about possibly through the actions of increasing levels of the various forms of somatostatin and the falls in growth hormone and somatomedin. Whatever the mechanisms involved it follows that as the rate of protein synthesis declines there should also be a corresponding decline in the rate of protein breakdown to ensure that the intracellular protein content remains essentially unchanged. In a number of model ageing systems a decline in the rate of protein breakdown has been clearly shown (McKay et al. 1980; Gracy et al., 1985; Wharton and Hipkiss, 1985; Carmichael and Hipkiss, 1989; Dice, 1989; Jahngen et al., 1990). However, while the rate of de novo synthesis of error protein declines corresponding to the overall total protein synthesis, the rate of formation of aberrant protein arising from postsynthetic origin does not fall. Hence the situation must eventually arise when the constitutive proteolytic apparatus is saturated with altered proteins thereby necessitating the induction of the stress response. However, recent research has shown that the stress response is slower in aged cells (Niedzwiecki et al., 1991), possibly because of decreased protein synthetic function, thereby allowing greater time for the deleterious interaction of the altered proteins with other cellular macromolecules and their aggregation in forms refractile to complete catabolism. It should be remembered that the stress response also involves the partial or complete inhibition of the synthesis of the 'regular' proteins normally synthesized by the cell which may further compromise proper physiological function.

PHYSIOLOGICAL CONTROL OF AGEING

It was shown some 60 years ago that it was possible to delay the onset of ageing and extend the mean and maximum life-spans (by up to 50%) of laboratory rodents by a process called calorie restriction, a feeding regime which involves restricting the calorie intake of the animals to about 60% of that of controls fed *ad libitum*. This process also seems to work in flies. However, there is no evidence that calorie restriction affects the timing of age-related phenomena or maximum life-span in humans. While the calorie restriction experiment has been repeated in many laboratories throughout the world, its significance has been questioned. For example, it is possible to argue that the control animals are eating themselves into an early grave as they become obese and inactive, whereas the restricted animals are smaller, much more mobile and thin. It should be remembered too that rats and mice in the wild might not normally be faced with unlimited availability of food, thus the *ad libitum* fed animals might not represent a proper control. However, it is clear that the onset of many age-related disease states such as atherosclerosis, cataractogenesis, autoimmune conditions and tumour formation, is significantly delayed in restricted animals, and not all of these conditions can be explained in simple terms by overeating. Similarly, delays in age-related declines in DNA repair (Werraarchkul *et al.* 1989) and protein degradation (Ishigami and Goto, 1990) have been reported in calorie-restricted animals suggesting that these processes may be important in maintaining molecular homeostasis during ageing.

Whilst the details by which calorie restriction extends life-span and delays ageing have not been fully explored, it is possible to outline a reasonable biochemical explanation. In the restricted animals circulatory glucose would not be continuously available from dietary sources but would have to be provided endogenously via increased intracellular protein degradation. This increased proteolytic requirement may increase the cellular levels of proteases and improve the removal of altered proteins and polypeptide fragments, including those deleterious to efficient cell function. Also the increased rate of general protein turnover will decrease the appearance of products of the slow spontaneous changes in structure (e.g. racemization, deamidation and isopeptide formation), the protein being degraded prior to the occurrence of the alteration.

Explanations, though speculative, of how calorie restriction affects the integrity of DNA might be found within the following observations. An increase in expression of any gene could improve its maintenance because it has been found that genes that are being transcribed have an increased likelihood of repair compared to those which are inactive. Therefore, increased expression of genes whose products are important in molecular maintenance, such as those involved in the proteolysis of aberrant proteins, may delay the fixation of damage in them and thereby postpone the onset of ageing. It should be remembered that at least one protein (the RAD6 gene product) may play a role in both DNA repair and the ubiquitinization of aberrant proteins. Hence it is at least conceivable that a system might exist for the simultaneous regulation of enzymes required for maintenance of the molecular integrity of both DNA and proteins. Additionally, lowered circulatory glucose levels in the restricted animals will decrease the incidence of nonenzymic glycosylation of proteins resulting in less aberrant polypeptide in general and in turn decreasing the load of endogenously generated mutagens following the proteolytic release of glycated (mutagenic) amino acids. Indeed both tumour incidence and somatic mutagenesis are decreased in restricted animals.

Genetic modulation of ageing

Each species has an apparent maximum life-span, and the approximate timing of onset of the deleterious changes associated with ageing is also common to all the individuals of any species. This has led to study of the genetics of ageing and to the concept of 'gerontogenes', i.e. genes which specifically determine ageing. However, as explained at the beginning of this chapter such ideas may be evolutionarily flawed. It is perhaps better to adopt an alternative view and to consider the genes essential for efficient physiological function up to the time when progeny are themselves capable of independent reproduction. Some of the functions of the genes for such longevity assurance could well be associated with the maintenance of molecular integrity (molecular homeostasis) involved either in the prevention of damage or its rapid repair. For example, the total anti-oxidant levels in the cells of long-lived species is higher than that present in the shorter lived animals. Similarly, DNA repair rates appear to correlate directly with maximum life-span in cultured fibroblasts obtained from a range of species (Warner et al. 1987; Kirkwood, 1989). Mouse fibroblasts spontaneously and frequently mutate to tumour cells in culture whereas the equivalent human cells show very low mutation rates. As oncogenesis is brought about by the activation of one or more oncogenes, then it follows that long-lived species may possess more or better tumour suppression genes to prevent the instigation or progression of cellular transformation. Such tumour suppression genes may also be thought to function in longevity assurance.

The progeroid syndromes, Werner's syndrome and progeria are autosomal recessive genetic traits associated with a decrease in longevity and premature or accelerated ageing. This again clearly points to the existence of specific gene functions essential for the delay in the occurrence of the ageing phenotype. As yet it is unknown what function is missing in these conditions, although in the case of Werner's syndrome the defective gene may be located on chromosome 8 (Goto et al., 1992). However, there are reports which show in Werner's syndrome an increase in the proportion of the thermolabile (i.e. altered) forms of at least two enzymes, glucose-6-phosphate dehydrogenase and Cu–Zn–superoxide dismutase as well as an increase in the amount of the glycated form of the latter (Tangiguchi et al., 1989). This has led to the speculation that there is an impairment in the removal of the altered form of the Cu–Zn–superoxide dismutase (and perhaps other altered proteins) in Werner's syndrome patients. Cockayne's syndrome is another rare form of premature ageing and here a defect in DNA repair has been reported, although it is not sure whether this is the primary cause.

There are a number of areas in which potential longevity assurance genes are being sought. The recently developed senescence accelerated mouse (SAM) (Kohno et al., 1985), especially following transgenic modification with candidate genes, will certainly provide a very useful tool in the exploration of the genetic determinants of longevity. The selection of long-lived mutants in insects is also currently yielding results at least as the phenotypic level, where longevity appears to be associated with increased expression of anti-oxidant enzymes such as superoxide dismutase. However, it should be remembered that even in the longest living forms the life-span is less than 1 year, a period in which some of the slow changes in macromolecular structure in longer living species would not be likely to occur.

ALZHEIMER'S DISEASE, OTHER NEURODEGENERATIVE DISORDERS AND AGEING

In this volume devoted to ageing and neurological changes it is appropriate to conclude with a brief consideration of some of general principles outlined above in relation to neurodegenerative conditions. In some cases of Alzheimer's disease alterations in the amino acid sequence of the amyloid precursor protein (APP) are seen which may be responsible for amyloid accumulation

(Chartier-Harlin *et al.*, 1991): but why does it take so long? However, as yet, alterations in the amino acid sequence of amyloid or its precursor appear absent in the majority of cases, therefore, alternative or additional explanations for the accumulation of the protein fragment must be found. If the amyloid is of neuronal origin (which is debated), are there changes occurring in cellular proteolytic systems during this time and can they be manipulated by intervention? For example, inhibition of such proteolysis by aluminium (Nixon *et al.*, 1990) may provide a link between the long suggested association between aluminium and Alzheimer's disease; model studies show that peptide fragments aggregate intracellularly if not rapidly catabolized (McKay and Hipkiss, 1985). The amyloid precursor protein is suggested to be a PEST protein and should therefore be a candidate for selective catabolism (Siman and Christoph, 1989). Indeed, recent studies suggest that there may be a proteolytic deficit (Matsumoto and Fujiwara, 1991), possibly lysosomal, in Alzheimer's disease which decreases the removal of partially degraded APP thereby allowing the accumulation A4 peptides and their subsequent aggregation due to their hydrophobic character. The accumulation of ubiquitinated neurofibrillary tangles in Alzheimer's disease brain (Tabaton *et al.* 1991) is also suggestive of a proteolytic deficit. A similar proposal has been made in Lewy body disease where aggregates of ubiquitinated proteins accumulate (Rechsteiner, 1988; Jentsch *et al.*, 1991; Mayer *et al.*, 1991); the attachment of ubiquitin to a protein may target it to a lysosome for destruction. But should lysosomal function be rate limiting to protein degradation the partially processed proteins may aggregate, as has been observed in reticulocytes (which have no lysosomes) synthesizing aberrant polypeptides (McKay and Hipkiss, 1985).

In the majority of Alzheimer cases no alteration in the APP primary structure has been found; this again implies that age-related changes are occurring in some function associated with the production or processing of APP (Marx, 1992). Indeed, it is still not clear whether the amyloid is of neuronal origin as APP is produced by cultured cells during normal metabolism (Haas *et al.*, 1992; Hardy and Mullan, 1992; Seubert *et al.*, 1992) and the β-peptide can be detected in biological fluids (Haas *et al.*, 1992; Hardy *et al.*, 1992; Seubert *et al.*, 1992). Small amounts of amyloid accumulate during normal ageing (i.e. non-Alzheimer's) implying that there may be increased APP production or a proteolytic deficit in a limited number of cells. In Down's syndrome there is no mutation in the amyloid precursor but again the A4 protein accumulates, possible due to its increased expression (via a gene dosage effect) and a comparatively early saturation of the activity which should degrade it. It is intriguing that APP is secreted by cultured human fibroblasts, that it is known as protease nexin-2 which can inhibit certain proteolytic activities, and whose synthesis is increased in senescent cells possibly under stress response control. It will be particularly interesting to find out if expression of APP is similarly regulated in the brain.

Generally, therefore, it may be that in Alzheimer's disease onset of amyloid accumulation is initiated by either increased synthesis of APP in response to cell stress, and/or insufficient proteolytic redundancy either because of a proteolytic defect present throughout life but not initially rate limiting to APP metabolism, or because of a decline in activity which is more rapid than normal. It will, therefore, be important to study the factors, endogenous or even exogenous in origin, which affect, directly or indirectly, the processing of APP. Whether and/or why A4 or amyloid cause neurodegeneration remain to be determined. The fact that in most cell types it has proved very difficult to detect the accumulation of proteolytic intermediates (fragments) suggests a considerable degree of intracellular proteolytic redundancy. The necessity for the evolution of such excess capacity further suggests that the substrates for such proteases and peptidases may be generally deleterious to efficient function and survival of the cell, and that their rapid removal is therefore advantageous to the organism. The fact that aggregates of proteins, often ubiquitinated, are observed in neurodegenerative conditions (Parkinson's disease, motor neuron disease and Lewy body disease) again suggests an association with incomplete proteolysis. But whether such incomplete proteins are causal to neuronal degeneration rather than another effect remains to be clearly established.

CONCLUSIONS

The fact that ageing is a universal phenomenon leading to the decline in efficiency and ultimate death of the individual is undisputed. It is also obvious that babies are born young, even from egg cells more than 30 years old or more; although there is a significant age-related increase in the risk of abnormality above 35 years. This allows us to ask questions about the processes which keep the egg cell genetically and phenotypically young in a 30-year-old body. Is it cellular specialization which ultimately limits the cell's ability for complete repair? This certainly is the case of the enucleate cells of the eye lens core where it appears that ageing begins immediately following loss of the nucleus. A comparison between the species in which the onset of cataractogenesis differs by decades may reveal which functions must be maintained to prevent crystallin aggregation and precipitation. In postmitotic nucleated cells such as nerve whose proliferation is repressed because of insufficient required growth factors, there is at least the potential for the repair, removal and replacement of damaged macromolecules, but this may become increasingly limited. It is not clear at present whether there is a change in some homoeostatic function which normally prevents accumulation of aberrant molecules. If so, this could occur by way of a quantum leap downwards in activity. Alternatively, there could be a continuous decline in activity arriving at a condition where the rate of the particular homoeostatic function is limited by the availability of enzyme, instead of the rate of formation of the substrate for that particular function as in the young condition. That is to say, inbuilt homoeostatic redundancy is important for longevity, with longer lived species maintaining redundancy for a longer time. Do long-lived species initially invest more of their resources in homoeostatic functions (Kirkwood and Rose, 1991) or is the rate of decline slower?

Only by the discovery of the underlying molecular bases of the ageing process in general can we hope to achieve a rational approach to the alleviation of Alzheimer's disease and much other age-related disease; perhaps 'molecular gerontology' would be a suitable term to describe such an endeavour.

REFERENCES

Adelman, R.C. and Dekker, E.E. (Eds) (1985). *Modification of Proteins during Aging*. Alan R. Liss, New York.

Bankmann, M., Prakash, L. and Prakash, S. (1992). Yeast RAD14 and human xeroderma pigmentosum group A DNA-repair genes encode homologous proteins. *Nature*, **335**, 555–64.

Barja de Ouiroga, G., Perez-Campo, R. and Lopez Torres, M. (1990). Anti-oxidant defences and peroxidation in liver and brain of aged rats. *Biochemical Journal*, **272**, 247–50.

Barnes, D.B. (1992). Damage limitation exercises. *Nature*, **359**, 12–13.

Baynes, J.W. and Monnier, V.M. (Eds) (1989). *The Maillard Reaction in Aging, Diabetes and Nutrition. Progress in Clinical and Biological Research*, Vol. 304. Alan R. Liss, New York.

Bittles, A.H. (1992). Evidence for and against the causal involvement of mitochondrial DNA mutation in mammalian ageing. *Mutation Research*, **275**, 217–25.

Carmichael, P.L. and Hipkiss, A.R. (1989). Age-related changes in proteolysis of aberrant crystallin in bovine lens cell-free preparations. *Mechanics of Ageing and Development*, **50**, 37–48.

Carmichael, P.L. and Hipkiss, A.R. (1991). Differences in susceptibility between crystallins and non-lenticular proteins to copper and H_2O_2-mediated peptide bond cleavage. *Free Radical Research Communications*, **15**, 101–10.

Chartier-Harlin, M-C., Crawford, F., Houlden, H. *et al.* (1991). Early onset of Alzheimer's disease caused by mutations at codon 717 of the beta-amyloid precursor gene. *Nature*, **353**, 844–6.

Dell'Orco, R.T. and Anderson, L.E. (1991). Decline of polyADP-ribosylation during *in vivo* senescence in human diploid fibroblasts. *Journal of Cellular Physiology*, **146**, 216–21.

Dice, J.F. (1989). Altered intracellular protein degradation in aging: a possible cause of proliferative arrest. *Experimental Gerontology*, **24**, 451–9.

Dice, J.F. (1990). Peptide sequences that target cytosolic proteins for lysosomal proteolysis. *Trends in Biochemical Science*, **15**, 305–9.

Doherty, F.J. and Mayer, R.J. (1992). *Intracellular Protein Degradation*. IRL Press at Oxford University Press, Oxford.

Driscoll, M. and Chalfie, M. (1992). The mec-4 gene is a member of a family of Carenorhabditis elegans genes that can mutate to induce neuronal degeneration. *Nature*, **349**, 588–93.

Ellis, R.J. and Van der Vies, S.M. (1991). Molecular chaperones. *Annual Review of Biochemistry*, **60**, 321–47.

Goto, M., Rubenstein, M., Weber, J. *et al.* (1992). Genetic linkage of Werner's syndrome to five markers on chromosome 8. *Nature*, **355**, 735–8.

Gracy, R.W., Yuksel, K.U., Chapman, M.L. *et al.* (1985), Impaired protein degradation may account for the accumulation of abnormal proteins in aging cells. In *Modifications of Proteins during Aging*, Adelman, R.C. and Dekker, E.E. (Eds), pp. 1–18. Alan R. Liss, New York.

Haas, C., Schlossmacher, M.G., Hung, A.Y. *et al.* (1992). Amyloid beta-peptide is produced by cultured cells during normal metabolism. *Nature*, **359**, 322–5.

Halliwell, B. and Aruoma, O.I. (1991). DNA damage by oxygen-derived species: its mechanism and measurement in mammalian systems. *FEBS Letters*, **281**, 9–19.

Hardy, J. and Mullan, N. (1992). Alzheimer's disease: in search of the soluble. *Nature*, **359**, 268–9.

Harley, C.B. (1991). Telomere loss: mititoc clock or genetic time bomb? *Mutation Research*, **256**, 271–82.

Harman, D. (1984). Free radical theory of aging: the 'free radical' diseases. *Age*, **7**, 111–31.

Hayflick, L. (1987). Origins of longevity. In *Modern Biological Theories of Aging*, Warner, H.R., Butler, R.N., Sprott, R.L. and Schneider, E.L. (Eds), pp. 21–37. Raven Press, New York.

Hunt, J.V., Dean, R.T. and Wolff, S.P. (1988). Hydroxyl radical production and autoxidative glycosylation; glucose autoxidation as the cause of protein damage in the experimental glycation model of diabetes mellitus and ageing. *Biochemical Journal*, **256**, 205–12.

Ishigami, A. and Goto, S. (1990). Effect of dietary restriction on the degradation of proteins in senescent mouse liver parenchymal cells in culture. *Archives of Biochemistry and Biophysics*, **283**, 362–6.

Jahngen, J.H., Lipman, R.D., Eisenhauer, D.A. *et al.* (1990). Aging and cellular maturation cause change in ubiquitin-eye lens protein conjugates. *Archives of Biochemistry and Biophysics*, **276**, 32–7.

Jentsch, S., Seufert, W. and Hauser, H-P. (1991). Genetic analysis of the ubiquitin system. *Biochimica Biophysica Acta*, **1089**, 127–39.

Kirkwood, T.B.L. (1989). DNA, mutation and aging. *Mutation Research*, **219**, 1–7.

Kirkwood, T.B.L. and Rose, M.L. (1991). Evolution of senescence: late survival sacrificed for reproduction. *Philosophical Transactions of the Royal Society of London B*, **332**, 15–24.

Kohno, A., Yonezu, T., Matsushita, M. *et al.* (1985). Chronic food restriction modulates the advance of senescence in the senescence accelerated mouse (SAM). *Journal of Nutrition*, **115**, 1259–66.

Lee, A.T. and Cerami, A. (1989). Nonenzymic glycosylation of DNA by reducing sugars. In *The Maillard Reaction in Aging, Diabetes and Nutrition. Progress in Clinical and Biological Research*, Baynes, J.W. and Monnier, V.M. (Eds), Vol. 304, pp. 291–9. Alan R. Liss, New York.

Legerski, R. and Peterson, C. (1992). Expression cloning of a human DNA repair gene involved in xeroderma pigmentosum group C. *Nature*, **359**, 70–3.

Lindahl, T. and Nyberg, B. (1972). The rate of depurinisation of native deoxyribonucleic acid. *Biochemistry*, **25**, 3610–18.

Marx, J. (1992). Alzheimer's debate boils over. *Science*, **257**, 1336–8.

Matsumoto, A. and Fujiwara, Y. (1991). Abnormal and deficient processing of beta-amyloid precursor protein in familial Alzheimer's disease lymphoblastoid cells. *Biochemical and Biophysical Research Communications*, **175**, 361–5.

Mayer, R.J., Arnold, J., Laszlo, L. *et al.* (1991). Ubiquitin in health and disease. *Biochimica Biophysica Acta*, **1089**, 141–57.

McKay, M.J., Daniels, R.S. and Hipkiss, A.R. (1980). Breakdown of aberrant proteins in rabbit reticulocytes decreases with cell age. *Biochemical Journal*, **188**, 279–83.

McKay, M.J. and Hipkiss, A.R. (1982). ATP-independent proteolysis of globin cyanogen bromide peptide fragments in rabbit reticulocyte cell-free extracts. *European Journal of Biochemistry*, **125**, 567–73.

McKay, M.J. and Hipkiss, A.R. (1985). The subcellular distribution and proteolysis of abnormal proteins in aging rabbit reticulocytes. In *Cellular and Molecular Aspects of Aging: The Red Cell as a Model*, Eaton, J.W., Konzen, D.K. and White, J.G. (Eds), pp. 29–41. Alan R. Liss, New York.

Minc-Golomb, D., Knobler, H. and Groner, Y. (1991). Gene dosage of CuZnSOD and Down's syndrome: diminished prostaglandin synthesis in human trisomy 21, transfected cells and transgenic mice. *EMBO Journal*, **10**, 2119–24.

Nackerdien, Z., Rao, G., Cacciuttolo, M.A. *et al.* (1991). *Chemical nature of DNA–protein cross-links produced in mammalian chromatin by hydrogen peroxide in the presence of iron or copper ions. Biochemistry*, **30**, 4873–9.

Niedzwiecki, A., Kongpachith, A.M. and Fleming, J.E. (1991). Aging affects expressing of 7-kDa heat shock proteins in Drosophilia. *Journal of Biology and Chemistry*, **266**, 9332–8.

Nixon, R.A., Clarke, J.F., Logvinenko, K.B. *et al.* (1990). Aluminium inhibits calpain-mediated proteolysis and induces neurofilament proteins to form protease-resistant high molecular weight complexes. *Journal of Neurochemistry*, **55**, 1950–9.

Parag, H.A., Raboy, B. and Culka, R.Q. (1987). Effect of heat shock on protein degradation in mammalian cells: involvement of the ubiquitin system. *EMBO Journal*, **6**, 55–61.

Poot, M. (1991). Oxidants and antioxidants in proliferative senescence. *Mutation Research*, **256**, 177–89.

Raff, M.C. (1992). Social controls on cell survival and cell death. *Nature*, **346**, 397–400.

Rattan, S.I.S. (1991). Protein synthesis and the components of protein synthetic machinery during cellular ageing. *Mutation Research*, **256**, 115–25.

Rechsteiner, M. (Ed.). *Ubiquitin*. Plenum Press, London, New York.

Richter, C., Park, J.W. and Ames, B.N. (1988). Normal oxidative damage to mitochondrial and nuclear DNA is extensive. *Proceedings of the National Academy of Sciences USA*, **85**, 6465–7.

Rogers, S., Wells R. and Rechsteiner, M. (1986). Amino acid sequences common to rapidly degraded proteins: the PEST hypothesis. *Science*, **234**, 364–8.

Rosenberger, R.F. (1991). Senescence and the accumulation of abnormal proteins. *Mutation Research*, **256**, 255–62.

Satoh, M.S. and Lindahl, T. (1992). Role of poly(ADP-ribose) formation in DNA repair. *Nature*, **356**, 356–8.

Saul, R.L., Gee, P. and Ames, B.N. (1987). Free radicals, DNA damage and aging. In *Modern Biological Theories of Aging*, Warner, H.R., Butler, R.N., Sprott, R.L. and Schneider, E.L., pp. 113–29. Raven Press, New York.

Scott, M.D., Meshnick, S.R. and Eaton, J.W. (1987). Superoxide dismutase-rich bacteria: paradoxical increase in oxidant toxicity. *Journal of Biology and Chemistry*, **262**, 3640–5.

Setlow, R.B. (1987). Theory presentation and background summary. In *Modern Biological Theories of Aging*, Warner, H.R., Butler, R.N., Sprott, R.L. and Schneider, E.L., pp. 177–82. Raven Press, New York.

Seubert, P., Vigo-Pelfrey, C., Esch, F. *et al.* (1992). Isolation and quantification of soluble Alzheimer's beta-peptide from biological fluids. *Nature*, **359**, 325–7.

Shibamato, T. (1989). Gentoxicity testing of Maillard reaction products. In *The Maillard Reaction in Aging, Diabetes and Nutrition. Progress in Clinical and Biological Research*, Baynes, J.W. and Monnier, V.M. (Eds), Vol. 304, pp. 359–76. Alan R. Liss, New York.

Siman, R. and Christoph, G. (1989). Beta-amyloid precursor is a PEST protein. *Biochemistry and Biophysics Research Communications*, **165**, 1299–304.

Stadtman, E.R. (1992). Protein oxidation and aging. *Science*, **257**, 1220–4.

Stephenson, R.C. and Clarke, S. (1989). Succinimide formation from aspartyl and asparaginyl peptides as a model for the spontaneous degradation of proteins. *Journal of Biology and Chemistry*, **264**, 6164–70.

Tabaton, M., Cammarata, S., Mancardi, G. *et al.* (1991). Ultrastructural localizatin of beta-amyloid, tau, and ubiquitin epitopes in extracellular neurofibrillary tangles. *Proceedings of the National Academy of Sciences USA*, **88**, 2098–102.

Taniguchi, N. Kinoshita, N., Arai, K. *et al.* (1989). Inactivation of erythrocyte CuZn–superoxide dismutase through nonenzymic glycosylation. In *The Maillard Reaction in Aging, Diabetes and Nutrition. Progress in Clinical and*

Biological Research, Baynes, J.W. and Monnier, V.M. (Eds), Vol. 304. Alan R. Liss, New York.

Varshavsky, A., Bachmair, A., Finlay, D. *et al.* (1988). The N-end rule of selective protein turnover; mechanistic aspects and functional implications. In *Ubiquitin*, Rechsteiner, M. (Ed.), pp. 287–324. Plenum Press, London, New York.

Vincent, V.L., Smith, R.A., Ma, S. and Cutler, R.G. (1987). Genomic 5-methyldeoxycytidine decreases with age. *Journal of Biological Chemistry*, **262**, 9948–51.

Vlassara, H., Brownlee, M. and Cerami, A. (1985). High affinity receptor-mediated uptake and degradation of glucose modified proteins: a potential mechanism for the removal of senescent molecules. *Proceedings of the National Academy of Sciences USA*, **82**, 3588–92.

Warner, H.R., Butler, R.N., Sprott, R.L. and Schneider, E.L. (Eds) (1987). *Modern Theories of Aging*. Raven Press, New York.

Werraarchkul, N., Strong, R., Wood, W.G. and Richardson, A. (1989). The effect of aging and dietary restriction on DNA repair. *Experimental Cell Research*, **181**, 197–204.

Wharton, S.A. and Hipkiss, A.R. (1985). Degradation of peptides and proteins of different sizes by homogenates of human MRC-5 lung fibroblasts; aged cells have a decreased ability to degrade shortened proteins. *FEBS Letters*, **156**, 249–53.

Wiztum, J.L. and Koschinsky, T. (1989). Metabolic and immunological consequences of glycation of low density lipoproteins. In *The Maillard Reaction in Aging, Diabetes and Nutrition. Progress in Clinical and Biological Research*, Baynes, J.W. and Monnier, V.M. (Eds), Vol. 304, pp. 219–34. Alan R. Liss, New York.

Yarom, R., Sapaznikov, D., Havivi *et al.* (1988). Premature aging changes in neuromuscular junctions of transgenic mice with an extra copy of human CuZnSOD gene: a model for tongue pathology in Down's syndrome. *Journal of Neurological Science*, **88**, 41–53.

Yen, T-C., Su, J-H., King, K-L. and Wei, Y-H. (1991). Ageing-associated 5kb deletion in human liver mitochondrial DNA. Biochemistry and Biophysics Research Communications, **178**, 124–31.

Carol Jagger
Department of Epidemiology and Public Health
and
James Lindesay
Department of Psychiatry
University of Leicester

3 THE EPIDEMIOLOGY OF SENILE DEMENTIA

INTRODUCTION

The discipline of epidemiology is concerned with the investigation and understanding of factors which relate to the occurrence, natural history and associations of diseases. More recently the specialized methods used in epidemiology have also been brought to bear on issues such as the evaluation of treatment programmes and service provision.

This chapter aims to describe both the epidemiological methods useful in research into dementia and the current state of our knowledge of its epidemiology in terms of the natural history and extent of dementing disorders and possible risk factors. There are particular problems with research into diseases such as dementia which are, as yet, not fully defined. We begin with a section highlighting these issues.

PARTICULAR PROBLEMS OF DEMENTIA RESEARCH

The majority of the problems faced in dementia research are in the areas of definition and the methods used for detecting the specific disorders. These will be dealt with in turn.

Definition

Dementia is an umbrella term for a variety of neuropsychological syndromes caused by a wide range of disorders such as Alzheimer's disease, cerebrovascular disease, Pick's disease, diffuse Lewy body disease, chronic alcohol abuse and neurosyphilis. Because of the cerebral pathology that underlies dementia, epidemiologists tend to favour a categorical approach to case definition; that is, individuals either have the disorder or else they do not (Mann, 1991). However, there are no reliable *ante-mortem* markers for many of the most important causes of dementia, so epidemiological studies have to rely on diagnoses based upon clinical symptoms alone. This presents problems, since it is necessary that case-finding procedures distinguish between dementia and other reasons for poor performance on cognitive function testing in the elderly, such as delirium, severe depression, low intelligence, mental handicap and chronic schizophrenia. To this end, various explicit diagnostic criteria for dementia have been drawn up; early attempts such as DSM-III proved unreliable because the criteria were open to interpretation, and they have been superseded by more refined case definitions in DSM-IIIR (American Psychiatric Association, 1987) and ICD10 (World Health Organization, 1987). Criteria for specific causes of dementia have also been devised, such as the NINCDS–ADRDA criteria of Neurological and Communicative Disorders and Stroke and the Alzheimer's Disease and Related Disorders Association in the USA (McKhann *et al.*, 1984).

It is important to bear in mind that, while the categorical approach to case definition in dementia is appropriate for some studies, such as investigations of external risk factors, genetic studies and trials of treatment, a dimensional, quantitative description of dementia may be preferred for other sorts of research, for example, studies of factors associated with severity or service need, or the relationship between dementia and age-associated memory impairment.

Detection

Since the prevalence (extent) of dementia is relatively low, particularly in the younger elderly, accurate estimation of the extent of disease requires a large study population. The amount of information required to diagnose cases correctly, and the need for highly trained specialists to administer assessments, means that if the whole population is assessed, considerable resources are wasted on collecting extensive data on large numbers of disease-free individuals. Over the last decade there has been an increased use of two-phase designs in dementia research, the first phase being a relatively short screening test on the whole population to identify those individuals who are definitely not suffering from dementia. This stage is often administered by a trained fieldworker. On the basis of their score on the screening test, the remainder are then assessed more fully, usually by a clinician. Newman *et al.* (1990) discuss the efficiency of the two-phase design to estimate the extent of mental disorders in a population and conclude that if the screen has good sensitivity and specificity and is cheap to administer compared to the full diagnostic procedure, then this design can result in appreciable gains in efficiency and improvements in case detection compared to a one-phase study (i.e. full diagnostic assessment of the whole population). However, this has to be weighed against the increased complexity of the data analysis which has to allow for the method of sampling. If further stratification is included in the design this might outweigh any savings in efficiency, although Newman *et al.* (1990) recommend the use of software such as SESUDAAN (Shah, 1981) for the analysis in these cases.

There is a considerable number of candidates for the first stage screening instrument, both involving testing of the subject and collecting information from an informant. The main ones used in modern epidemiological studies of dementia will be discussed here, and information on others may be found in Israel *et al.* (1984).

The Mini-Mental State Examination (MMSE) of Folstein *et al.* (1975) is the most widely used screening instrument and, as with many others, was originally devised to assess cognitive impairment in clinical situations. The MMSE consists of 19 items with a total score of 30, lower scores denoting increased impairment. The items cover orientation, registration and recall, calculation and language. The test as a whole has now been translated into a number of different languages and the culturally specific items appear to have been successfully substituted.

Various cut-points have been recommended in order to discriminate between cases and noncases of cognitive impairment. The original cut-point derived on inpatient samples was 23/24 and this was also used by O'Connor *et al.* (1989a) in their study in Cambridge. Other recent studies in UK community populations (Brayne and Calloway, 1989; Clarke *et al.*, 1991) have lowered this to 21/22 and some US studies have discriminated further by using 17 and below to indicate severe cognitive impairment. Analysis of the MMSE against a clinician's diagnosis using Receiver Operating Characteristic (ROC) curves found that a cut-point of 18/19 was optimal for the detection of moderate and severe dementia (Jagger et al., 1992a) and 21/22 when mild dementia was included. With a cut-point of 21/22 the sensitivity of the MMSE for detecting moderate and severe dementia has been found to lie between 83% (Brayne and Calloway, 1989) and 100% (Clarke et al., 1991) with a specificity around 85%. Both sensitivity and specificity are considerably reduced if milder dementia is taken into account.

Although the MMSE has good sensitivity for detecting dementia at the more severe end of the spectrum, is short and relatively easy to administer and has been successfully translated, problems have arisen with misclassification of specific subgroups of individuals. A low level of education, extreme age, manual social class, visual impairments and to some extent manual dexterity have all been implicated in causing subjects to be misclassified as cases, although findings have been somewhat equivocal (Fillenbaum et al., 1988; Jorm et al., 1988; O'Connor et al., 1989b; Brayne and Calloway, 1990; Blessed et al., 1991; Ganguli et al., 1991; Jagger et al., 1992b). To overcome the educational bias, Uhlmann and Larson (1991) have developed education-specific cut-points for the MMSE, whilst Bleeker et al. (1988) have done the same for age. Jagger et al. (1992a) found that dropping the four items which required visual and manual ability (reading and writing a sentence, copying a drawing and folding a piece of paper) considerably improved the overall performance of the test. However, the extent to which the results show true associations between these factors and cognitive impairment is still unclear.

The Clifton Assessment Schedule (CAPE) of Pattie and Gilleard (1979) has both a behaviour rating scale and an Information/Orientation (IO) subtest, the latter covering memory and orientation in time and place. The IO subtest has been used predominantly in the UK (Morgan et al., 1987; Brayne and Calloway, 1989; Clarke et al., 1991), as opposed to the MMSE which has, until late, been mostly a US screening tool. The IO subtest is shorter than the MMSE, with only 12 items, none of which require pencil or paper. A score of seven or below was originally suggested to define severe cognitive impairment, but later work on community populations suggests that eight or below has a higher sensitivity (95%) with little reduction in specificity (96%) for detecting moderate and severe dementia (Brayne and Calloway, 1989; Clarke et al., 1991). Although doubts have been cast upon the ability of the IO subtest to detect dementia accurately (Black et al., 1990), comparison of the IO subtest and the MMSE over their full range with ROC analysis (Jagger et al., 1992a) found that the IO subtest performs better than the full MMSE for moderate and severe dementia and has a slightly worse performance, though not significantly so, for mild and worse dementia. From this analysis, a cut-point of 11/12 appears optimal for the detection of mild, moderate and severe dementia and this demonstrates the 'ceiling' effect evident with shorter tests.

Another short screening instrument for cognitive impairment that has been used in surveys of elderly people is the Organic Brain Syndrome (OBS) scale of the Comprehensive Assessment and Referral Evaluation (CARE) schedule (Gurland et al., 1977; 1984). The CARE, a semi-structured schedule taking around 1.5 hours to complete, was developed in a series of studies of elderly people in London and New York. It is made up of items dealing with psychiatric disorder, physical health, social problems, and supports and services received. A clinically trained interviewer is not a prerequisite for administering the CARE, although the interview incorporates interviewer observations and judgements rather than those of a qualified informant. By means of latent class analysis of all of the items, 38 'homogenous-items' scales have been derived, of which the OBS scale is one of the most widely used and validated in both community and residential samples of the elderly. The OBS scale has been used and validated as a screen for cognitive impairment in community surveys of the elderly (Lindesay et al., 1989; Livingston et al., 1990), and versions of the scale with modified wording, number and order of the homogenous items have been developed, used and validated in various settings; for example, the SHORT-CARE in general practice (Macdonald, 1986), and the Brief Assessment Schedule (BAS) in residential homes (Mann et al., 1984). The shortened scales do not include a physical examination or informant information, making diagnoses of specific dementing disorders impossible.

A number of informant questionnaires now exist which aim to overcome some of the difficulties met by cognitive testing of elderly subjects. The older Blessed Dementia Scale (BDS) (Blessed et al., 1986) consists of 11 questions covering the everyday activities of the subject. The more recently developed Informant Questionnaire on Cognitive Decline in the Elderly (IQCODE) of Jorm et al. (1991a) has 26 items and specifically asks informants to rate the change in the subject's memory over the previous 10 years. The Détérioration Cognitive Observée (DECO) of Ritchie and Fuhrer (1992) has 19 items dealing with changes over the past year in a variety of behaviours as observed by someone who has known the subject closely for at least 3 years.

Rating scales using informants overcome the issues of the influence of education, age and social class on cognitive tests, and all appear to perform as well as existing cognitive scales, although extensive application in community populations has not yet been undertaken. Informant questionnaires do, however, presuppose that a suitable person is available and willing to answer questions. With up to 50% of elderly over the age of 75 years living alone in the UK and the increased mobility of families, a qualified informant may not always be easy to trace. This notwithstanding, these types of scales or combinations of cognitive tests and informant observations may well produce more accurate screening tools in the near future.

The choice of the diagnostic (second stage) instrument in two-stage studies is of paramount importance if there is to be any comparability between studies. The main instruments in use and under development at the present time are the Geriatric Mental State (GMS) of Copeland et al. (1976) from which AGECAT has developed, the Cambridge Mental Disorders of the Elderly (CAMDEX) of Roth et al. (1988), the previously mentioned CARE, the newer Structured Interview for the diagnosis of Dementia of the Alzheimer type, Multi-infarct dementia and dementias of other aetiology (SIDAM) of Zaudig et al. (1991) and the Canberra Interview for the Elderly (CIE) from the Social Psychiatry Research Unit in Canberra (1992). Some of these use a form of standardized interview schedule from which a clinician arrives at a diagnosis according to specified criteria (CARE, CAMDEX) whilst others (AGECAT, SIDAM, CIE) use an algorithm to combine the information and reach a diagnosis. In the case of AGECAT and CIE this stage is performed by a computer.

As with the CARE, the GMS was developed from a transatlantic study comparing psychiatric disorders in the elderly in London and New York (Gurland et al., 1983). The GMS has many items in common with both the Present State Examination (PSE) and the Present Status Schedule (PSS), two psychiatric interviews aimed at younger adults. Interviews take around 30–40 minutes and reliability across different interviewers has been found to be high although ratings of the same subject at different time points is more variable. This latter observation may suggest that the GMS is sensitive to minor changes in cognitive function. AGECAT, the computerized algorithm applied to GMS items, was developed with the aim of ensuring reliability of diagnosis across interviewers. Although it has been widely used, AGECAT cannot produce diagnoses of specific dementing disorders and may disagree with a clinician's diagnosis as it fails to take into account factors other than the mental state of the patient. Work is being undertaken on this aspect, including collecting information from an informant by means of the History and Aetiology Schedule (HAS).

In contrast, the CAMDEX procedure includes both a physical examination and an interview with an informant as well as a present and past medical and psychiatric history and various laboratory tests. Interviews typically last between 1.5 and 2 hours including the informant interview. Although its main use has been with clinicians undertaking the interviews, it has been administered by trained nurses. Taking all the information into account and using specific diagnostic criteria for rating the severity of the dementia, the interviewer comes to a primary clinical diagnosis of specific dementing disorders including Alzheimer's disease (AD), multi-infarct dementia (MID), mixed AD/MID and dementia secondary to other causes. Allowance is made for depression both as a primary diagnosis and secondary to dementia, and O'Connor et al. (1990) found few problems with diagnoses by the CAMDEX in subjects with coexisting dementia and depression. The large cognitive section in the CAMDEX, the CAMCOG, includes the MMSE, and the Blessed scale is also included in the informant's part. Work is currently underway to incorporate the CAMCOG scores and scores on three other scales within the CAMDEX measuring organicity, depression and MID, into a computerized algorithm for diagnosis. Few reliability and validity studies have been carried out on other than hospital populations, but these have shown good results.

The newly developed SIDAM is a brief schedule taking 30 minutes for the diagnosis of dementia and cognitive impairment according to DSM-IIIR and ICD10 criteria. Like GMS/AGECAT and CARE, it does not involve a physical examination but consideration is made in part of the assessment of information from an informant. It aims mainly to differentiate 'normal' from 'demented' subjects rather than classification into specific dementing disorders. With these aims its early reliability and validity results are promising. This instrument is available in a number of languages, as are all the other schedules discussed here.

The most recent instrument to be developed is the CIE, which draws on the wide experience of the Social Psychiatry Research Unit in Canberra, and attempts to overcome a number of the problems of the other diagnostic schedules. Specifically designed to be administered by a lay person, it uses cognitive testing, informant reports and interviewer ratings of concentration and confusion to reach a diagnosis of dementia or depression compatible with DSM-IIIR and the draft ICD10 criteria. Reliability on a small-scale sample has been shown to be high, but validity testing and its use in community populations has not yet been reported.

EPIDEMIOLOGICAL METHODS IN DEMENTIA RESEARCH

Since the diagnosis of dementia can only be made with any degree of certainty at autopsy, epidemiological methods used with other well-defined diseases may be inappropriate. All epidemiological investigations require that the study population defining those at risk of the disease be selected with care and attention. First the choice of population for the study of dementia will be considered.

Choice of study population

Since most dementia occurs in the elderly, studies often wish to concentrate resources on this age group. However, this assumes that some mechanism (in the form of a list) exists which allows identification of elderly by age. In developed countries this may be as inclusive as in parts of Scandanavia where countrywide registers exist, or more usually electoral rolls or general practitioner registers. In the developing world where these sources may not exist, or in the developed world in inner city areas where the sources are known or suspected to be under-inclusive, preliminary enumeration by 'door-knocking' methods may be required first to obtain an accurate sampling frame (Veras and Murphy, 1991).

Wherever feasible, the sampling frame should include institutionalized subjects to avoid underestimation of the extent of dementia. Areas with no residential care for the elderly should endeavour to determine to where the institutionalized elderly are migrating. The use of psychiatric registers for ascertainment of cases is not to be encouraged as these rarely include all cases, in particular those in residential and nursing homes. Care should be taken when using general practitioner lists as sampling frames, as long-term psychiatric inpatients are deregistered after varying lengths of time. In the UK, inaccurate general practitioner lists through migration are less of a problem in older age groups, and overinflation through the inclusion of patients who have died and not been removed should decrease with the requirement to meet targets for the annual screening of over 75 year olds by general practitioners. Within inner city areas however, general practitioner lists are likely to be of questionnable accuracy as a sampling frame for some time to come.

The main study designs used in dementia research are those applicable to any epidemiological investigation. The advantages and disadvantages of their use in investigating the extent of dementia in a population are discussed below.

Cross-sectional studies

Cross-sectional studies are commonly used to measure the extent of a disease in a population at a particular time. The prevalence rate of a disease is defined as the number of cases with the disease at a point in time divided by the number in the population at risk of acquiring the disease. Sometimes studies measure the extent of disease over short periods, for example, 6 months, and from these a *period prevalence* can be calculated similarly. Since these rates are usually obtained from samples of the population at risk, they are only *estimates* of the true prevalence, and the precision of this estimate is indicated by the associated 95% confidence intervals.

These studies can also assess the extent of unmet need in populations. With regard to risk factors, however, this design can only be used to generate hypotheses by investigating associations between the prevalence and particular subgroups defined by, for example, gender and social class. Since all measurements are taken at a single point in time, the causal pathway cannot be inferred. The comparison of prevalence rates from studies across geographic populations may provide a valuable insight into the causes of disease although comparisons can only be made sensibly if the case definition is the same. For dementia this is more problematic than for other non-psychiatric diseases, although cross-cultural studies are at present in the planning stage.

Cross-sectional (or prevalence) studies need to assess the disease status of a large population. For dementia the problems this brings have been discussed in some detail earlier with regard to the use of two-stage design. These studies are becoming more common and have been used recently by O'Connor *et al.* (1989a), Brayne and Calloway (1989), Clarke *et al.* (1991) and Heeren *et al.* (1991). The use of simple random samples from larger populations is less ideal as the very elderly, in whom dementia is more prevalent, will tend to be relatively underrepresented, and prevalence rates in these older groups will have much wider confidence intervals. A better approach is to stratify the population by age, and sample the age groups using different sampling fractions, for example, 1 in 20 of the 75–79 year olds, 1 in 10 of those aged 85 years and over. This will result in greater precision of the rates for the very elderly. Examples of prevalence studies using this sampling method are those of Brayne and Calloway (1989), Morgan *et al.* (1987) and Campbell *et al.* (1983).

In large-scale health studies where mental health may not be the only criterion, it is tempting to use one of the many short screening tests for cognitive impairment to measure the prevalence of mental impairment. Although these tests are often highly sensitive, this condition is not optimal for accurate estimation of prevalence (Hand, 1987). Black *et al.* (1990) have suggested that some of the low prevalence rates reported may be due to the insensitivity of some of the short screening tests, but where a disease such as dementia has a relatively low prevalence it is much more likely that the high reported rates are due to tests with low specificity (Jagger *et al.*, 1992c).

Cohort studies

Cohort studies (or longitudinal studies) follow up a group of individuals over time in order to investigate prospectively the development of the disease. The group of individuals are usually defined by some common attribute, for example, occupation or year of birth, but more often place of residence. From cohort studies the *incidence* (or more accurately the *incidence rate*) of the disease can be ascertained, i.e. the number of subjects developing the disease in a specified time period divided by the size of the population at risk. As subjects are followed up over time, the predictive validity of the classification of dementia can be examined and aetiological factors identified.

Longitudinal cohort studies to determine the incidence of dementia are still relatively rare in comparison with cross-sectional (prevalence) studies. The main reasons for this are the enormous problems of designing and executing any longitudinal study, but specific problems arise when the study population is elderly and the disease in question has no well-defined onset, as with dementia. Continual monitoring of a population is impossible, so longitudinal studies aim at specific times for reassessment: 1, 2, sometimes 5 or 10 years. Although response rates to health surveys in the elderly have been very good historically, Murphy (1991) cites evidence that rates may be beginning to fall. Refusal due to 'oversurveying' may be an increasing concern in the UK with the annual screening of the elderly within general practice now underway (Jagger *et al.*, 1992d). Reasons for decreasing the time intervals between reassessments are mainly to ensure more accurate date of onset and to minimize loss to follow-up through death or migration. The latter is less likely to be a problem in the elderly than the former, although some geographic populations may lose subjects to institutions out of the area.

Designing a cohort study requires a delicate balancing act between the minimization of loss to follow-up through migration and death and the maximization of 'customer satisfaction' in terms of response rates. It needs little reiteration that such studies are very costly and this, together with the other design issues, has resulted in few accurate estimates of the incidence of dementia. Despite this, there are a number of incidence studies currently underway, mostly of a multicentre design so that sufficient 'events' of the disease can be amassed. To encourage further multicentred research and the meta-analysis of single-centre studies, the EURODEM group have set up a protocol for future incidence studies (Launer, 1992).

Case-control studies

For diseases with a low incidence a cohort study may require an impractically long follow-up time to amass sufficient incident cases. In these situations it is quicker and less costly to use a case-control study design. Case-control studies begin with a representative set of cases of the disease and a set of controls without the disease belonging to the same population from which the cases arose. Retrospective information about factors of interest thought to be associated with the disease (exposures) are elicited from cases and controls. Association between disease and exposure is measured by calculation of the *odds-ratio*, the ratio of the odds of disease in the exposed and nonexposed groups, which approximates the *relative risk* of disease, or ratio of incidence in the exposed and nonexposed groups. Furthermore, direct estimation of the *attributable risk* or amount of disease in the population which can be explained by the exposure of interest, is possible. Case-control studies also allow for the control of confounding factors, that is factors which are associated both with the exposure being investigated and the disease under study.

Despite low cost and time relative to cohort studies, case-control studies may suffer from a number of problems which potentially bias any results obtained. Firstly, cases should be incident cases rather than prevalent ones to avoid *survivorship bias* with cases who have had the disease longer being less likely to survive and therefore eligible for selection. This poses the same problem as discussed earlier in defining an incident case of a disease whose onset is insidious. Also, all cases in the community should be available for selection into the study. Defining incident cases in this setting is subject to general practitioners recognizing and referring cases, and evidence has been found (Williamson *et al.*, 1964; O'Connor *et al.*, 1988) to show that general practitioners miss a large percentage of cases; this may result in *case-ascertainment bias* if the cases being detected differ in the risk factors of interest. *Referral bias* may also be present if practitioners chose not to refer certain patients, perhaps the very old or frail, for inclusion into the study.

On the subject of choice of controls, these are often matched in order to produce subjects as comparable as possible to the cases. It is important to realize that any factor matched for cannot be investigated for association with the disease, thus overmatching should be avoided. It is generally sufficient to match on age, sex and perhaps area of residence, although the latter should be avoided if environmental factors or those associated with socioeconomic group are being studied. Any retrospective information should be collected in the same way from both cases and controls to avoid *recall bias*.

To overcome some of these biases a design known as a nested case-control study may be employed. This is a case-control study embedded within a cohort study. When a case becomes incident, a control is drawn from all in the cohort alive at that time and at risk of developing the disease. Information about factors of interest is collected at the start of the cohort study ensuring that cases and controls do not selectively recall events. To overcome the problem of small numbers of cases and the subsequent missing of clinically significant associations, the EURODEM incidence group has proposed a collaborative study and designed a protocol to allow for pooling of results from several nested case-control studies which are included in the ongoing incidence studies mentioned previously (Launer *et al.*, 1992).

PREVALENCE AND INCIDENCE OF DEMENTIA

Due to the problems of follow-up and accurate measurement of onset of dementia, the vast majority of studies in the past have been conducted to measure the prevalence rather than the incidence of dementing disorders. Jorm *et al.* (1987) list 47 prevalence studies of dementia or cognitive impairment on community samples undertaken worldwide between 1945 and 1985, and there have been at least a further dozen reported since these. Jorm *et al.* (1987) tried to compare the studies quantitively and found that studies of rural communities, those assessing the total population as opposed to a random sample and the inclusion of mild dementia in the assessment, tended to report lower rates of dementia overall. Further modelling of those studies with adequate age breakdowns resulted in a model of the prevalence–age curve with prevalence rates doubling every 5 years. Preston (1986) earlier had fitted a similar model to much fewer studies and found rates doubled around every 6 years.

The EURODEM group have undertaken a similar re-analysis of studies of the prevalence of dementia but have used much more stringent criteria (Hofman *et al.*, 1991). Studies had to be conducted in Europe between 1980 and 1990, dementia had to be defined by DSM-III criteria or equivalent and institutional residents were included in the samples. There was some heterogeneity of rates by age but the application of a similar model-fitting method to that of Jorm *et al.* (1987) resulted in a prevalence–age curve which differed between the sexes and levelled off after the age of 85 years (unpublished data). Table 3.1 shows the estimated rates by age group and sex from this analysis.

Table 3.2 demonstrates the difference between this and the previous analyses of prevalence studies. The study by Ritchie *et al.* (1991) was a repeat of the Jorm *et al.* (1987) analysis but including only post-1980 studies. The levelling off at older ages is shown here too, although the rates at each age are somewhat lower, perhaps because of the wide geographical spread of the studies used.

Integrating results from over a wide geographical area can be misleading due to the varying ratios of AD to MID found worldwide and the different prevalence–age curves for the specific disorders. Another factor which comes to play, particularly in less developed countries, is the differing survival patterns. Jorm *et al.* (1987) found that the prevalence of MID doubled with every 5.3 years of age, whilst for AD doubling occurred with every 4.6 years.

Table 3.1 Estimated prevalences (%) by age group for men and women from the EURODEM re-analysis.

Age group (years)	Median age (years)	Estimated prevalence (%) (95% CI)	
		Men	Women
65–69	67.5	2.1 (1.2,3.4)	1.1 (0.7,1.8)
70–74	72.5	3.5 (2.4,5.0)	3.0 (2.4,4.3)
75–79	77.5	6.1 (4.3,8.4)	6.9 (5.0,9.4)
80–84	82.0	10.0 (7.3,13.6)	12.8 (9.5,17.0)
85–89	87.0	17.4 (13.0,22.9)	21.7 (16.6,27.9)
90–94	91.5	27.7 (20.3,36.7)	30.6 (23.7,38.5)

CI = confidence interval.

Table 3.2 Estimated prevalences (%) for both sexes combined from the EURODEM model (unpublished data) and those of Jorm, Preston and Ritchie *et al.*

Age group (years)	Median age (years)	Estimated overall prevalence (%)			
		Preston (1986)	Jorm (1987)	Ritchie *et al.* (1991)	EURODEM (unpublished)
65–69	67.5	1.8	1.4	1.4	1.5
70–74	72.5	3.3	2.8	2.6	3.2
75–79	77.5	6.3	5.6	4.7	6.6
80–84	82.0	11.7	10.5	8.1	11.8
85–89	87.0	22.0	20.8	14.9	20.5
90–94	91.5	41.3	38.6	25.7	29.9

Age-adjusted rates for AD were significantly higher for females than males, whilst for MID overall rates were higher for males than females. This latter finding has also been confirmed by the EURODEM group (Rocca *et al.*, 1991a). In addition most European studies show a significant excess of AD cases over MID; Japanese, Chinese and Russian an excess of MID, and Finnish and US studies show no significant difference (Jorm *et al.*, 1987). The 'norm' in present studies appears to be an overall rate of dementia in those aged 65 years and over of between 4 and 7% although a recent study in East Boston, USA reported rates of 11.6%, these being mainly AD (Evans *et al.*, 1989).

In contrast to the large number of prevalence studies, Jorm (1990) lists only 12 studies of the incidence of senile dementia in old age and only half of these separated out the specific dementing disorders. Although differences in rates are extremely likely with the range of diagnostic criteria used, some global conclusions can be made, albeit tentatively. Certainly, and not surprisingly, the incidence of dementia rises sharply with age from around 0.3% at age 65 years to around 3.5% at age 85 years. There is some evidence that the incidence rates of AD level off in the very old, but the small number of events combined with small population size at these ages make the confidence intervals on estimates at these ages very wide indeed. A more recent study in Japan (Fukunishi *et al.*, 1991) confirms the overall rates by age but shows no levelling off of AD at older ages. With both the dearth of incidence studies in the past and the change in diagnostic criteria over time, there is little evidence available for any changes in incidence rates over time. Only the Lundby study in Sweden has such long-term incidence data and Rorsman *et al.* (1986) report no significant difference in the incidence rates between 1947–57 and 1957–72. Over the next few years the EURODEM group will be reporting the results of incidence studies undertaken in a number of European countries using a standard protocol which will overcome some of the problems of differing diagnostic criteria and the low power of individual studies.

RISK FACTORS FOR DEMENTIA

The assessment of factors which give rise to an increased risk of developing dementia can lead to a better understanding of the mechanisms which cause the disease, as well as suggesting strategies which might be adopted for primary prevention. The majority of evidence for and against specific risk factors for both AD and MID is derived from case-control studies. Much more research has been done on risk factors for AD than for MID, mainly because the prevalence of MID is low relative to AD within the USA and Europe where the majority of case-control and longitudinal studies have been conducted. A further reason for the dearth of research into risk factors for MID has been that a consensus on definitions and diagnosis is still far away and a number of potential risk factors are involved in defining cases (e.g. hypertension).

Jorm (1990) reviews the risk factors for AD and MID separately. Advanced age has been consistently associated with an increased risk of both AD and MID. Gender has shown less conclusive associations. Other sociodemographic variables such as social class or level of education have had little investigation with regard to incidence, although Lammi et al. (1989) found that low education level was associated with later mental disability, and both Boller et al. (1991) and Aronson et al. (1990) found a greater rate of cognitive dysfunctioning in those with poor verbal fluency. The latest evaluation of suspected risk factors comes from a series of papers prepared by the EURODEM Risk Factors Research Group, who have undertaken a comprehensive re-analysis of eleven case-control studies (Van Duijn et al., 1991b). Although the problems of spurious significant associations due to bias from case-control studies has already been discussed, a number of these were overcome in restricting the analysis to only those studies where data were collected symmetrically for cases and controls. Certain analyses were restricted further to only those case-control pairs who were concordant for relationship of informant to case/control. Furthermore, although both prevalent and incident cases were included in the studies, specific analyses were restricted to incident cases to reduce the likelihood of survivorship bias.

The genetic component in the development of dementia has been investigated predominantly by the proxy of family history of dementia, often restricted to first degree relatives to avoid biases in recall and survival. For both vascular dementia and AD a positive family history has been shown to produce an increased risk in the subject by a number of studies. The EURODEM re-analysis (Van Duijn et al., 1991a) confirmed an increased risk of both early and late onset cases (defined as under/over 70 years) although the association for late onset cases was weaker.

Other familial disease has been implicated in AD and MID, most notably Down's syndrome and Parkinson's disease in AD and stroke in MID. The collaborative re-analysis showed a significantly increased risk of AD with a family history of Down's syndrome overall, with the individual studies having relative risks of above unity though not reaching significance. As the prevalence of Down's syndrome is low this is compatible with the low power of the individual studies. Both family history of Down's and Parkinson's disease showed increased risks of AD even in the absence of a family history of dementia, suggesting that these factors increase the risk of AD regardless of the presence of others. Evidence for association with diseases such as haematological malignancies has been equivocal and needs further investigation.

A variety of previous medical conditions has been evaluated for AD with the major finding being previous head trauma resulting in loss of consciousness. Jorm (1990) reviews it as still only a possible risk factor and the EURODEM group (Mortimer et al., 1991) still urge caution in interpreting the significant results. The latter analysis reports consistently increased risk of AD for trauma with loss of consciousness in all studies although the effect appears significant only in men. The Dutch study (Hofman et al., 1989) demonstrated an increased risk of AD for trauma less than 10 years before onset of dementia after adjustment for both family history of dementia and level of education. However, there appears little evidence from this or from Mortimer et al. (1991) that those with a family history of dementia are at any more risk after head trauma than those with no family history.

A potentially interesting increased risk of AD in subjects with a history of depression was found by the EURODEM group (Jorm et al., 1991b). As the study used medical records any recall bias is eliminated, and as the increased risk was observed before onset of AD the finding is unlikely to be due to the dementia. However, other biases cannot be ruled out and this factor merits further investigation from prospective studies.

Diabetes does not appear to have a significant association with AD, a number of studies showing risks around unity, although Meyer et al. (1988) found cases of vascular dementia to have significantly more diabetes than controls. Meningitis and encephalitis, heart disease and kidney disease are classed by Jorm (1990) as requiring further investigation in AD whilst thyroid disease, herpes infection, stomach ulcers, arthritis and allergies are dismissed as unlikely risk factors on the evidence so far. The EURODEM group found some tentative associations between AD and both hypothyroidism and epilespy (Breteler et al., 1991). Severe headaches and migraine were found to confer a reduced risk of AD although all of these significant results may well be due to recall bias or 'data dredging'. Hypertension has been implicated with MID, although this is often hampered by its presence being required for a positive diagnosis.

The majority of factors in the area of dietary and environmental factors have stemmed from links with exposure to aluminium or drug abuse. Those associated with aluminium such as antacid use and dietary intake of aluminium appear to have little evidence, confirmation of significant findings being based on ecological correlations and assessment of dementia based on reports from death certificates (known to be an unreliable source of dementia prevalence) or computed tomographic (CT) scans without examination of the subject. Drug abuse, on the other hand, has more evidence in its favour. Phenaticin abuse has been found by Murray et al. (1971) to result in an increased risk of dementia, although various case-control studies have failed to replicate the findings, possibly due to the low power. High alcohol consumption, despite being a plausible risk factor for both AD and MID, has shown no excess risk of AD from the EURODEM analysis (Graves et al., 1991a).

Smoking, on the other hand, is showing more evidence of associations with AD and MID. With MID, smoking appears to be associated with an increased risk of dementia whilst for AD it appears to have a protecting effect (Graves et al., 1991a). These results for AD may well be due to selection or survival biases, particularly in the systematic classification of smokers to diagnoses other than AD although the protective effect of smoking has also been found in Parkinson's disease (Marttila and Rinne, 1980; Haack et al., 1981) and may suggest a joint aetiology of these two diseases.

Occupational exposures such as use of solvents and vibratory tools have been investigated in a few studies with no startling findings. As with other exposures the size of studies required to pick up a moderate effect of many of these occupational exposures is much larger than has been achieved thus far. The collaborative re-analysis (Graves et al., 1991b) validated the earlier negative findings, although the focus was not on particular high-risk occupations and detailed exposure measurement.

The positive association between Down's syndrome and AD has resulted in research into parental age as a possible risk factor. Of the later studies (post-1980) listed by Jorm (1990) as evaluating maternal age, only two found a significantly higher mean age for cases over that of controls. It has been suggested that the incidence curve for Down's is U-shaped with both young and old maternal ages being associated with an increased risk, and the collaborative re-analysis (Rocca et al., 1991b) adds weight to this. Paternal age has been investigated less frequently than maternal age and findings are both negative and positive.

In summary, most of the risk factors have been assessed by case-control studies due to the paucity of longitudinal studies, particularly for MID. The EURODEM incidence studies now underway with a standard protocol for data collection (Launer *et al.*, 1992) should provide more conclusive evidence on many of these risk factors without the problems of recall, selection or survival biases inherent in case-control studies. At the moment there is little scope for public health interventions in any of the areas.

CONCLUSIONS

The picture of the onset and progression of dementia and how best it can be alleviated is far from complete. Whilst the 1960s to early 1980s saw an epidemic of individual, uncoordinated prevalence studies, in the late 1980s some researchers began to realize that much more could be accomplished by an integrated approach with studies using common protocols. The EURODEM prevalence and incidence groups have been at the forefront of this line of investigation and the rewards should be reaped, in terms of tighter incidence rates by age and risk factor assessment, in the next few years.

Another line of research which should add more pieces to the jigsaw is that of cross-cultural studies. The now famous studies of Japanese migrants in the USA added much to the research into risk factors for coronary heart disease. The same could be true for dementia. Although migrant populations tend to be much younger than the indigenous population, some minorities now have significant numbers of elderly people. For example, within Leicester an ideal population would be the Asian population, where comparisons with a Caucasian elderly group and a nonmigrant group from India may provide valuable evidence on risk factors, onset and how different cultures cope with the disease. One of the main problems in mounting such a study is the diagnostic instrument to be used. Research is urgently needed on the acceptability and diagnostic accuracy of translated versions of the usual diagnostic schedules. Although culturally equivalent items can be substituted in batteries, as has been done in the Mini-Mental State, it is difficult to test whether these items are diagnostically equivalent.

However, despite these potentially fruitful lines of research, the changing age structure of elderly populations with increased survival and the enhanced levels of health and social welfare experienced in early life by the newer elderly cohorts, will provide uncertainties for researchers and service providers for some time to come.

REFERENCES

American Psychiatric Association (1987). *Diagnostic and Statistical Manual of Mental Disorders*, 3rd edition revised. American Psychiatric Association, Washington DC.

Aronson, M.K., Ooi, W.L., Morgenstern, H. *et al.* (1990). Women, myocardial infarction, and dementia in the very old. *Neurology*, **40**, 1102–6.

Black, S.E., Blessed, G., Edwardson, J.A. and Kay, D.W.K. (1990). Prevalence rates of dementia in an ageing population: are low rates due to the use of insensitive instruments? *Age and Ageing*, **19**, 84–90.

Bleeker, M.L., Bolla-Wilson, K., Kawas, C. and Agnew, J. (1988). Age-specific norms for the Mini-Mental State Exam. *Neurology*, **38**, 1565–8.

Blessed, G., Tomlinson, B.E. and Roth, M. (1986). The association between quantitative measures of dementia and senile change in the cerebral grey matter of elderly subjects. *British Journal of Psychiatry*, **114**, 797–811.

Blessed, G., Black, S.E., Butler, T. and Kay, D.W.K. (1991). The diagnosis of dementia in the elderly. A comparison of CAMCOG (the cognitive section of the CAMDEX), the AGECAT program, DSM-III, the Mini-Mental State Examination and some short rating scales. *British Journal of Psychiatry*, **159**, 193–8.

Boller, F., Becker, J.T., Holland, A.L. *et al.* (1991). Predictors of decline in Alzheimer's disease. *Cortex*, **27**, 9–17.

Brayne, C. and Calloway, P. (1989). An epidemiological study of dementia in a rural population of elderly women. *British Journal of Psychiatry*, **155**, 214–19.

Brayne, C. and Calloway, P. (1990). The association of education and socioeconomic status with the Mini-Mental State Examination and the clinical diagnosis of dementia in elderly people. *Age and Ageing*, **19**, 91–6.

Breteler, M.M.B., Van Duijn, C.M., Chandra, V. *et al.* (1991). Medical history and the risk of Alzheimer's disease: a collaborative re-analysis of case-control studies. *International Journal of Epidemiology*, **20** (Suppl. 2), S36–S42.

Campbell, A.J., McCosh, L.M., Reinken, J. and Allan, B.C. (1983). Dementia in old age and the need for services. *Age and Ageing*, **12**, 11–16.

Clarke, M., Jagger, C., Anderson, J. *et al.* (1991). The prevalence of dementia in a total population: a comparison of two screening instruments. *Age and Ageing*, **20**, 396–403.

Copeland, J.R.M., Kelleher, M.J., Kellett, J.M. *et al.* (1976). A semi-structured clinical interview for the assessment of diagnosis and mental state in the elderly: The Geriatric Mental State Schedule. I. Development and reliability. *Psychological Medicine*, **16**, 89–99.

Evans, D.A., Funkenstein, H.H., Albert, M.S. *et al.* (1989). Prevalence of Alzheimer's disease in a community population of older persons. *Journal of the American Medical Association*, **262**, 2551–6.

Fillenbaum, G.G., Hughes, D.C., Heyman, A. *et al.* (1988). Relationship of health and demographic characteristics to Mini-Mental State Examination score among community residents. *Psychological Medicine*, **18**, 719–26.

Folstein, M.F., Folstein, S.E. and McHugh, P.R. (1975). 'Mini-Mental State': a practical method for grading the cognitive state of patients for the clinician. *Journal of Psychiatric Research*, **12**, 189–98.

Fukunishi, I., Hayabara, T. and Hosokawa, K. (1991). Epidemiological surveys of senile dementia in Japan. *International Journal of Social Psychiatry*, **37**, 51–6.

Ganguli, M., Ratcliff, G., Huff, J. *et al.* (1991). Effects of age, gender and education on cognitive tests in a rural elderly community sample: norms from the Monongahela Valley Independent Elders Survey. *Neuroepidemiology*, **10**, 42–52.

Graves, A.B., Van Duijn, C.M., Chandra, V. *et al.* (1991a). Alcohol and tobacco consumption as risk factors for Alzheimer's disease: a collaborative re-analysis of case-control studies. *International Journal of Epidemiology*, 20 (Suppl. 2), S48–S57.

Graves, A.B., Van Duijn, C.M., Chandra, V. *et al.* (1991b). Occupational exposure to solvents and lead as risk factors for Alzheimer's disease: a collaborative re-analysis of case-control studies. *International Journal of Epidemiology*, **20** (Suppl. 2), S58–S61.

Gurland, B.J., Copeland, J.R.M., Kuriansky, J. *et al.* (1983). *The Mind and Mood of Ageing*. Crown Helm, London.

Gurland, B., Golden, R.R., Teresi, J.A. and Challop, J. (1984). The SHORT-CARE: an efficient instrument for the assessment of depression, dementia and disability. *Journal of Gerontology*, **39**, 166–9.

Gurland, B., Kuriansky, J., Sharpe, L. *et al.* (1977). The Comprehensive Assessment and Referral Evaluation (CARE) – rationale, development and reliability. *International Journal of Aging and Human Development*, **8**, 9–42.

Haack, D.G., Baumann, R.J., McKean, H.E. *et al.* (1981). Nicotine exposure and Parkinson disease. *American Journal of Epidemiology*, **114**, 191–200.

Hand, D.J. (1987). Screening vs prevalence estimation. *Applied Statistics*, **36**, 1–7.

Heeren, T.J., Lagaay, A.M., Hijmans, W. and Rooymans, H.G.M. (1991). Prevalence of dementia in the 'oldest old' of a Dutch community. *Journal of the American Geriatrics Society*, **39**, 755–9.

Hofman, A., Schulte, W., Tanja, T.A. *et al.* (1989). History of dementia and Parkinson's disease in 1st-degree relatives of patients with Alzheimer's disease. *Neurology*, **39**, 1589–92.

Hofman, A., Rocca, W.A., Brayne, C. *et al.* (1991). The prevalence of dementia in Europe: a collaborative study of the 1980–1990 findings. *International Journal of Epidemiology*, **20**, 736–48.

Israel, K., Kozaveric, D. and Sartorius, N. (1984). *Source Book of Geriatric Assessment*. Karger, Basle.

Jagger, C., Clarke, M. and Anderson, J. (1992a). Screening for dementia – a comparison of two tests using Receiver Operating Characteristic (ROC) analysis. *International Journal of Geriatric Psychiatry*, **7**, 659–66.

Jagger, C., Clarke, M., Anderson, J. and Battcock, T. (1992b). Misclassification of dementia by the Mini-Mental State Examination – are education and social class the only factors? *Age and Ageing*, **21**, 404–11.

Jagger, C., Clarke, M., Anderson, J. and Battcock, T. (1992c). Dementia in Melton Mowbray – a validation of earlier findings. *Age and Ageing*, **21**, 205–10.

Jagger, C., Clarke, M. and Anderson, J. (1992d). Incidence of dementia in Melton Mowbray – a proposed study and its problems. *Neuroepidemiology*, **7** (Suppl. 1), 57–60.

Jorm, A.F. (1990). *The Epidemiology of Alzheimer's disease and related disorders*. Chapman and Hall, London.

Jorm, A.F., Korten, A.E. and Henderson, A.S. (1987). The prevalence of dementia: a quantitative integration of the literature. *Acta Psychiatrica Scandinavica*, **76**, 465–79.

Jorm, A.F., Scott, R., Henderson, A.S. and Kay, D.W.K. (1988). Educational level differences on the Mini-Mental State: the role of test bias. *Psychological Medicine*, **18**, 727–31.

Jorm, A.F., Scott, R., Cullen, J.S. and MacKinnon, A.J. (1991a). Performance of the Informant Questionnaire on Cognitive Decline in the Elderly (IQCODE) as a screening test for dementia. *Psychological Medicine*, **21**, 785–90.

Jorm, A.F., Van Duijn, C.M., Chandra, V. *et al.* (1991b). Psychiatric history and related exposures as risk factors for Alzheimer's disease: a collaborative re-analysis of case-control studies. *International Journal of Epidemiology*, **20** (Suppl. 2), S43–S47.

Lammi, U-K., Kivela, S-L., Nissinen, A. *et al.* (1989). Mental disability among elderly men in Finland: prevalence, predictors and correlates. *Acta Psychiatrica Scandinavica*, **80**, 459–68.

Launer, L.J. (1992). Overview of incidence studies of dementia conducted in Europe. *Neuroepidemiology*, **11** (Suppl. 1), 2–13.

Launer, L.J., Brayne, C., Breteler, M.M.B. *et al.* (1992). Epidemiologic approach to the study of dementing disease: a nested case-control study in European incidence studies of dementia. *Neuroepidemiology*, **11** (Suppl. 1), 114–18.

Lindesay, J., Briggs, K. and Murphy, E. (1989). The Guy's/Age Concern Survey. Prevalence rates of cognitive impairment, depression and anxiety in an urban elderly community. *British Journal of Psychiatry*, **155**, 317–29.

Livingston, G., Sax, K., Willison, J. *et al.* (1990). The Gospel Oak Study stage II: the diagnosis of dementia in the community. *Psychological Medicine*, **20**, 881–91.

Macdonald, A.J.D. (1986). Do general practitioners 'miss' depression in elderly patients? *British Medical Journal*, **292**, 1365–7.

Mann, A. (1991). Epidemiology. In *Psychiatry in the Elderly*, Jacoby, R. and Oppenheimer, C. (Eds). Oxford University Press, Oxford.

Mann, A.H., Graham, N. and Ashby, D. (1984). Psychiatric illness in residential homes for the elderly: a survey in one London Borough. *Age and Ageing*, **13**, 257–65.

Marttila, R.J. and Rinne, U.K. (1980). Smoking and Parkinson's disease. *Acta Neurologica Scandinavica*, **62**, 322–5.

McKhann, G., Drachman, D., Folstein, M. *et al.* (1984). Clinical diagnosis of Alzheimer's disease: report of the NINCDS–ADRDA Work Group, Department of Health and Human Services task Force on Alzheimer's disease. *Neurology*, **34**, 939–44.

Meyer, J.S., McClintic, K.L., Rogers, R.L. *et al.* (1988). Etiological considerations and risk factors for multi-infarct dementia. *Journal of Neurology, Neurosurgery and Psychiatry*, **51**, 1489–97.

Morgan, K., Dalloso, H.M., Arie, T, *et al.* (1987). Mental health and psychological well-being among the old and very old living at home. *British Journal of Psychiatry*, **150**, 808–14.

Mortimer, J.A., Van Duijn, C.M., Chandra, V. *et al.* (1991). Head trauma as a risk factor for Alzheimer's disease: a collaborative re-analysis of case-control studies. *International Journal of Epidemiology*, **20** (Suppl. 2), S28–S35.

Murphy, E. (1991). Surveying old people: some practical problems. *International Journal of Geriatric Psychiatry*, **2**, 1–2.

Murray, R.M., Greene, J.G. and Adams, J.H. (1971). Analgesic abuse and dementia. *Lancet*, **ii**, 242–5.

Newman, S.C., Shrout, P.E. and Bland, R.C. (1990). The efficiency of two-phase designs in prevalence surveys of mental disorders. *Psychological Medicine*, **20**, 183–93.

O'Connor, D.W., Pollitt, P.A., Hyde, J.B. *et al.* (1988). Do general practitioners miss dementia in elderly patients? *British Medical Journal*, **297**, 1107–10.

O'Connor, D.W., Pollitt, P.A., Hyde, J.B. *et al.* (1989a). The reliability and validity of the Mini-Mental State in a British Community Survey. *Journal of Psychiatric Research*, **23**, 89–96.

O'Connor, D.W., Pollitt, P.A. Treasure, F.P. *et al.* (1989b). The influence of education, social class and sex on Mini-Mental State scores. *Psychological Medicine*, **19**, 771–6.

O'Connor, D.W., Pollitt, P.A. and Roth, M. (1990). Coexisting depression and dementia in a community survey of the elderly. *International Psychogeriatrics*, **2**, 45–53.

Pattie, A.H. and Gilleard, C.J. (1979). *Manual of the Clifton Assessment Procedures for the Elderly (CAPE)*. Hodder and Stoughton Educational, Sevenoaks.

Preston, G.A.N. (1986). Dementia in elderly adults: Prevalence and institutionalisation. *Journal of Gerontology*, **41**, 261–7.

Ritchie, K. and Fuhrer, R. (1992). A comparative study of the performance of screening tests for senile dementia using Receiver Operating Characteristics analysis. *Journal of Clinical Epidemiology*, **45**, 627–37.

Ritchie, K., Kildea, D. and Robine, J.M. (1991). A reconsideration of the relationship between age and the prevalence of senile dementia based on a meta-analysis of recent data. Proceedings of Euromedicine, Montpellier.

Rocca, W.A., Hofman, A., Brayne, C. *et al.* (1991a). The prevalence of vascular dementia in Europe: facts and tragments from 1980–1990 studies. *Annals of Neurology*, **30**, 817–24.

Rocca, W.A., Van Duijn, C.M., Clayton, D. *et al.* (1991b). Maternal age and Alzheimer's disease: a collaborative re-analysis of case-control studies. *International Journal of Epidemiology*, **20** (Suppl. 2), S21–S27.

Rorsman, B., Hagnell, O. and Lanke, J. (1986). Prevalence and incidence of senile and multi-infarct dementia in the Lundby study: a comparison between time periods 1947–1957 and 1957–1972. *Neuropsychobiology*, **15**, 122–9.

Roth, M., Huppert, F.A., Tym, E. and Mountjoy, C.Q. (1988). *The Cambridge Examination for Mental Disorders of the Elderly*. Cambridge University Press, Cambridge.

Social Psychiatry Research Unit, NH and MRC, Australian National University. (1992). The Canberra Interview for the Elderly: a new field instrument for the diagnosis of dementia and depression by ICD-10 and DSM-III-R. *Acta Psychiatrica Scandinavica*, **85**, 105–13.

Shah, B.V. (1981). *SESUDAAN: Standard Errors Program for Computing of Standardized Rates from Sample Survey Data*. Research Triangle Institute, Research Triangle Park, NC.

Uhlmann, R.F. and Larson, E.B. (1991). Effect of education on the Mini-Mental State Examination as a screening test for dementia. *Journal of the American Geriatrics Society*, **39**, 876–80.

Van Duijn, C.M., Clayton, D., Chandra, V. *et al.* (1991a). Familial aggregation of Alzheimer's disease and related disorders: a collaborative re-analysis of case-control studies. *International Journal of Epidemiology*, **20** (Suppl. 2), S13–S20.

Van Duijn, C.M., Stijnen, T.S. and Hofman, A. (1991b). Risk factors for Alzheimer's disease: overview of the EURODEM collaborative re-analysis of case-control studies. *International Journal of Epidemiology*, **20** (Suppl. 2), S4–S27.

Veras, R.P. and Murphy, E. (1991). The ageing of the Third World: tackling the problems of community surveys. Part II: A community survey of the elderly population in Rio de Janeiro: A methodological approach. *International Journal of Geriatric Psychiatry*, **6**, 629–37.

World Health Organization. (1987). *ICD-10. Clinical descriptions and diagnostic guidelines (1986 draft for field trials)*. World Health Organization, Geneva.

Williamson, J., Stockoe, I.H., Gray, S. *et al.* (1964). Old people at home: their unreported needs. *Lancet*, **i**, 1117–20.

Zaudig, M., Mittelhammer, J., Hiller, W. *et al.* (1991). SIDAM – A structured interview for the diagnosis of dementia of the Alzheimer type, multi-infarct dementia and dementias of other aetiology according to ICD-10 and DSM-III-R. *Psychological Medicine*, **21**, 225–36.

Adrienne Little
Maudsley Hospital
and
Alistair Burns
University of Manchester
Withington Hospital

4 MONITORING CHANGE IN ALZHEIMER'S DISEASE

INTRODUCTION

Studies of the progression of Alzheimer's disease (AD) have enormous potential. They should develop our understanding of the natural history of AD and how this differs from normal ageing, allowing us to distinguish between stages and subtypes of the disorder and to identify risk factors which may be aetiologically significant. Alongside these theoretical gains are benefits for clinical practice – improving the advice we are able to offer patients and carers about prognosis, developing methods of accurate and early diagnosis, developing measures to monitor the impact of interventions and providing a rational basis for planning services. Research has gone some way to achieving these goals, but studies of change are beset by serious methodological difficulties which have limited their value. We begin by examining these difficulties and then consider what studies of change can tell us about AD.

METHODS OF MONITORING CHANGE IN ALZHEIMER'S DISEASE

Most researchers assume that the best way to study progression is by following up a sample of people with AD over time. However, longitudinal studies are extremely expensive, tying up large numbers of personnel and subjects over a considerable time. Their expense can be justified only if they are more effective than cheaper alternatives. However, longitudinal designs are beset by serious methodological difficulties. Unless these difficulties can be overcome, longitudinal research may be misleading as well as expensive. La Rue (1987) identified three types of methodological difficulties (Table 4.1) — factors limiting the extent to which results can be generalized to other populations ('threats to external validity'); factors which reduce the power of the study; and factors which confound the changes shown by obscuring or exaggerating them ('threats to internal validity').

Longitudinal studies and their methodological difficulties

Recruitment bias and selective attrition
Results can be generalized only if the sample is representative of the population of interest. Collecting and maintaining a representative sample is extremely difficult. Studies of normal elderly people demonstrate that subjects (particularly volunteers) are relatively elite, i.e. are healthier, more able and of higher socioeconomic status than the elderly population as a whole (Busse and Maddox, 1985). Samples may become less representative over time because of

Table 4.1 Principal methodological difficulties of longitudinal studies.

Methodological difficulty	Examples
1. Threats to external validity	
Recruitment bias at baseline	Stringent inclusion criteria
	Volunteer samples
Selective attrition during follow-up	Refusal
	Death
	Tracing difficulties
2. Threats to the power of the design	
Inadequate sample size	Attrition
3. Threats to internal validity	
Intervening events during follow-up	Bereavement
	Physical illness
	Institutionalization
Measurement change ('instrumentation bias')	Personnel changes
Impact of repeated measurement	Practice effects
Insensitivity of measure to change	Floor and ceiling effects
	Regression to the mean

selective attrition, i.e. the differential loss of the more impaired subjects (Norris, 1985).

Most longitudinal studies of AD (Table 4.2a–e) recruit very restricted samples. Many adopt stringent selection criteria with comprehensive screening in order to ensure accurate diagnosis. Some collect relatively mild cases, often recruited from volunteers. Unsurprisingly, samples can be very different from people found in ordinary clinical practice. For example, the Washington study (described in Table 4.2c) (Berg *et al.*, 1988) gathered 43 subjects who have been followed up over six years. These were recruited from media and local advertisements to ensure 'mild' cases. All were white, the average age at entry was 71 years and the average number of years spent in education was over 12 (Botwinick *et al.*, 1986). Results from these very selected samples may not be typical of patients with AD as a whole.

Substantial numbers of subjects will be lost during follow-up. For example, the Washington study had lost almost half of their original sample by 2.5 years (Berg *et al.*, 1987). With relatively mild subjects, loss is often due to refusal or difficulties in tracing people who have moved. With more impaired subjects and longer follow-up intervals, loss is more likely to be due to death, institutionalization or an inability to complete the assessments. At 5 years, only half of the surviving subjects from the Washington study had data (Berg *et al.*, 1988) and by 7 years, only six of the original 43 could be assessed (Botwinick *et al.*, 1988). The cause of loss is important. Norris (1985) suggests that among normal elderly samples, loss due to death introduces more bias than loss due to refusal. The Washington study suggests that loss produces less distortion among samples of people with AD than for normal elderly people. They found surprisingly few differences between subjects who remained in their study and those who were lost for whatever reason (Berg *et al.*, 1988; Botwinick *et al.*, 1988). This suggests that selective attrition is not a particular problem for studies of change in AD. However, their results may also indicate that the measures they included were particularly poor predictors of outcome.

Table 4.2a Studies of short-term changes in cognition in Alzheimer's disease.

Study	Population	Sample	Duration	Data points	Control group	Measure	Significance of change
Walton (1958)[a]	HI	12	6 weeks	4	F	WMS	+
Kendrick (1972)[a]	HI	38	6 weeks	2	N, F	DCT, SLT	NS
Hodkinson (1973)[a]	HA	257	4 weeks	3	N, CS	MTS	+
Stonier (1974)[a]	HI	29	6 weeks	6	N	MTS, TBSMQ	+
Cowan et al. (1975)[a]	HA	26–32	1–3 months	3	F	PALT, DCT,	+
Kendrick and Moyes (1979)[a]	HI	28	6 weeks	2	N, F	BGT	+
Thompson and Blessed (1987)[a]	HDP	27	7 days	2	F	DCT, OLT	*
Teng et al. (1989)	OP	54	4 weeks	5	None	AMTS	*
Taylor et al. (1991)	HI, HDP	16	2 weeks	3	MID	Battery	?
						Battery	

AMTS = Abbreviated Mental Test Score. BGT = Bender Gestalt Test. DCT = Digit Copy Test. MTS = Mental Test Score. OLT = Object Learning Test. PALT = Paired Associate Learning Test. SLT = Synonym Learning Test. TBMSQ = Tooting Bec Mental Status Questionnaire. WMS = Weschler Memory Scale. HA = hospital admissions. HDP = hospital day patients. HI = hospital inpatients. OP = outpatients. CS = confusional status. F = functional illness. MID = multi-infarct dementia. N = normal controls. + = significant difference between changes shown by dementia and control groups. NS = no significant differences between groups nor within group. * = significant improvement by dementia group. ? = not reported.
[a] May contain subjects with dementia other than Alzheimer's disease.

Table 4.2b Studies of cognitive changes in Alzheimer's disease over 6 months or longer.

Study	Population	Sample	Duration (months)	Data points	Control group	Measure	Significance of change
Whitehead (1977)[a]	HA	15	12	2	Other HA	Battery	+, **
Brull et al. (1979)	HI, OP	42	48	6	None	Battery	**
Naguib and Levy (1982)	HI	10	24	2	None	MTS	**
Reisberg et al. (1983)[b]	OP	41	24	2	None	MSQ	**
Rabins et al. (1984)	HA	13	24	2	PD, F	MMSE	+, **
Mayeux et al. (1985)	OP, HI	50	6–48	8	None	MMSE	?
Botwinick et al. (1986)[b]	V	18	48	4	N	Battery	+, **
Little et al. (1986)	HI, OP	26	6	5	None	PALT	**
Berg et al. (1987)[b]	V	26	30	3	N	SPMSQ, FHT	+, **
Uhlmann et al. (1987)[a]	OP	115	12–24	2	None	MMSE	NS
Becker et al. (1988)	V	56	12	2	N	Battery	+, **
Berg et al. (1988)[b]	V	43	15–66	2–5	N	Battery	+, **
Katzman et al. (1988)	NH, OP, V	161	12–72	Variable	None	IMC	**
Thal et al. (1988)	OP	40	15–55	Variable	None	IMC	?
Yesavage et al. (1988)	V	30	6	2	None	MMSE	**
Ortof and Crystal (1989)	OP	54	12	Variable	None	IMC	?
Huff et al. (1990)	OP	53	12	2	N	MMSE	?
Rebok et al. (1990)	OP	51	24	5	N	Battery	+, **
Teri et al. (1990)	OP	106	Up to 36	2–6	None	MMSE	**
Burns et al. (1991)	HI, HA, HDP, OP	85	12	2	None	CAMCOG, MMSE, AMTS	**

AMTS = Abbreviated Mental Test Score. CAMCOG = cognitive scales of the Cambridge Mental Disorders of the Elderly schedule. FHT = Face–Hand Test. IMC = Information Memory Concentration Test (from the Blessed Dementia Scales). MMSE = Mini-Mental State Examination. MSQ = Mental Status Questionnaire. MTS = Mental Test Score. PALT = Paired Associate Learning Test. SPMSQ = Short Portable MSQ. HA = hospital admissions. HDP = hospital day patients. HI = hospital inpatients. NH = nursing home residents. OP = outpatients. V = volunteers. F = functional illness. PD = pseudodementia. N = normal controls. + = significant difference between changes shown by dementia and control groups. NS = no significant differences between groups nor within groups. ** = significant decline by dementia group. ? = not reported.
[a] May contain subjects with dementia other than Alzheimer's disease.
[b] Includes 'mild' dementia.

Table 4.2c Studies of clinical change in Alzheimer's disease.

Study	Population	Sample	Duration (months)	Data points	Control group	Measure	Outcomes[c] D (%)	S (%)	I (%)
USA–UK									
Gurland et al. (1982)[a,b]	S	27	12	2	None	Global Clinical rating	37	48	15
Washington									
Berg et al. (1984)[b]	V	42	12	2	None	CDR	50	50	0
Berg et al. (1987)[b]	V	26	30	3	N	CDR	72	18	0
Berg et al. (1990)[b]	V	15–19	34	3	None	CDR	?	?	?
Botwinick et al. (1986)[b]	V	18	48	4	N	CDR	67	33	0
Berg et al. (1988)[b]	V	17–20	66	5	N	CDR	90	0	10
Botwinick et al. (1988)[b]	V	4	84	6	None	CDR	50	0	50
New York									
Reisberg et al. (1985, 1986)[a,b]	OP	83	36–48	2	None	GDS	12	84	4
	(a) Very mild	40					5	95	0
	(b) Mild	30					10	80	10
	(c) Moderate	10					40	60	0
	(d) Moderate severe	3					33	67	0
Flicker et al. (1991)[b]	V	32	24	2	N	GDS	72	?	128
Pao Alto									
Yesavage et al. (1988)	V	30	6	2	None	GDS	?	?	?

CDR = Clinical Dementia Rating. GDS = Global Deterioration Scale. OP = outpatients. S = community survey. V = volunteers. N = normal controls. ? = not reported.

[a] May contain subjects with dementia other than Alzheimer's disease.
[b] Includes 'mild' dementia.
[c] Proportion of subjects with dementia rated as follow-up as: D = declined. S = stable. I = improved.

Table 4.2d Studies of behaviour and self-care changes in Alzheimer's disease.

Study	Population	Sample	Duration (months)	Data points	Control group	Measure	Significance of change
Whitehead (1977)[a]	HA	15	12	2	Other HA	Nurse ratings of self-care	+, **
Gilleard and Pattie (1978)[c]	HI, EMI	69	18	2	None	SGRS	**
Hersch et al. (1978)[a]	HI	32	18	6	F	LPRS	+, **
Berg et al. (1987)[b]	V	26	30	3	N	DRS	+, **
Uhlmann et al. (1987)[a]	OP	115	12–24	2	None	Informant ratings of self-care from DRS	NS
Becker et al. (1988)	V	56	12	2	None	Informant ratings of self-care from DRS	**
Huff et al. (1990)	OP	53	12	2	N	DRS	?

DRS = Dementia Rating Scale (from the Blessed Dementia Scales). LPRS = London Psychogeriatric Rating Scale. SGRS = Stockton Geriatric Rating Scale. EMI = elderly mentally infirm home residents. HA = hospital admissions. HI = hospital inpatients. OP = outpatients. V = volunteers. F = functional illness. N = normal controls. + = significant difference between changes shown by dementia and control groups. NS = no significant differences between groups nor within groups. ** = significant decline in dementia group. ? = not reported
[a] May contain subjects with dementia other than Alzheimer's disease.
[b] Includes 'mild' dementia.
[c] Includes subjects with diagnoses other than dementia.

Table 4.2e Studies of change of multi-dimensional scales in Alzheimer's disease.

Study	Population	Sample	Duration (months)	Data points	Control group	Measure	Significance of change
Rosen et al. (1984)	OP	10	12	2	N	ADAS	**
Huff et al. (1987)	OP	77	3–60	2	PSD	BDS	+
Kramer-Ginsberg et al. (1988)	V	60	12	3	N	ADAS	+
Yesavage et al. (1988)	V	30	6	2	None	ADAS	**

ADAS = Alzheimer's Disease Assessment Scale. BDS = Blessed Dementia Scales. OP = outpatients. V = volunteers. N = normal controls. PSD = presenile dementia. + = significant difference between changes shown by dementia and control groups. ** = significant decline by dementia group.

Impact of attrition on power

Obviously the final sample size must be adequate to detect patterns of change and to examine any hypotheses of interest (Overall, 1987). Attrition will reduce the sensitivity of the study unless many times the final required number of subjects are recruited. This is extremely expensive. Authors have adopted various strategies to accommodate missing data without necessarily losing subjects. Some substitute scores by using median values or assuming worse performance levels (Berg *et al.*, 1990). Others employ statistical models such as regression analysis which can cope with varying data over variable follow-up intervals (e.g. Ortof and Crystal, 1989; Teri *et al.*, 1990).

Difficulties measuring change

Measures must be sensitive to the progression of AD but reliable, i.e. insensitive to short-term fluctuations, changes in testers etc. Traditionally, studies have relied upon clinical and psychometric measures developed to discriminate between people with and without dementia. Very few of these have been validated as measures of change. The demands of quantifying change are very different from those of discriminating between groups at a single point of time. Several studies show that good diagnostic discriminators make poor measures of change. Kaszniak *et al.* (1986) examined five standardized neuropsychological measures firstly as discriminators between diagnostic groups with and without AD and secondly as discriminators between the differential changes shown by these two groups over time. They concluded that 'the relative efficiency in tracking AD patient deterioration is generally opposite (to the) . . . efficiency in initial group discrimination' (p. 423). Thus, the most effective diagnostic discriminator (a test of memory) was the least sensitive measure of change, whilst the most sensitive measure of change (a test of language) was the least efficient diagnostic discriminator. Later studies confirm these results (Huff *et al.*, 1990; Flicker *et al.*, 1991).

The process of developing a diagnostic discriminator inevitably undermines its sensitivity to change. The ideal diagnostic discriminator includes a restricted range of items, sensitive to the particular level and type of impairments characteristic of referrals for diagnosis. Often this demands a scale which is sensitive to mild or 'early' impairment and so must include predominantly difficult items. A difficult scale has a 'high floor'. It discriminates well amongst less impaired people but is insensitive to the impairments and changes shown as people become more impaired. Conversely, a scale which includes predominantly easy items will have a 'low ceiling' making it insensitive to impairment and changes amongst less impaired people. There is no single measure which discriminates throughout the range of impairments shown by people with dementia. Many neuropsychological tests are useful measures of short-term changes (e.g. as monitors of the impact of intervention). However, they rapidly become too difficult as subjects become too impaired for the floor of the test. As a result many will refuse or fail to score (e.g. Botwinick *et al.*, 1988). Most mental status questionnaires are brief and sensitive only to moderate impairment. They often present floor *and* ceiling effects (Reisberg *et al.*, 1983; Berg *et al.*, 1990; Salmon *et al.*, 1990). For example, the New York study (Table 4.2c, Reisberg *et al.*, 1983) has followed up a sample of people with dementia over 2 years. Those classified as moderately impaired appear to show the most decline on the ten item mental status questionnaire (with an average decline of three points). In contrast, mildly or severely impaired subjects show relatively little change (with an average decline of one point or less).

The impact of floor and ceiling effects is complicated if the type as well as the level of impairment changes as AD progresses. Two models describe sequences of qualitative change. The Piagetian model describes AD as a reversal of the pattern of cognitive development in childhood (Ajuriaguerra and Tissot, 1968; Constantinidis *et al.*, 1978). In the earlier stages, people with dementia lose formal operational thinking. This is followed in turn by disintegrating concrete thought and finally a loss of pre-operational thinking. Reisberg *et al.* (1989) independently suggest that the loss of functional ability mirrors the development sequence of childhood and proceeds at a similar pace. For example, people with dementia will successively lose their abilities to dress, to bath and to be continent. The information processing model describes the progression of cognitive impairment in AD as a reversal of the process of skill acquisition (Jorm, 1986). Here, the earlier stages of dementia are characterized by a loss of controlled information processing, i.e. processing which requires conscious effort. This produces difficulties in novel tasks, for example, learning new information. As dementia progresses, difficulties with automatic processing develop producing impairments of overlearned skills, for example, recognizing familiar information. These models suggest that measures of different types of impairment will be sensitive to changes during different stages of AD. Thus measures of new learning might be sensitive to early change (and thereby to diagnosis), whilst measures of the familiar skills such as language, would be more sensitive measures of change as dementia progresses. This would account for the finding of Kaszniak *et al.* (1985) of differential sensitivity to change and diagnosis described earlier.

It is difficult to disentangle measurement artefact from differential pattern of change. Several studies suggest that people with dementia show more decline in some areas than others (described later). This may reflect the natural history of AD, with some abilities being more affected by the disease than others. Alternatively, it may reflect the differential sensitivity of the measures included to the underlying changes in ability. There is conflicting advice about how to select a measure of change. Some authors recommend measures which have established correlation with indices of neuropathology and should therefore be sensitive to progression in pathology (Riege and Metter, 1988; Galasko *et al.*, 1991). The Mini-Mental State Examination (MMSE) (Folstein *et al.*, 1975) and the Dementia Rating Scale (DRS) (Blessed *et al.*, 1968; Perry *et al.*, 1978) correlate moderately well with anatomical pathology at *post-mortem* and have been widely employed to monitor change. Unfortunately, there is no consensus as to the best method of measuring neuropathological change particularly in life (Friedland *et al.*, 1988). This has limited the development of clinical indicators of pathology. Other authors recommend measures which are relatively resistant to normal age change, such as vocabulary (La Rue, 1987). Change on these measures is more likely to be abnormal. However, there is no evidence that these functions are more sensitive to the progression of AD. In general, any measure of long-term change must include a broad spectrum of items sensitive to different types and levels of impairment. Inevitably, this means a lengthy assessment with probable difficulties ensuring compliance, unless the measure can be structured in such a way as to tailor the difficulty level to each subject's current level of impairment (e.g. Little *et al.*, 1986).

Unfortunately, the difficulties of measuring change do not end with selecting measures. Performance can change for reasons other than the progression of dementia. Some factors depress performance and exaggerate decline (e.g. intercurrent illness). Other factors obscure decline (e.g. improvement with practice). People with dementia show practice effects over intervals as long as 2 months (Little *et al.*, 1986; Teng *et al.*, 1989) as well as over brief intervals

(Thompson and Blessed, 1987). Practice effects can be minimized by employing different versions of the measures at each assessment. Other period effects cannot be eliminated but must be monitored. There are also numerous statistical difficulties analysing change. Most serious are regression effects, whereby the error inherent in an unreliable measure is compounded when this measure is repeated to monitor change. As a result, people who perform relatively well at baseline may appear to decline, whilst those who perform relatively poorly may appear to improve. Baltes *et al.* (1972) have demonstrated the extent of regression effects in longitudinal studies of normal ageing. These difficulties can be overcome by selecting reliable measures and employing base-free measures of change, for example, by analysing follow-up performance and covarying baseline score rather than computing the difference between the two (Uhlmann *et al.*, 1987).

Given these serious difficulties measuring change, it is not surprising that recent studies have adopted different measurement models. Drachman *et al.* (1990) and Stern *et al.* (1987, 1990) explore AD progression in terms of the time taken to reach predetermined 'clinical endpoints' which correspond to clinically significant events (e.g. becoming incontinent) or preselected levels of performance (e.g. cognitive test score). However, many endpoints are constrained by factors outside AD itself (e.g. becoming incontinent or institutionalized) so will be poor indicators of disease progression.

Indirect methods of monitoring change in Alzheimer's disease
There are several methods of examining progression indirectly which are relatively inexpensive, quick and avoid many of the methodological difficulties of longitudinal designs.

Cross-sectional comparisons
Progression can be inferred from differences between groups defined by stage of impairment, e.g. by comparing 'early' and 'late' cases or 'mild', 'moderate' and 'severe' subgroups. This begs the question that AD progresses along the dimensions defined by these stages.

Two scales have been developed to classify people by stage of AD: the Clinical Dementia Rating (CDR) from the Washington study and the Global Deterioration Scale (GDS) from the New York study (Table 4.3). These define specific stages by level and type of impairment. There is some overlap, but the two scales do not correspond. Thus the CDR 'mild' dementia overlaps with the GDS 'mild' and 'moderate' stages. Berg *et al.* and Reisberg *et al.* (see Tables 4.2b and 4.2c) present evidence to justify their assumption that these stages form ordinal scales of AD progression. Longitudinal studies confirm that stages predict outcome. Thus very few people classified as showing little or no evidence of dementia decline, whereas most or all of those classified as moderately or severely demented show poor outcome. People who decline appear to progress through the stages. Reisberg *et al.* (1989) suggest that the GDS stage of 'moderate dementia' corresponds to the point at which a clinical diagnosis of dementia can be made with confidence. They suggest that the impairments defined by earlier stages ('very mild' and 'mild') correspond to 'incipient dementia'. People at these stages show outcomes similar to the general elderly population. They estimate the course of AD along the GDS with an incipient stage lasting 7 years, a middle stage of moderate to severe impairment lasting 6 years, and a final stage of very severe impairment which can last 6 or more years. Finally, they have confirmed the ordinal structure of the GDS with Guttman scale analysis.

Table 4.3 Methods of staging clinical changes in Alzheimer's disease.

	Clinical Dementia Rating	Global Deterioration Scale
Stages	1. Healthy 2. Questionable dementia 3. Mild dementia 4. Moderate dementia 5. Severe dementia	1. No cognitive decline 2. Very mild 3. Mild 4. Moderate 5. Moderately severe 6. Severe 7. Very severe
Rater	Clinician	Clinician
Content	1. Six scales – three cognitive and three self-care 2. Individual scales are rated according to descriptions of performance typical of each stage 3. Overall rating made according to predetermined criteria, emphasizing memory scale rating 4. Sum of ratings on six scales yields a quantitative score ('sum of boxes')	1. Stages defined by performance levels on two cognitive tests 2. Description of changes in cognition, self-care, affect and personality typical of each stage
Source	Informant and patient	Not specified
Inter-rater reliability	0.89* 0.74–0.91†	Not reported
Concurrent validity	1. DRS 0.74 0.53/0.59** 2. SPMSQ 0.84* 0.50/0.68**	MMSE 0.92¶

* Hughes *et al.* (1982). DRS = Dementia Rating Scale. (Blessed *et al.* 1968).
† Berg *et al.* (1990). SPMSQ = Short Portable Mental Status Questionnaire. (Pfeiffer 1975).
** Berg *et al.* (1988) MMSE = Mini-Mental State Examination. (Folstein *et al.* 1975).
¶ Reisberg *et al.* (1986a).

Informant reports of change
Using informants to describe progression overcomes the difficulties of assessing often anxious or uncooperative patients. However, informant reports may have poor reliability and validity. For example, it is notoriously difficult to establish accurately when dementia begins. Jorm and Korten (1988) and Jorm *et al.* (1989) have developed a standardized scale to quantify informant ratings of cognitive decline. Informants rate the extent of change in several abilities over the previous 10 years. These ratings correlate well with measures of cognitive impairment and care need, but Jorm *et al.* do not offer evidence to validate them as measures of decline. However Uhlmann *et al.* (1987) suggest that

informants can accurately assess AD progression. They compared measured changes in cognitive performance and behaviour over 1 to 2 years, with informant ratings of retrospective change in cognitive ability, self-care, physical health and interpersonal skills. Informant ratings correlated moderately and significantly with measures of change and also predicted mortality 1 year later.

Deterioration indices

If AD has an uneven course, with some abilities affected earlier or to a greater extent than others, change can be estimated from patterns of current performance. Performance on measures which appear resistant to dementia ('hold tests') can be compared with performance on measures sensitive to dementia ('don't hold tests'). Alternatively, performance on 'hold tests' can be used to estimate premorbid ability on 'don't hold tests'. For example, reading ability correlates moderately well with measured IQ among well samples. Reading appears to decline little, if at all, in the early stages of dementia. Rough estimates of IQ based upon current reading ability can be compared with performance on IQ tests (Nelson and O'Connell, 1978). (Sociodemographic variables can similarly be used to estimate premorbid IQ, although less accurately.)

However, these deterioration indices are as good as their estimates of premorbid level. This depends fundamentally upon the 'hold tests' being resistant to dementia. This is questionable and can be established only by longitudinal studies. Earlier deterioration indices (based upon patterns of current performance on IQ tests) have proved disappointing diagnostic discriminators (Woods and Britton, 1985). Reading ability can decline in AD, albeit generally in the later stages (Hart, 1988). This will depress premorbid function and obscure the extent of decline.

Are longitudinal studies necessary?

There are many advantages to monitoring progression indirectly. However, these indirect models face problems, not least overcoming widespread doubts about their credibility. Do indirect methods accurately monitor change?

Recent evidence cautiously suggests that at least some methods of indirectly monitoring change provide comparable results to longitudinal designs. Mann *et al.* (1989) estimated the rate of cognitive decline shown by patients with AD, by dividing their current performance by the estimated duration of the disease (based upon informant reports). They compared these estimated rates of decline with changes measured over 1 year. Correlations were significant and substantial with coefficients of 0.8), suggesting the indirect estimate did accurately monitor progression. However, this is based upon a very small sample (10). Botwinick *et al.* (1988) compared the cognitive changes shown by subjects from the Washington study as they progressed along the CDR stages with cross-sectional comparisons of the performance of subjects at different stages. The performance of subjects at different stages was significantly different, whether based on cross-sectional or longitudinal comparisons. There were no differences between the performance of subjects classified cross-sectionally at a particular stage and the performance of those who had progressed to that stage in the longitudinal study. They conclude that 'unless the focus is on individual subjects' change, or the rate of change, . . . cross-sectional data of SDAT progression provide the same basic information as longitudinal data' (p. 496).

However, Botwinick *et al.* (1988) provide an important caveat to their conclusion, i.e. 'at least for performance on behavioural tests' (p. 496). This study suggests that direct and indirect methods produce different pictures of

AD progression for other types of measure, i.e. clinical ratings of specific symptoms and performance on a brief Mental Status Questionnaire (Berg *et al.*, 1990). Here, people classified as severely impaired cross-sectionally show significantly less clinical impairment than those who progress longitudinally to this stage. Thus, the indirect method would underestimate the severity of progression. Berg *et al.* (1990) attribute this to recruitment bias. Studies of AD would generally include subjects who are relatively less impaired in the population of AD sufferers, for example, by excluding people in institutions. Thus even subjects classified at baseline as 'severely' impaired are unlikely to show levels of impairment characteristic of very advanced dementia. However, longitudinal studies attempt to follow-up all subjects, retaining people as they become institutionalized. Recruitment bias may have less impact upon cognitive tests than clinical measures, because cognitive tests are more vulnerable to floor effects. If there is little room for severely impaired subjects to show further cognitive decline, differences between cross-sectional and longitudinal comparisons may be obscured.

This suggests that longitudinal studies are necessary, at least to validate the results of indirect designs and possibly to monitor change accurately in certain areas. To date, most studies of AD progression have relied upon longitudinal methods. These are reviewed below. However, the progression of AD occurs in the context of normal ageing, and some of the functions affected by AD are also sensitive to age itself. Disentangling normal and abnormal changes can be difficult, particularly at the earlier stages of AD.

STUDIES OF CHANGE IN 'NORMAL AGEING'

Schaie (1983) and Salthouse (1991) review studies of psychological change in normal ageing. Most have examined cognitive change. Despite an enormous number of cross-sectional studies comparing old and young, and a smaller number of longitudinal studies monitoring change with age, there is no clear model of what, when or how abilities change. It seems that normal ageing does involve some cognitive change, but changes are modest, specific to certain functions, occur rarely below the age of 70 years, and vary from person to person.

Cross-sectional comparisons of old and young subjects may overestimate age change because of cohort differences. Thus younger cohorts may well perform better because of improved educational opportunities etc. However, longitudinal studies may underestimate change because of the impact of period effects such as selective attrition or practice. The most satisfactory model for examining change is a cross-sequential design, combining cross-sectional and longitudinal studies. Here, different cohorts are monitored across several measurement occasions. For example, two cohorts (born in 1900 and 1910) could be monitored over 10 years (from 1980 to 1990). Change within each cohort provides an estimate of age effects (from age 80 to 90 years and age 70 to 80 years). The difference between the cohorts in 1980 and 1990 measures cohort effect. The impact of period effects is estimated by time-lag comparisons of the two cohorts at the same age (comparing the baseline scores of the 1900 cohort with the follow-up scores of the 1910 cohort).

Two large studies have employed cross-sequential designs (Table 4.4). These establish substantial and significant cohort differences, confirming that cross-sectional comparisons of young and old people will often exaggerate age change. Both report significant but modest age effects, occurring only in the oldest groups and restricted to specific measures. For example, in the Seattle

Table 4.4 Cross-sequential studies of cognitive change in normal ageing

	Hamburg study Riegel et al. (1967) Riegel and Riegel (1972)	Seattle study Schaie (1983, 1988)
Began	1956	1956
Initial sample size	202	128
Age at baseline	55–74+ years	22–70 years
Composition	'Community residents representative of the population'	'Drawn from a health care plan' 'Disproportionately high socioeconomic status'
Follow-up	5 years	21 years
Measurement points	4	
Measures	1. Wechsler Adult Intelligence Scale 2. Multiple Choice Verbal Tests	1. Thurstone Primary Mental Abilities 2. Test of Behavioural Rigidity

study, cohort differences were seven times as large as age change. Age changes were restricted to specific measures and only shown by some people in their 70s and 80s. Even amongst the oldest subjects (aged 80 and over), half showed little or no evidence of any decline.

Most studies have emphasized the variability and specificity of age changes. Even cross-sectional studies (with relatively large age differences) generally report average scores for their oldest subjects which are within one standard deviation of the average for the youngest group. In other words, many people in their 70s and 80s perform better than the average level for people in their 20s. Some abilities, particularly measures of crystallized ability or acquired knowledge such as vocabulary, show very little age difference or change. Age effects are most marked on measures assessing 'fluid abilities', for example, learning, reasoning and nonverbal skills.

Thus the impact of normal age change upon studies of AD progression will depend upon the age range of the sample, the length of follow-up and the measures included. It is likely to be negligible with relatively young subjects, for short follow-up periods and on measures of crystallized ability. However, age effects may contribute to the longer term changes shown by people in their 70s and 80s, particularly on measures of fluid ability.

STUDIES OF CHANGE IN ALZHEIMER'S DISEASE

Tables 4.2a–e collate the principal UK and US studies. This is not an exhaustive review. Measures selected include cognitive tests, clinical scales, informant ratings of behaviour and self-care, and multidimensional scales assessing different functions. Samples vary from small to substantial. Some studies simply describe change, in terms of performance level or by classifying subjects in outcome groups. Other studies have examined the significance of change, usually by comparing people with AD with control groups. Almost all studies confirm that people with AD show significantly different patterns of change relative to controls, with relatively little change over brief periods but significant decline over follow-up periods of 6 months or longer. It is more useful to examine specific questions about the rate, variability and predictability of these changes.

How rapidly does Alzheimer's disease progress?

Many studies have estimated the rate of progression by calculating the average change in performance per year (or month). These annual rates of change (or ARC) have several uses. They offer a method for comparing results of different studies with different follow-up intervals. The ARC shown by different groups of subjects can be compared to examine the significance of variables as potential predictors of outcome. Clinically, ARC provide norms to evaluate the significance of the changes shown by individual patients. Table 4.5 summarizes recent studies which have reported ARC (or given results in such a way as to allow the reviewer to compute ARC).

The ARC reported for some measures are remarkably consistent, for example, the Alzheimer's Disease Assessment Scale (ADAS) or Information Memory Concentration Test (IMC). Studies report very different estimates of progression for other measures, for example, the MMSE. Galasko et al. (1991) suggest that these discrepancies reflect sampling differences. Studies reporting low ARC on the MMSE may include relatively mild subjects, whilst those reporting higher ARC include more impaired groups. Certainly, Berg et al. (1987) and Reisberg et al. (1983) show that ARC vary according to severity of dementia. Generally, the more severely impaired subjects show faster rates of decline, although floor effects may limit the changes shown by the most severely impaired groups particularly on brief mental status questionnaires (Table 4.5). However, it is striking that the MMSE appears more sensitive to severity of impairment than the IMC. Katzman et al. (1988) compared rates of IMC change for four different samples. The baseline IMC scores range considerably (from 5.1 to 16.3). However, the ARC ranged little (from 3.8 to 4.8). Katzman et al. (1988) conclude that ARC were 'surprisingly consistent and independent of subjects' age, education and residence' (p. 384). However, they did find that ceiling effects influenced IMC changes, with the most severely impaired subjects showing little decline. They excluded these when estimating ARC. The MMSE samples a broad range of cognitive abilities and may be more sensitive to advanced impairment than the relatively restricted IMC. As a result, the MMSE would be more influenced by sampling differences.

How specific are the changes?

Many studies include several measures of the same or different abilities and compare how people change on these. As discussed earlier, it is difficult to establish whether people show greater decline on some measures than others because of the differential sensitivity of measures to change or because of the developmental course of dementia. Another difficulty is that measures cannot be compared directly. A decline of 'x' points on one measure is not necessarily equivalent to a decline of 'x' points on another because measures vary in length and scaling (Jorm, 1990). As a result, it is misleading to compare ARC or significance of changes on different measures, although many authors have done so. Different measures can be validly compared in several ways. Some authors compare 'effect size', that is, the magnitude of performance change relative to variability (e.g. Kaszniak et al., 1986; Rebok et al., 1990). Others transform performance on different scales to a common scale with standardized

Table 4.5 Annual rates of change shown in Alzheimer's disease

Measure	Study	Annual rate of change[a]
ADAS	Rosen *et al.* (1984)	7.8[b]
	Kramer-Ginsberg *et al.* (1988)	7.1 ± 9.8
	Yesavage *et al.* (1988)	8.3[b]
AMTS	Burns *et al.* (1991)	1.1[b]
BDS	Huff *et al.* (1987)	7.6[b]
CAMCOG	Burns *et al.* (1991)	12.3[b]
DRS	Berg *et al.* (1987)	
	(a) Mild CDR	0.9[b]
	(b) Moderate CDR	2.9[b]
	(c) Severe CDR	7.4[b]
	Huff *et al.* (1990)	1.5[b]
DRS (self-care)	Becker *et al.* (1988)	0.9[b]
IMC	Katzman *et al.* (1988)	4.4 ± 3.6
	Thal *et al.* (1988)	4.5 ± 0.5
	Ortof and Crystal (1989)	4.1 ± 3.0
	Salmon *et al.* (1990)	3.2 ± 3.0
Mattis Dementia Rating Scale	Salmon *et al.* (1990)	11.4 ± 11.1
MMSE	Rabins *et al.* (1984)	4.5[b]
	Uhlmann *et al.* (1986)	2.2 ± 5.0
	Becker *et al.* (1988)	1.8[b]
	Yesavage *et al.* (1988)	4.2 ± 4.8
	Huff *et al.* (1990)	2.9[b]
	Salmon *et al.* (1990)	2.8 ± 4.3
	Teri *et al.* (1990)	2.8[b]
	Burns *et al.* (1991)	0.5[b]
MSQ	Reisberg *et al.* (1983)	
	(a) Very mild GDS	0.6[b,c]
	(b) Mild GDS	0.36[b]
	(c) Moderate GDS	1.43[b]
	(d) Moderately severe GDS	0.5[b]
SPMSQ	Berg *et al.* (1987)	
	(a) Mild CDR	1.37[b]
	(b) Moderate CDR	1.25[b]
	(c) Severe CDR	2.5[b]

ADAS = Alzheimer's Disease Assessment Scale. AMTS = Abbreviated Mental Test Score. BDS = Blessed Dementia Scales. CAMCOG = cognitive scales of the Cambridge Mental Disorders of the Elderly schedule. CDR = Clinical Dementia Rating. DRS = Dementia Rating Scale (from BDS). GDS = Global Deterioration Scale. IMC = Information Memory Concentration Test (from BDS). MMSE = Mini-Mental State Examination. MSQ = Mental Status Questionnaire. SPMSQ = Short Portable MSQ.
[a] Annual rate of change given as average points per year ± standard deviation.
[b] No standard deviation available.
[c] Change represents improvement in performance.

scores (e.g. Botwinick *et al.*, 1986; Berg *et al.*, 1988; Yesavage *et al.*, 1988; Rebok *et al.*, 1990; Tinklenberg *et al.*, 1990). Finally, change can be expressed as a proportion of the length of the scale or baseline performance (e.g. Hersch *et al.*, 1978; Botwinick *et al.*, 1986; Huff *et al.*, 1990; Tinklenberg *et al.*, 1990), although Jorm (1990) suggests that this does not overcome the difficulties of comparing scales because it assumes, unjustifiably, that all measures have a true zero point.

People with dementia appear to show more change on some measures than others. For example, the effect sizes associated with measures of cognitive ability vary considerably, for example, from 4.3 to 18.8 (Kaszniak *et al.*, 1986) or from 3.9 to 48.1 (Rebok *et al.*, 1990). Kaszniak *et al.* and Rebok *et al.* agree that subjects show most decline on measures of language, least on measures of memory. However, Botwinick *et al.* (1986) examined change as a proportion of baseline performance and found that a memory test was the most sensitive measure from a battery of 16 tests, including several measures of language. Measures of psychomotor performance also showed relatively great decline. Botwinick *et al.*'s study included less impaired subjects than those of Kaszniak *et al.* or Rebok *et al.* This may account for these discrepant findings if, as discussed earlier, measures of memory are more sensitive to change early in AD, whilst measures of language are more sensitive to later changes.

A few studies have compared change on measures of different domains. Generally, people with dementia appear to show relatively more decline on cognitive measures than on behavioural or clinical ratings. For example, Yesavage *et al.* (1988) standardized and compared the changes shown on the cognitive and noncognitive items from the ADAS. The ARC cognitive items were consistently higher (0.2–0.8) than the ARC for noncognitive items (0.1–0.4). Reisberg *et al.* (1983) similarly report higher ARC for cognitive measures than ratings of clinical change (again using standardized scores).

Subjects also show different patterns of change within a measure. Yesavage *et al.* (1988) compared the ARC on standardized scores for individual items from three measures of cognitive performance. The ARC showed a decline ranging from 0.1 to almost 0.9 points. Again, items assessing language appear to show greater decline than those assessing memory. However, even language items show variable declines with ARC ranging from 0.2 (word-finding ability) to 0.7 (the combined language items from the MMSE). Tinklenberg *et al.* (1990) also report a relatively greater decline for language than memory items within the MMSE. Subjects declined by an average of 17% on particular language items (carrying out a three-stage command) but showed virtually no change on some memory items (recalling a three item list). Similar patterns of differential change are also evident within measures of behaviour (Hersch *et al.*, 1978). This suggests that the structure of scales as measures of change may be very different from the structure of scales as measures of performance at a single point. Tinklenberg *et al.* (1990) compared the results of a factor analysis of baseline MMSE performance with a factor analysis of changes over a year on the same scale. The cross-sectional analysis provided a two-factor solution, whilst a more complex five-factor structure described patterns of change.

These studies suggest that the progression of AD is complex and specific. This implies that change must be monitored with very precise measures of particular functions rather than by global assessments. Overall change on the MMSE (for example) will mask relative stability of some functions and decline of others.

How consistent is the rate of change?

Two studies have compared change during successive follow-up periods to examine whether people with dementia continue to progress at a constant rate. Unfortunately, their results conflict. On the one hand, Thal *et al.* (1988) report that 'most but not all subjects' (p. 1088) progress at a constant rate over up to eight successive 6-month periods on the IMC. Unfortunately, they do not provide details to substantiate this claim. Salmon *et al.* (1990) examine change on the IMC and two similar measures. They report little correlation between the rates of decline shown during the first and second years of follow-up. At best, the ARC on the DRS correlated moderately ($r = 0.3$) but this relationship was not statistically significant. It is possible that these apparently conflicting findings reflect sampling differences. Thal *et al.*'s sample appears less impaired at baseline. It may be that less impaired subjects do indeed show more variable progression (see below). Salmon *et al.* suggest that their results reflect the variable progression of AD with some patients remaining stable whilst others decline. However, the relative absence of progression could be attributed to various diagnostic and measurement artefacts including floor and ceiling effects. This is taken up by Yesavage and Brookes (1991) who propose a 'tri-linear model' to describe the patterns of changes shown over time in AD. They describe decline as proceeding through three stages: an initial period of stability, followed by decline and then a final period of stability. Unfortunately, they do not advise how to disentangle measurement artefacts from real stability of underlying progression.

Do people with Alzheimer's disease vary in how they change?

Reisberg *et al.* (1989) claim that their studies describe a relatively consistent picture of AD progression with an inevitable decline through a series of defined clinical stages over a specified time scale. Most studies confirm the general pattern of progressive decline but highlight variability. Thus not all people with dementia progress at the same rate or show the same pattern of change. It may be that undue emphasis has been placed upon variability of outcome, ignoring the more obvious and consistent findings of progressive decline. However, variability offers an opportunity to understand the nature of AD. Variability has been explored in two ways.

Some studies classify subjects on the basis of the changes shown, for example, as declining, stable or improving. Most subjects do decline but some more than others and some may remain stable or even improve. Table 4.2 summarizes the variability of clinical change. If the very mild and mild subjects from Reisberg *et al.* (1985, 1986a, b) are excluded (since they recommend applying the GDS rating of moderate dementia as the cut-off point for clinical dementia) between 33% and 90% of subjects decline. In other words, up to two-thirds of people may improve or show little change. Table 4.6 summarizes studies classifying change on cognitive measures. Here, between 29 and 90% of subjects are classified as declining. Again, about two-thirds may improve or change little. People classified as showing little or no clinical change also appear to show little or no decline in cognitive performance (Botwinick *et al.*, 1986) or on informant ratings (Berg *et al.*, 1987). Examination of Tables 4.2c and 4.6 suggest that the proportion of subjects classified as declining depends upon the length of follow-up and sample composition. Studies reporting relatively few subjects showing decline tend to include brief follow-up intervals and samples with relatively mild or early dementia (e.g. Brull *et al.*, 1979; Gurland *et al.*, 1982).

Table 4.6 Variability of cognitive change in Alzheimer's disease.

Study[a]	Sample (with dementia available at follow-up)	Duration (months)	Outcome[b] Severe decline (%)	Decline (%)	No change or improvement
Brull et al. (1979)	41	6	←——— 29 ———→		71
Naguib and Levy (1982)	10	24	←——— 50 ———→		50
Mayeux et al. (1985)	6–58	36	←——— 86 ———→		14
Ortof and Crystal (1989)	54	12	20	70	10
Burns et al. (1991)	84	12	20	44	36

[a] For full details of studies, please refer to Table 4.2b.
[b] Proportion of subjects with dementia rated as showing 'severe decline', 'decline' or 'no change'/'improvement' during follow-up.

Variability is also highlighted by the ranges of ARC reported (Table 4.5). Katzman et al. (1988) included the largest sample. They report a standard deviation for ARC (3.6) which is almost as large as the ARC itself (4.4). Teri et al. (1990) give confidence intervals for ARC on the MMSE. Ninety-five per cent of their subjects show change which fall within a very wide band: from an improvement of two points to a decline of over seven (on a measure scaled 0–30). Again, length of follow-up appears to be an important determinant of outcome variability. Teri et al. found that outcomes were very variable over brief follow-up periods (4 months or less) but were more consistent with time. However, there is no strong evidence that less impaired people show more variable ARC (e.g. Salmon et al., 1990).

Two explanations have been proposed to account for this variability of progression. On the one hand, it may be an artefact, attributable to diagnostic error or period effects. Thus subjects who fail to decline may have been incorrectly diagnosed, precluded from showing decline because of floor effects or may have effectively improved in performance because of intervening events (e.g. the treatment of depression or physical illness). For example, Ortof and Crystal (1989) examined the five subjects from their sample of 54 who showed no decline over 1 year. They were able to attribute the absence of decline for three subjects to intervening events. They suggested that a fourth case was 'atypical', leaving just one subject for whom no explanation could be found. Others attribute the variability of outcome to the inherent variability of dementia. This variability may be dimensional. Three studies examine the distribution of ARC for cognitive performance (Thal et al., 1988; Ortof and Crystal, 1989; Burns et al., 1991b). These distributions approach a normal curve, supporting the hypothesis of dimensional variability. Botwinick et al. (1988) suggest that the dimension underlying the distribution of outcomes is speed of decline. They suggest that everyone with AD will decline, but people vary in the rate of progression. They continued to follow-up over 7 years those subjects who had shown little or no decline during earlier follow-ups. By the end of the study, most had died or shown some clinical decline (although often slight). Only two of their original sample of 42 showed no evidence of clinical decline over 7 years. However, Botwinick et al. suggest that even these had shown some evidence of decline on cognitive measures. Alternatively, variability may reflect qualitatively distinct subtypes of dementia, for example 'benign and malignant' forms.

How predictable is this variability?

Several studies have attempted to identify variables which predict outcomes and might therefore indicate particular sub-types of AD or describe the dimensions underlying variability. Some studies have directly tested hypotheses by comparing outcomes for subjects classified at baseline by potential predictors, for example, depression (Reifler *et al.*, 1986), neuropsychiatric symptoms (Mayeux *et al.*, 1985), hearing impairment (Uhlmann *et al.*, 1986). Others adopt a less powerful strategy and compare outcome groups on a wide range of baseline variables (e.g. Mann *et al.*, 1989). Table 4.7 summarizes the range of variables which have been examined as predictors of change. Most, but not all, studies find that severity and type of baseline impairment significantly predict outcome. Thus, people who are more impaired and also show particular impairments (notably language) show greater decline. It is uncertain whether these particular impairments indicate qualitatively distinct subtypes or simply reflect severity itself (Jorm, 1985; Drachman *et al.*, 1990). Thus people may develop language impairment as their AD progresses. Sociodemographic variables consistently show little relationship to outcome. Studies examining clinical or neuroradiological variables have inconsistent results.

Table 4.7   Variables examined as potential predictors of change in Alzheimer's disease.

Baseline performance
 Severity of impairment, e.g. baseline score
 Type of impairment, e.g. language
  'frontal'
  'parietotemporal'

Sociodemographic variables
 Age
 Sex
 Education

Clinical variables
 History, e.g. age at onset
   duration
   family history
 Physical health
 Neuropsychiatric symptoms, e.g. depression
        psychosis
        extrapyramidal features

Neuroradiological variables
 Lateral ventricular size
 Volumetric assessments

The most useful studies adopt statistical models which examine the strength as well as the significance of the relationship between predictor and outcome, and which disentangle the inter-relationships between potential predictors. Four studies illustrate different models to examine the prediction of change. Berg *et al.* (1987) examine performance on the Short Portable Mental Dementia

Rating Scale (DRS) Status Questionnaire (SPMSQ) and the Face–Hand Test (FHT) as predictors of outcome groups classified by clinical change, using stepwise discriminant function analysis. No variable independently predicted outcome, and even combining all three, correctly classified only 46% of subjects. In contrast, Drachman *et al.* (1990) found that cognitive impairment could be a useful predictor of outcome. They included a broad range of variables (baseline performance, sociodemographic and clinical) as predictors of 'clinical end points' selected to identify clinically significant decline (for example, becoming incontinent, institutionalized or self-care dependent). They examined the relationship between variables and outcome categories by univariaté and multivariate life-table analysis. The best individual predictor of outcome was a measure of cognitive impairment. When measures were combined multivariately, only cognitive performance significantly predicted outcome. They explored the strength of this relationship by classifying subjects by level of cognitive performance at baseline (using a measure of psychomotor speed). The majority of the more impaired subjects had a poor outcome at 3 years: 89% were self-care dependent, 66% incontinent and 65% institutional-ized. The less impaired subjects showed more variable outcome with only 50% being activities of daily living (ADL) dependent, 41% incontinent and 31% institutionalized. In contrast, Teri *et al.* (1990) offer evidence for the value of clinical variables as predictors. They compared 16 clinical variables as predic-tors of MMSE change by stepwise regression analysis. They expressed the value of variables as predictors by comparing the estimated ARC for subjects with and without each factor. The estimated decline shown by subjects without any significant behavioural or health problems was 2.8 points per year. Only three of the 16 variables significantly predicted change – alcohol abuse, agitation and neurological symptoms. Subjects with these problems showed greater decline, for example, those with evidence of alcohol abuse declined by an estimated 7.8 points per year. Finally, Huff *et al.* (1990) adopted a similar model to examine sociodemographic variables and clinical symptoms as predictors of DRS change. Only one variable independently predicted progression (naming visually presented objects). This alone accounted for 22% of variance in change score. Subjects with naming impairment at baseline declined by an average of 3.8 points per year, in comparison with a decline of 0.4 points per year for those without any language impairment. A multivariate model (including severity at baseline, age, education, emotional lability and naming ability) accounted for 40% of outcome variance.

Galasko *et al.* (1991) conclude their review of recent studies examining prediction of outcome by describing results as disappointing: 'the variability of clinical findings and rate of progression have not been explained' (p. 939). Why are results generally disappointing? Some difficulties relate to methodology. Many studies have included relatively mildly impaired subjects. This is the most difficult group to diagnose with confidence, and mild or early impairment may be the least predictable stage of AD. Outcomes appear more consistent and potentially more predictable with more severely impaired groups. Studies often examine outcomes over relative short time periods. Again, short-term outcomes may be inherently more variable and less predictable (e.g. Teri *et al.*, 1990). More fundamentally, if the progression of AD is multidimensional, it may be impossible to predict gross change. Thus if different functions change at different rates (as appears likely) it is necessary to examine the prediction of very specific changes. For example, several studies have attempted to predict DRS change. Stern *et al.* (1987) could not significantly predict global change in DRS score with a broad range of clinical variables. Subsequently Stern *et al.*

(1990) attempted to predict change on four dimensions of DRS performance, i.e. cognitive, personality, apathy/withdrawal and self-care. As before, they were unable to predict change significantly on two scales (personality and apathy/withdrawal). However, clinical variables did predict cognitive and self-care decline, but very specifically. Family history and psychotic symptoms significantly predicted cognitive decline, whereas extrapyramidal symptoms significantly predicted change on self-care. This suggests that it may be necessary to examine a broad range of very specific predictors. For example, Huff *et al.* (1990) found that naming visually presented objects significantly predicted outcome, whilst other measures of language impairment showed little or no relationship (including reading comprehension, writing, auditory comprehension).

OTHER METHODS OF ASSESSING CHANGE

Neuroimaging techniques have been used to assess longitudinal change in AD. They obviously provide different information to that of cognitive tests: structural imaging such as computed tomography (CT) or magnetic resonance imaging (MRI) give assessments of structural change while positron emission tomography (PET) and single photon emission tomography (SPET) assess blood flow and measures of metabolism.

Relatively little work has been performed on longitudinal assessments of patients with AD for a number of reasons. Longitudinal studies have their own inherent methodological problems as outlined previously. In addition, neuroimaging has an inherent variability and difficulties in interpreting the results are well recognized. The difficulty of placing the head in precisely the same position over time and problems with other aspects of imaging have been outlined elsewhere (Burns *et al.*, 1991b).

Table 4.8 outlines longitudinal studies which have examined changes which have occurred in studies looking at CT scans. Progression is the norm and generally this is greater than that which occurs in normal controls. De Carli *et al.* (1990) recently reviewed the literature on the discriminatory potential of CT in AD and normal ageing. Some longitudinal studies of CT scans on individuals 1 year apart achieved 100% separation of patients from controls.

Barclay *et al.* (1984) showed progressive changes in cerebral blood flow using SPET and found the patients with AD showed deterioration over time. Rogers *et al.* (1986) showed that in patients with vascular dementia, cerebral blood flow declined before the onset of symptoms whereas in patients with AD blood flow did not decline until after the subject was symptomatic. Philpot *et al.* (1991) were able to localize changes in blood flow using SPET over 12 months and found that significant deteriorations in frontal and parietal areas occurred. Studies with PET have demonstrated the preservation of parietal lobe metabolism over time (Jagust *et al.*, 1988). Clearly, these studies have important implications for monitoring progression of the disease but should not be done in isolation and should always be related to clinical variables.

Neurophysiological measures have also been employed to look at changes over time. St Clair *et al.* (1988) examined 12 patients with AD over 1 year and found changes in the P3 wave form which corresponds to neuropsychological deterioration. One group showed progressive changes while in another the decline was slower. Helkala *et al.* (1991) used the electroencephalogram (EEG) to predict subsequent decline showing that an abnormal EEG early in the course of the disorder was associated with deterioration of cognitive function in particular in praxis and speech.

Table 4.8 Longitudinal computed tomographic scan changes in dementia of the Alzheimer type.

Study	Number	Mean age (years)	Follow-up	Findings
Naguib and Levy (1982)	10	76.2	18–36 months	Two subgroups emerged – stable ventricles with little cognitive deterioration, increasing ventricular size with cognitive deterioration
Gado et al. (1982)	45	71.0	12 months	Volumetric measures more sensitive to change than linear measures. Changes greater in patients compared to controls
Brinkman et al. (1984)	5	60.6	15–35 months	Four of the five patients had increases greater than the normative values suggested
Luxenberg et al. (1987)	12 male 6 female	62.8 (male) 70.8 (female)	6–60 months	Rate of lateral ventricular enlargement discriminated male patients from controls
de Leon et al. (1989)	50	71.2	36 months	Ventricular volume increase: 9% in patients, 2% in controls
Burns et al. (1991)	63	79.3	12 months	Ventricular enlargement correlated with cognitive deterioration

Based on a table in Burns et al. (1991a).

CONCLUSIONS

Essential to a diagnosis of AD is that deterioration should occur over time. There is no shortage of information about progression in AD as the number of studies involved attest. The main difficulty is in the interpretation of the results. Longitudinal studies are expensive and complicated. However, they are essential to the issue and there is no substitute for prospective clinical evaluation of a large number of cases. Other models of analysis should be considered but only employed if they are shown to be superior to conventional longitudinal designs.

It is now well recognized that AD is not an homogenous condition. Thus, progression of AD should not be expected to be uniform and significant variability should be anticipated. Studies suggest that different neuropsychological functions deteriorate at different rates and, as such, this has been taken as evidence of subgroups of the disorder. However, to confine analysis to purely cognitive indices implies an overly narrow view of the disease. Inevitably cognitive measures have taken precedence in the study of progression and search for predictors of decline. We need to redraw this by developing methods of monitoring other aspects of AD change. Multidimensional assessments which include measures of activities of daily living and other noncognitive features may provide 'truer' pictures of progression. Detailed analysis of individual features (whether they be cognitive or noncognitive) should reveal valuable information about various aspects of progression and may help to tease apart individual subtypes of the disorder.

Given that progression in AD is such a fundamental principal on which the diagnosis and model of the disorder is based, it is disappointing that only recently have studies looked at this issue in detail. Studies which amalgamate potential aetiological factors, detailed longitudinal assessment and perhaps adjuvant investigations such as neuroimaging, will be essential to untangle the issues involved.

REFERENCES

Ajuriaguerra, J. de and Tissot, R. (1968). Some aspects of psychoneurologic disintegration in senile dementia. In *Senile Dementia*, Muller, C. and Ciompi, L. (Eds). Huber, Berne.

Baltes, P.B., Nesselroade, J.R., Schaie, K.W. and Labourie, E.W. (1972). On the dilemma of regression effects in examining ability- level-related differentials in ontogenetic patterns of intelligence. *Developmental Psychology*, **6**, 78–84.

Barclay, L., Zemcov, A., Blass, J.P. and McDowell, F. (1984). Rates of decrease of cerebral blood flow in progressive dementias. *Neurology*, **34**, 1555–60.

Becker, J.T., Huff, J., Nebes, R.D. *et al.* (1988). Neuropsychological function in Alzheimer's disease. *Archives of Neurology*, **45**, 263–8.

Berg, L., Danzinger, W.L., Storandt, M. *et al.* (1984). Predictive features in mild senile dementia of the Alzheimer's type. *Neurology*, **34**, 563–9.

Berg, G., Edwards, D.F., Danzinger, W.L. and Berg, L. (1987). Longitudinal changes in three brief assessments of SDAT. *Journal of the American Geriatrics Society*, **35**, 205–12.

Berg, L., Miller, J.P., Storandt, M. *et al.* (1988). Mild senile dementia of the Alzheimer type: 2 – Longitudinal assessment. *Annals of Neurology*, **23**, 477–87.

Berg, L., Smith, D.S., Morris, J.C. *et al.* (1990). Mild senile dementia of the

Alzheimer type: 3 – Longitudinal and cross-sectional assessment. *Annals of Neurology*, **28**, 648–52.

Blessed, G., Tomlinson, B.E. and Roth, M. (1968). The association between quantitative measures of dementia and of senile change in the cerebral grey matter of elderly subjects. *British Journal of Psychiatry*, **114**, 797–811.

Botwinick, J., Storandt, M. and Berg, L. (1986). A longitudinal behavioural study of senile dementia of the Alzheimer type. *Archives of Neurology*, **43**, 1124–7.

Botwinick, J., Storandt, M., Berg, L. and Boland, S. (1988). Senile dementia of the Alzheimer type. *Archives of Neurology*, **45**, 493–6.

Brinkman, S., Largen, J. (1984). Changes in brain ventricular size with repeated CAT Scans in suspected Alzheimer's disease. *Am. J. Psychiatry*, **141**, 81–3.

Brull, J., Wertheimer, J. and Haller, E. (1979). Evolutive profiles in senile dementia. A psychological and neuropsychological longitudinal study. *Bayer-Symposium VII: Brain Function in Old Age*. Springer-Verlag, Heidelberg.

Burns, A., Jacoby, R., Berg, R. *et al.* (1991a). CT in Alzheimer's disease. *Biological Psychiatry*, **29**, 383–90.

Burns, A., Jacoby, R. and Levy, R. (1991b). Progression of cognitive impairment in Alzheimer's disease. *Journal of the American Geriatrics Society*, **39**, 39–45.

Busse, E.W. and Maddox, G.L. (1985). *The Duke Longitudinal Studies of Normal Ageing 1955–1980*. Springer, New York.

Constantinidis, J., Richard, J. and de Ajuriaguerra, J. (1978). Dementias with senile plaques and neurofibrillary tangles. In *Studies in Geriatric Psychiatry*, Isaacs, A.D. and Post, F. (Eds). John Wiley and Sons, Chichester.

Cowan, D.W., Copeland, J.R.M., Kelleher, M.J. *et al.* (1975). Cross-national study of diagnosis of the mental disorders: A comparative psychometric assessment of elderly patients admitted to mental hospitals in Queens County, New York and the former borough of Camberwell, London. *British Journal of Psychiatry*, **126**, 560–70.

De Carli, C., Kaye, J. and Morowitz, B. (1990). Critical analysis of the use of computer assisted transversive axial tomography to study human brain in ageing and dementia. *Neurology*, **40**, 872–3.

Drachman, D.A., O'Donnell, B.F., Lew, R.A. and Swearer, J.M. (1990). The prognosis in Alzheimer's disease. *Archives of Neurology*, **47**, 851 6.

Folstein, M.F., Folstein, S.E. and McHugh, P.R. (1975). 'Mini-Mental State' – A practical method for grading the cognitive stage of patients for the clinician. *Journal of Psychiatric Research*, **12**, 189–98.

Flicker, C., Ferris, S.H. and Reisberg, B. (1991). Mild cognitive impairment in the elderly: Predictors of dementia. *Neurology*, **41**, 1006–9.

Friedland, R.P. Horwitz, B. and Koss, E. (1988). Measure of disease progression in Alzheimer's disease. *Neurobiology of Ageing*, **9**, 95–7.

Gado, M., Hughes, C., Danzinger, W. and Chi, D. (1983). Aging, dementia and brain atrophy: A longitudinal CT study. *American Journal of Neuroradiology*, **4**, 699–702.

Galasko, D., Corey-Blom, J. and Thal, L.J. (1991). Monitoring progression in Alzheimer's disease. *Journal of the American Geriatrics Society*, **39**, 932–41.

Gilleard, C.J. and Pattie, A.H. (1978). The effect of location on the elderly mentally infirm: Relationship to mortality and behavioural deterioration. *Age and Ageing*, **7**, 1–6.

Gurland, B.J., Dean, L.L., Copeland, J. *et al.* (1982). Criteria for the diagnosis of dementia in the community elderly. *Gerontologist*, **22**, 180–5.

Hart, S. (1988). Language of dementia: a review. *Psychological Medicine*, **18**, 99–112.

Helkala, E.-L., Laulumaa, V., Soininen, H. *et al.* (1991). Different patterns of cognitive decline related to normal or deteriorating EEG in a 3-year follow-up study of patients with Alzheimer's disease. *Neurology*, **41**, 529–32.

Hersch, E.L., Kral, V.A. and Bruce-Palmer, R. (1978). Clinical value of the London Psychogeriatric Rating Scale. *Journal of American Geriatrics Society*, **26**, 348–54.

Hodkinson, H.M. (1973). Mental impairment in the elderly. *Journal of the Royal College of Physicians*, **7**, 305–17.

Huff, F.J., Belle, S.H., Shim, Y.K. *et al.* (1990). Prevalence and prognostic value of neurologic abnormalities in Alzheimer's disease. *Dementia*, **1**, 32–40.

Huff, F.J., Growdon, J.H., Corkin, S. and Rosen, T.J. (1987). Age at onset and rate of progression of Alzheimer's disease. *Journal of the American Geriatrics Society*, **35**, 27–30.

Hughes, C.P., Berg, L., Danzinger, W.L. *et al.* (1982). A new clinical scale for the staging of dementia. *British Journal of Psychiatry*, **140**, 566–72.

Jagust, W.J., Friedland, R.P., Budinger, T.F. *et al.* (1988). Longitudinal studies of regional cerebral metabolism in Alzheimer's disease. *Neurology*, **30**, 909–12.

Jorm, A.F. (1985). Subtypes of Alzheimer's dementia: A conceptual analysis and critical review. *Psychological Medicine*, **15**, 543–55.

Jorm, A.F. (1986). Controlled and automatic information on processing in senile dementia: A review. *Psychological Medicine*, **16**, 77–88.

Jorm, A.F. (1990). Some pitfalls in data analysis. In *Advances in Neurology, Vol. 51: Alzheimer's disease*, Wartman, R.J. (Ed.). Raven Press, New York.

Jorm, A.F. and Korten, A.E. (1988). Assessment of cognitive decline in the elderly by informant interview. *British Journal of Psychiatry*, **152**, 209–13.

Jorm, A.F., Scott, R. and Jacomb, P.A. (1989). Assessment of cognitive decline in dementia by informant questionnaire. *International Journal of Geriatric Psychiatry*, **4**, 35–9.

Kaszniak, A.W., Fox, J., Gandell, D.L. *et al.* (1978). Predictors of mortality in presenile and senile dementia. *Annals of Neurology*, **3**, 246–52.

Kaszniak, A.W., Wilson, R.S., Fox, J.H. and Stebbins, G.T. (1986). Cognitive assessment in Alzheimer's disease: Cross-sectional and longitudinal perspectives. *Canadian Journal of Neurological Sciences*, **13**, 420–3.

Katzman, R., Brown, T., Thal, L.J. *et al.* (1988). Comparison of rate of annual change of mental test score in four independent studies of patients with Alzheimer's disease. *Annals of Neurology*, **24**, 384–9.

Kendrick, D.C. (1972). The Kendrick battery of tests: Theoretical assumptions and clinical uses. *British Journal of Social and Clinical Psychology*, **11**, 373–86.

Kendrick, D.C. and Moyes, I.C.A. (1979). Activity, depression, medication and performance on the Revised Kendrick Battery. *British Journal of Social and Clinical Psychology*, **18**, 341–50.

Kramer-Ginsberg, E., Mohs, R.C., Aryan, M. *et al.* (1988). Clinical predictors of course of Alzheimer patients in a longitudinal study: A preliminary report. *Psychopharmacology Bulletin*, **24**, 458–62.

La Rue, A. (1987). Methodological concerns: Longitudinal studies of dementia. *Alzheimer Disease and Associated Disorders*, **1**, 180–92.

de Leon, M., George, A., Reisberg, B. *et al.* (1989). Alzheimer's disease. Longitudinal CT studies of ventricular change. *American Journal of Radiology*, **152**, 1257–62.

Little, A.G., Volans, P.J., Hemsley, D.R. and Levy, R. (1986). The retention of new information in senile dementia. *British Journal of Clinical Psychology*, **25**, 71–2.

Luxenberg, J., Harby, J., Creasey, H. *et al.* (1987). Rate of ventricular enlargement in dementia of the 'Alzheimer' type correlates with rate of neuropsychological deterioration. *Neurology*, **37**, 1135–49.

Mann, U.M., Mohr, E. and Chase, T.N. (1989). Rapidly progressive Alzheimer's disease. *Lancet*, **ii**, 799.

Mayeux, R., Stern, Y. and Spanton, S. (1985). Heterogeneity in dementia of the Alzheimer type: Evidence of subgroups. *Neurology*, **35**, 453–61.

Naguib, M. and Levy, R. (1982). C.T. scanning in senile dementia: A follow-up of survivors. *British Journal of Psychiatry*, **141**, 618–20.

Nelson, M.E. and O'Connell, A. (1975). Dementia: the estimation of premorbid intelligence levels using the new adult reading test. *Cortex*, **14**, 234–44.

Norris, F.H. (1985). Characteristics of older non-respondents over five waves of a panel study. *Journal of Gerontology*, **40**, 627–36.

Ortof, E. and Crystal, H.A. (1989). Rate of progression of Alzheimer's disease. *Journal of the American Geriatrics Society*, **37**, 511–14.

Overall, J.E. (1987). Estimating sample size for longitudinal studies of age-related cognitive decline. *Journal of Gerontology*, **42**, 137–41.

Perry, E.K., Tomlinson, B.E., Blessed, G. *et al.* (1978). Correlation of cholinergic abnormalities with senile plaques and mental test scores in senile dementia. *British Medical Journal*, **ii**, 1457–9.

Pfeiffer, E. (1975). A Short Portable Mental Status Questionnaire for the assessment of organic brain deficit in elderly patients. *Journal of the American Geriatrics Society*, **23**, 433–41.

Philpot, M., Costa, D.C., Durval, C. *et al.* (1991). Single photon emission tomography in Alzheimer's disease: A longitudinal study of changes in relative regional cerebral blood flow. *International Journal of Geriatric Psychiatry*, **6**, 767–74.

Rabins, P.V., Merchant, A. and Nestadt, G. (1984). Criteria for diagnosing reversible dementia caused by depression: Validation by two-year follow-up. *Journal of Psychiatry*, **144**, 488–92.

Rebok, G., Brandt, J. and Folstein, M. (1990). Longitudinal cognitive decline in patients with Alzheimer's disease. *Journal of Geriatric Psychiatry and Neurology*, **3**, 91–7.

Reifler, B.V., Larson, E., Teri, L. and Poulsen, M. (1986). Dementia of the Alzheimer type and depression. *Journal of the American Geriatrics Society*, **34**, 855–9.

Reisberg, B., Ferris, S., Anand, R. *et al.* (1985). Clinical assessment of cognition in the aged. In *Dementia in the Elderly*, Shamoian, C.A. (Ed.). American Psychiatric Press, Washington DC.

Reisberg, B., Ferris, S.H. and Crook, T. (1982). Signs, symptoms and course of age-associated cognitive decline. In *Alzheimer's Disease: A Report of Progress in Ageing*, Corkin, S. (Ed.), Vol. 19. Raven Press, New York.

Reisberg, B., Ferris, S.H., de Leon, M.J. *et al.* (1989). The stage specific temporal course of Alzheimer's disease: Functional and behavioural concomitants based upon cross-sectional and longitudinal observation. *Alzheimer's Disease and Related Disorders*, **317**, 23–41.

Reisberg, B., Ferris, S.H., Franssen, E. *et al.* (1986a). Age-associated memory impairment: The clinical syndrome. *Developmental Neuropsychology*, **2**, 401–12.

Reisberg, B., Ferris, S.H., Shulman, E. *et al.* (1986b). Longitudinal course of normal ageing and progressive dementia of the Alzheimer type: A prospective study of 106 subjects over a 3–6 year mean interval. *Progress in Neuropsychopharmacology and Biological Psychiatry*, **10**, 571–8.

Reisberg, B., Shulman, E., Ferris, S.H. *et al.* (1983). Clinical assessments of age-associated cognitive decline and primary degenerative dementia: Prognostic concomitants. *Psychopharmacology Bulletin*, **19**, 734–9.

Riege, W.H. and Metter, E.J. (1988). Cognitive and brain imaging measures of Alzheimer's disease. *Neurobiology of Ageing*, **9**, 69–86.

Riegel, K.F. and Riegel, R.M. (1972). Development, drop and death. *Developmental Psychology*, **6**, 306–19.

Riegel, K.F., Riegel, R.M. and Meyer, G. (1967). Socio-psychological factors of ageing: A cohort-sequential analysis. *Human Development*, **10**, 27–56.

Rogers, R.L., Meyer, J.S., Mortel, K.F. *et al.* (1986). Decreased cerebral blood flow precedes multi-infarct dementia, but follows senile dementia of Alzheimer type. *Neurology*, **36**, 1–6.

Rosen, W.G., Mohs, R.C. and Davis, K.L. (1984). A new rating scale of Alzheimer's disease. *American Journal of Psychiatry*, **141**, 1356–64.

Salmon, D.P., Thal, L.J., Butters, N. and Heindel, W.C. (1990). Longitudinal evaluation of dementia of the Alzheimer type: A comparison of three standardised mental status examinations. *Neurology*, **40**, 1225–30.

Salthouse, T.A. (1991). *Theoretical Perspectives on Cognitive Ageing*. Lawrence Erlbaum Associates, Hillsdale.

Schaie, K.W. (1983). *Longitudinal Studies of Adult Psychological Development*. Guildford Press, New York.

St Clair, D., Blackburn, I., Blackwood, D. and Tyrer, G. (1988). Measuring the course of Alzheimer's disease: A longitudinal study of neuropsychological function and changes in P3 event-related potential. *British Journal of Psychiatry*, **152**, 48–54.

Stern, Y., Hesdorffer, D., Sano, M. and Mayeus, R. (1990). Measurement and prediction of functional capacity in Alzheimer's disease. *Neurology*, **40**, 8–14.

Stern, Y., Mayeux, R., Sano, M. *et al.* (1987). Predictors of disease course in patients with probable Alzheimer's disease. *Neurology*, **37**, 1649–53.

Stonier, P.D. (1974). Score changes following repeated administration of mental status questionnaire. *Age and Ageing*, **3**, 91–6.

Taylor, R., Gilleard, C.J. and McGuire, R.J. (1991). Short-term cognitive fluctuation in multi-infarct dementia and dementia of the Alzheimer type. *International Journal of Geriatric Psychiatry*, **6**, 497–500.

Teng, E.L., Wimer, C., Roberts, E. *et al.* (1989). Alzheimer's dementia: Performance on parallel forms of the dementia assessment battery. *Journal of Clinical and Experimental Neuropsychology*, **11**, 899–912.

Teri, L., Hughes, J.P. and Larson, E.B. (1990). Cognitive deterioration in Alzheimer's disease: Behavioural and health factors. *Journal of Gerontology: Psychological Sciences*, **45**, 58–63.

Thal, L.J., Grundman, M. and Klauber, M.R. (1988). Dementia: Characteristics of a referral population and factors associated with progression. *Neurology*, **38**, 1083–90.

Thompson, P. and Blessed, G. (1987). Correlation between the 37 item Mental Test score and Abbreviated 10 item Mental Test Score by psychogeriatric day patients. *British Journal of Psychiatry*, **151**, 206–9.

Tinklenberg, J., Brooks, J.O., Tanke, E.D. *et al.* (1990). Factor analysis and preliminary validation of the Mini-Mental State Examination from a longitudinal perspective. *International Psychogeriatrics*, **2**, 123–34.

Uhlmann, R.F., Larson, E.B. and Buchner, D.M. (1987). Correlations of Mini-Mental State and Modified Dementia Rating Scale to measure of transitional health status in dementia. *Journal of Gerontology*, **42**, 33–6.

Uhlmann, R.F., Larson, E.B. and Keopsell, T.D. (1986). Hearing impairment and cognitive decline in senile dementia of the Alzheimer type. *Journal of the American Geriatrics Society*, **34**, 207–10.

Walton, D. (1958). The diagnostic and predictive accuracy of the Wechsler Memory Scale in psychiatric patients over 65. *Journal of Mental Science*, **104**, 1111–18.

Whitehead, A. (1977). Changes in cognitive functioning in elderly psychiatric patients. *British Journal of Psychiatry*, **130**, 605–8.

Woods, R.T. and Britton, P.G. (1985). *Clinical Psychology with the Elderly*. Croom-Helm, Beckenham.

Yesavage, J.A. and Brooks, J.O. (1991). On the importance of longitudinal research in Alzheimer's disease. *Journal of the American Geriatrics Society*, **39**, 941–4.

Yesavage, J.A., Poulsen, S.L., Sheilch, J. and Tanke, E. (1988). Rates of change of common measures of impairment in senile dementia of the Alzheimer type. *Psychopharmacology Bulletin*, **24**, 531–4.

Adrian M. Owen

Department of Experimental Psychology
University of Cambridge
and
Section of Old Age Psychiatry
Institute of Psychiatry
London

5 COMPUTERIZED ASSESSMENT OF COGNITIVE FUNCTION IN AGEING AND DEMENTIA

INTRODUCTION

In recent years, computerized testing procedures have become increasingly popular in the assessment of cognitive dysfunction in dementia and related neuropsychiatric disorders. In this chapter the main technological developments in this field will be described and their relevance to both clinical assessment and experimental research discussed.

The advantages of computer systems over more traditional means of assessment will be considered in the context of recent studies that have adopted this technological approach. Specifically, the sensitivity of computerized tests to cognitive changes in dementia and to the effects of pharmacological intervention will be addressed. In addition, comparative studies of human neurosurgical populations and animals with selective neurochemical lesions using analogous computerized tests will be described. The role of such comparisons in defining the specificity of cognitive deficits in dementia and in identifying the underlying neural substrates responsible will be discussed.

Finally, in order to illustrate these points, one particular computerized paradigm, adapted for use with both humans and experimentally lesioned primates, will be described in detail, illustrating how the innovative use of existing computer technology can be used to define the neural and neurochemical basis of specific neuropsychological deficits.

TECHNOLOGICAL CONSIDERATIONS

Hardware

With the widespread availability of computing technology, it is now possible for most research groups to design, implement and standardize computerized psychological testing procedures for routine use in the clinic. The choice of microcomputers is considerable. In recent years the Acorn BBC Master computer has proved to be a popular choice offering high-resolution colour graphics at relatively low cost. However, with the rapid decrease in the cost of computing technology and the development of more powerful and flexible systems, a new

Adrian M. Owen and much of the work discussed in this chapter is supported by a Major Award from the Wellcome Trust to Drs T.W. Robbins, B.J. Everitt and B.J. Sahakian. I would like to thank Drs O.P. Almeida, A.C. Roberts and T.W. Robbins for critical reading of this manuscript.

generation of personal computers (or PCs) have entered the neuropsychological arena. In particular, the IBM PCs (including IBM 'compatibles' or 'clones') are now widely available and have a number of advantages over the more basic Acorn BBC system. As well as increasing overall processing speed, test stimuli can be presented and responses measured with millisecond accuracy. In addition, large amounts of data can be stored on the computer's hard disk and more easily transferred between the neuropsychological test programs and popular statistical and graphics packages.

In relation to dementia, one important attribute of computer technology is the availability of peripheral systems which allow the patient to interact directly with the computer. Many alternative response media are available including single touch key pads, mice, joysticks, tracker balls and light-pens. In recent years, touch sensitive screens have proved to be extremely valuable in assessing patients with neurodegenerative disorders since they enable the subject to respond directly by touching stimuli presented on the monitor (Morris et al., 1988; Sahakian et al., 1988, 1990; Downes et al., 1989). The main advantage of this method is that the stimulus material which guides the decision of the subject is identical to the cues which guide the response. Thus, the patient is not required to divide their attention between the stimulus and the response, an important consideration given that demented patients are known to be impaired on such tasks (Baddley et al., 1986; Morris, 1986). In addition, Carr et al. (1986) found that cognitively impaired elderly patients preferred using a touch sensitive screen to a board with illuminated response buttons.

For reaction time studies, single touch key pads may be used in combination with a touch sensitive screen to provide separate and accurate measures of reaction time (i.e. the time to remove the hand from the key pad) and movement time (i.e. the time between moving the hand from the pad and touching the screen) (see Downes et al., 1989; Sahakian et al., 1990).

Software
In principle, it should be possible for most research groups to design and program neuropsychological tests according to their own specific require-ments. On the Acorn BBC machine, BBC BASIC is a simple but powerful programming language with a versatile graphics system. For IBM compatible PCs, various packages exist to simplify programming in a number of high level languages including BASIC (e.g. Microsoft QuickBASIC) and C (e.g. Microsoft Quick C).

Alternatively, some existing computerized neuropsychological test packages are commercially available. The main advantage of these systems is that they may already have been extensively used on a number of patient and control populations and relevant data may previously have been published.

For example, the Bexley–Maudsley Automated Psychological Screening Battery (Acker and Acker, 1982) includes tests of visual–spatial memory and spatial orientation, a symbol–digit coding task (similar to the Digit Symbol subtest of the Wechsler Adult Intelligence Scale (WAIS) and a test of concept formation based on the Wisconsin Card Sorting Test, WCST (Grand and Berg, 1948; Milner, 1964). This system was originally programmed for the now largely redundant Commodore PET computer but a version for the Apple II microcomputer has also been produced.

In the evolving world of computing hardware, the most useful neuropsycho-logical tests are likely to be those designed to run on popular 'industry standard' machines such as the IBM PC and compatible systems.

For example, the Cambridge Neuropsychological Test Automated Battery* (CANTAB) is a set of three computerized neuropsychological test batteries designed to test various aspects of visual memory, attention, working memory and planning. In a fourth battery, five parallel versions of many of the tests are supplied which may be useful for longitudinal studies in which subjects are retested on a number of occasions. The tests have been designed and programmed to run on both an Acorn BBC Master microcomputer (using a high-resolution Microvitec Touchtech 501 touch sensitive monitor) and an IBM (or compatible) PC (using a variety of IBM compatible touch sensitive screens). The CANTAB tests were developed by Dr T.W. Robbins and colleagues at the University of Cambridge and at the Institute of Psychiatry, London.

In recent years the CANTAB test batteries have been used extensively to assess cognitive function in a number of clinical groups including patients with dementia of the Alzheimer type (DAT; Sahakian *et al.*, 1988, 1990, 1991; Sahgal *et al.*, 1991, 1992), depression (Abas *et al.*, 1990), Parkinson's disease (Morris *et al.*, 1988; Downes *et al.*, 1989), Korsakoff's syndrome (Joyce and Robbins, 1991), multiple system atrophy (Robbins *et al.*, 1992) and patients with localized excisions of the frontal and temporal lobes (Owen *et al.*, 1990, 1991).

THE ADVANTAGES OF COMPUTERIZED TESTS

Experimentally, computerized testing procedures have many practical and theoretical advantages over more conventional testing methods. For example, response latencies can be measured to millisecond accuracy, which may be important in sophisticated reaction time studies. However, they are also more flexible than traditional neuropsychological techniques with data being recorded, processed and scored automatically during the testing session.

Moreover, computer systems greatly improve the accuracy with which the testing situation can be controlled, isolating the factors of interest and reducing experimental 'noise' which is frequently difficult to achieve in a clinical environment. For example, both stimulus presentation time and intertrial intervals may be held constant for each trial and, more importantly, for each subject. Conversely, they can be precisely and systematically varied to examine the relationship between these factors and performance.

In addition, computers can accurately record and analyse many aspects of performance simultaneously, providing a componential analysis of the behaviour being assessed. In particular, measures of response latency and response accuracy may be combined in order to examine the processes comprising particular cognitive operations in great detail (e.g. response latency for correct responses versus incorrect responses). This is essential, for example, in information processing studies of dementia where it may be necessary to record simultaneous information about the speed and accuracy of the patient.

The detailed analyses produced by computerized systems also increase the accuracy with which 'task difficulty' can be determined and equilibrated across different paradigms. This is particularly important in the assessment of dementia since failure on one task may often reflect a general, nonspecific effect of task difficulty. By comparing performance across a number of tasks of equal complexity, the specificity of observed deficits can be more accurately determined.

Another advantage of computer-controlled tests is that they can be designed

*Paul Fray Ltd, 4, Flint Lane, Ely Road, Waterbeach, CB5 9QZ.

so that each testing session is administered in a more systematic and objective way than may be possible in a typical clinical setting. For example, the difficulty of a task may be automatically adjusted according to strict and predefined criteria. In this way, tests may be tailored to suit the abilities of each individual, shortening test sessions and minimizing the experience of failure in the severely impaired patient. In a similar way, computer tests can easily be 'fixed' (in terms of the number of successes and failures) such that the subjective experience of being tested is equivalent for each patient.

Finally, using precise computer control, a consistent amount of positive and negative feedback can be given to each subject, increasing inter-rater and test–retest reliability and making computer systems ideal for multicentred trials.

Of course, everything has its price and computerized neuropsychological assessment is no exception. Computer-controlled tests are in general, more expensive and less portable than their more conventional 'paper and pencil' counterparts. Individual items such as touch sensitive monitors are awkward to carry and easily damaged. However, in the near future falling computer prices and the increased availability of truly portable computers or 'laptops' may reduce the importance of these differences.

Computers are also limited in the types of test material to which they are suited. For example, the advantages of a computerized version of a verbally administered test such as the Mini-Mental State Examination (Folstein *et al.*, 1975) are not obvious.

In summary, despite the obvious practical considerations computerized neuropsychological tests have many advantages over more conventional testing methods in terms of improved control over the testing situation and an enormous increase in the depth and breadth of information provided.

THE APPLICATIONS OF COMPUTERIZED TESTS

The relative precision and sensitivity of computerized neuropsychological techniques makes them valuable tools for investigating small, sometimes quite subtle, behavioural alterations which may not be detected using more conventional 'paper and pencil' tests. For example, in a recent longitudinal study of elderly depressed patients, performance on several traditional tests such as the Mini-Mental State Examination (Folstein *et al.*, 1975) and the Kendrick Object Learning Test (Kendrick, 1985) improved significantly on recovery, although residual deficits were detected using computerized tests of memory and learning (Abas *et al.*, 1990). In recent years, computerized neuropsychological testing has become commonplace in a number of research centres and has been successfully applied in many experimental and clinical areas, in particular for:

1. Charting the course of cognitive deficits in dementia and related neurodegenerative disorders
2. Assessing the effects of pharmacological intervention in dementia and other neurodegenerative disorders
3. Distinguishing between different neuropsychiatric disorders
4. Imaging studies
5. Comparative assessment of cognitive dysfunction in experimentally lesioned animals and dementia
6. Comparative assessment of cognitive dysfunction in dementia and patients with localized neurosurgical excisions

Much of this work has been carried out at Cambridge University, the Institute of Psychiatry in London and related research centres using tests from the CANTAB neuropsychological test battery. The results of several of the more important studies will be described below.

Longitudinal and cross-sectional studies of cognitive dysfunction in dementia
Computer-controlled tests are particularly well suited for following the course of many neurological diseases including DAT. Thus, assessments at regular intervals can provide reliable indications of whether the underlying neurological condition is changing, and if so, in what way.

In a recent 5-year study, Sahakian et al. (unpublished observations) reassessed 12 patients with mild DAT annually using a number of computer-controlled tests from the CANTAB battery (Morris et al., 1987). Marked differences in visual memory performance were observed between each assessment with the most significant deterioration occurring between the second and third years.

Less powerful cross-sectional studies have also been successfully used to chart the course of cognitive dysfunction in dementia. For example, Sahgal et al. (1991) compared mnemonic and attentional processes in groups of patients with mild or moderate DAT, defined according to their scores on the Mini-Mental State Examination (Folstein et al., 1975). Both groups of DAT patients were significantly impaired on three computerized tests of memory (pattern recognition, delayed matching to sample and paired associative conditional learning) but not on a visual search, matching to sample test of attention. In addition, in the tests of delayed matching to sample and paired associates conditional learning, more severe impairments were observed in those DAT patients who were later in the course of the disease than in those with more mild clinical symptoms.

In a parallel study, visuospatial memory was compared in groups of patients with mild and moderate DAT using computerized tests of spatial recognition, spatial span and spatial working memory (Sahgal et al., 1992). Whilst equivalent deficits were observed in the tests of spatial working memory and spatial recognition only the spatial span task was able to distinguish between the two DAT groups.

The effects of pharmacological intervention
Computerized data are likely to provide the most sensitive indices of the extent to which medication enhances or compromises a patient's mental efficiency. For example, Lange et al. (1992) tested a group of patients with idiopathic Parkinson's disease (PD) on a comprehensive battery of automated tests of learning, memory, planning and attention whilst either 'on' or 'off' levodopa medication. Controlled withdrawal of medication interfered with aspects of performance on three tests known to be sensitive to frontal lobe dysfunction (Owen et al., 1990, 1991) but not on tests of visual recognition memory and paired associative conditional learning assumed to depend on more posterior structures.

Despite the previous resistance of cognitive decline in dementia to pharmacological intervention, several recent studies have used computer-controlled tests of cognitive function to examine the effects of experimental drug treatments in patients with DAT. For example, subcutaneously injected nicotine has been shown to produce marked improvements in discriminative sensitivity and reaction times but not short-term memory in both DAT patients with mild to moderate symptoms and healthy adults using a novel computerized test of attention and information processing (Sahakian *et al.*, 1989).

In a recent double-blind, placebo-controlled crossover trial of patients with DAT treated with the tetrahydroaminoacridine (THA) and lecithin (Eagger *et al.*, 1991a, b) a comprehensive battery of computerized tests was used to assess the effects of the drug as well as more conventional tests of intellectual function. Small but significant improvements were observed on two of the CANTAB computerized tests of attentional ability (Sahakian *et al.*, 1991) although significant improvements were also noted in the Mini-Mental State Examination and the abbreviated mental test score (Hodkinson, 1972).

Comparisons between dementia and other neuropsychiatric conditions

In assessing cognitive dysfunction, the efficacy of a test lies not only in its ability to detect and measure impairments in particular populations of patients but also in its ability to distinguish between those populations. The relative sensitivity and accuracy of computer tests increases the probability that subtle group differences will be reliably detected.

In several recent studies, specific patterns of impairment have been identified in a number of patient groups using a computerized test of simultaneous and delayed matching to sample (Sahakian *et al.*, 1988). Patients are shown a complex abstract pattern in the centre of the computer screen and are then required to match it to one of four choice patterns appearing below the target either simultaneously or after a brief, but variable (0–16 second) delay (Figure 5.1).

Patients with mild DAT exhibited a delay-dependent deficit in choice accuracy but were unimpaired in the simultaneous condition where there is no mnemonic component. In contrast, a group of medicated patients with idiopathic PD showed a delay-*independent* deficit in the delayed matching to sample test and were also significantly impaired in the simultaneous matching condition. On this basis, the cognitive deficits in patients with DAT and PD were differentially described in terms of mnemonic and attentional processes, respectively.

By comparison, the same paradigm has also been used to describe specific patterns of deficit in groups of patients with other neurological and psychiatric disorders. For example, nondemented patients with the progressive neurodegenerative condition multiple system atrophy (MSA), have been shown to be significantly impaired in the simultaneous condition but show normal delayed matching performance (Robbins *et al.*, 1992), the exact opposite of the pattern shown by patients early in the course of DAT. Similarly, using the same task, a unique pattern of prolonged response latencies and errors has been identified in elderly depressed patients, when compared to patients with DAT (Abas *et al.*, 1990).

Imaging studies

Single photon emission tomography (SPET) has recently been used to compare regional cerebral blood flow (rCBF) in relation to cognitive performance in 35 patients with DAT and 35 healthy matched controls. (O'Brien *et al.*, 1992.) In the DAT group, significant correlations were observed between rCBF and many of the neuropsychological measures, assessed using the CAMCOG cognitive subcomponent of the Cambridge Mental Disorders of the Elderly (CAMDEX) schedule (Roth *et al.*, 1986). In particular, memory correlated with left temporal activity whilst praxis, perception object assembly and block design correlated with right parietal activity. A subgroup of 20 DAT patients also received a

Presentation phase

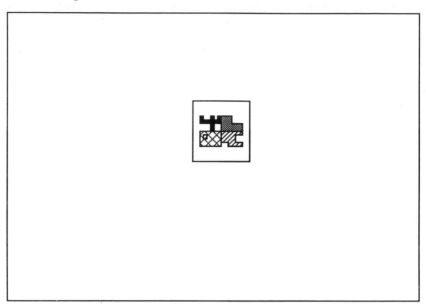

Response phase

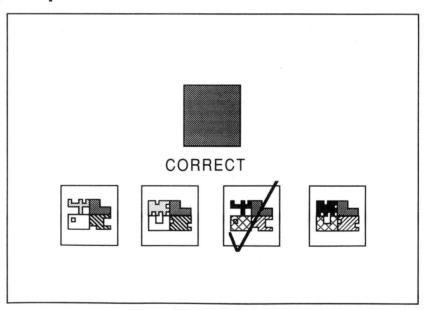

Fig. 5.1 The computerized simultaneous and delayed matching to sample test. In this example, the target stimulus has been correctly identified from among three distractor stimuli after a brief (0–16 second) delay.

number of computerized tests from the CANTAB automated test battery (Morris et al. 1987). Performance accuracy on the simultaneous and delayed matching to sample paradigm described above (Sahakian et al., 1988) correlated significantly with posterior temporal and parietal lobe activity, particularly in the right hemisphere (O'Brien et al., personal communication). Thus, it is possible that the severe deficit in visual short-term memory shown by DAT patients performing this test reflects dysfunction of temporal and parietal lobe structures, a possibility consistent with the patterns of neuropathological and neurochemical changes seen in the condition (Tomlinson, 1984).

Additionally, Abas et al. (1990) have reported a significant correlation between ventricular–brain ratio (VBR), calculated from mechanical planimetry of CT scans (Jacoby and Levy, 1980) and impaired latency for correct responses on the same computerized delayed matching to sample procedure in a group of elderly depressives.

Comparative assessment of cognitive dysfunction in experimentally lesioned animals and dementia

The specific neural or neurochemical basis of cognitive dysfunction in dementia and related progressive neurodegenerative diseases is particularly difficult to define since extensive primary and secondary pathological changes may preclude such conclusions from being drawn at *post-mortem*. Direct comparison of behavioural or cognitive deficits in patients with dementia and animals with selective neurochemical or neuroanatomical lesions can help to ascertain whether specific neuronal changes are causal to or correlates of impaired cognition.

Unlike human neuropsychology, animal studies have employed computer-controlled testing procedures for many years because of the better control they offer over stimulus presentation, the recording of responses and the programming of feedback contingencies. However, in general, even the relatively complex neuropsychological paradigms designed to assess cognitive dysfunction in nonhuman primates are not sufficiently sensitive for use with human subjects.

In recent years however, several traditional animal experimental tasks have been adapted using advanced computing technology to enable direct comparisons to be made between human and animal studies. For example, the computerized delayed matching to sample procedure described above (Sahakian et al., 1988; Sahgal et al., 1991) was derived directly from an existing paradigm originally designed to define the neural substrates of visual memory in monkeys (Sahgal and Iverson, 1978; Mishkin, 1982). Recent animal studies have established that performance on this test is critically dependent on cortical structures deep within the temporal lobes rather than on the limbic structures as originally thought (Squire and Zola-Morgan, 1991; Gaffan, 1992).

These findings confirm that the severe deficit in delayed matching to sample performance observed in patients with DAT reflects dysfunction of temporal lobe structures and is again consistent with the neuropathological and neurochemical changes seen in this condition (Tomlinson, 1984).

A computerized test based indirectly on Olton's radial arm maze (Olton, 1982), which has been used extensively in animal neuropsychology, has also been developed to assess spatial working memory performance in human patients (Morris et al., 1988; Owen et al., 1990). In the human version of the task, subjects are required to 'search through' a number of coloured boxes on the screen to find blue 'tokens', whilst avoiding those boxes in which a token has already been found. Importantly, subjects can search through the boxes in any order they wish although the number of boxes visited before a token is found is determined (unknown to the subject) by the computer. Thus, each subject receives the same degree of feedback prior to making an error.

Significant deficits on this task have been observed in both mildly and moderately demented DAT patients although the two groups were not differentially impaired (Sahgal *et al.*, 1992). Using analogous tasks in animal lesion studies, spatial working memory has been shown to depend crucially on both hippocampal (Olton, 1982) and frontal (Passingham, 1985) structures.

Comparative assessment of cognitive dysfunction in dementia and patients with localized neurosurgical excisions

The neuroanatomical basis of cognitive dysfunction in dementia may also be investigated by comparison with groups of nondemented patients with well-defined, neurosurgical excisions. In this regard, computer-controlled tests are particularly well suited since task difficulty may be systematically varied to allow direct comparisons to be made between high functioning controls, patients with selective impairments of specific abilities and patients with more global deficits in cognition.

For example, the self-ordered searching task described above has previously been used to explore the neuroanatomical substrates of spatial working memory in human neurosurgical patients (Owen *et al.*, 1990). Like patients with DAT, a group of frontal lobe patients was significantly impaired on this test in terms of the number of search errors. However, the frontal lobe patients were shown to be less efficient in the use of a strategy known to improve performance, suggesting that at least some of their impairment in spatial working memory arises secondarily from a more fundamental deficit in the use of organizational strategies. A similar pattern of impairment on this task has recently been reported in a group of patients with alcoholic Korsakoff syndrome (Joyce and Robbins, 1991). In contrast to both groups, patients with DAT are not impaired in terms of their strategy for approaching this task suggesting that their impairment represents a purer memory deficit. This may reflect the involvement of hippocampal (cf. Olton, 1982) rather than frontal lobe (cf. Passingham, 1985) structures.

In a similar way, a modified (but formally similar) version of the computerized delayed matching to sample procedure described above (see Fig. 5.1) has recently been used to compare visual short-term memory performance in patients with localized excisions of the frontal lobes, patients with temporal lobe excisions and patients who had undergone unilateral amygdalo hippocampectomy (Owen *et al.*, unpublished observations). Whilst frontal lobe patients were unimpaired on this task, significant deficits in the delayed but not simultaneous condition were observed in both groups of patients with more posterior lesions, a pattern similar to that previously observed in patients with DAT (Sahakian *et al.*, 1988; Sahgal *et al.*, 1991). This study supports the results of animal lesion studies discussed above (Squire and Zola-Morgan, 1991; Gaffan, 1992) suggesting again that short-term visual memory impairment in patients with DAT reflects dysfunction of temporal lobe structures.

Summary
In recent years, computerized methods of cognitive assessment have been successfully applied in a number of clinical and experimental areas. In dementia, specific patterns of memory impairment have been identified even early in the course of the disease which are clearly distinct from those observed

in related neuropsychiatric populations. Computerized tests have also been employed in both longitudinal and cross-sectional studies of dementia to redefine the characteristic decline in intellectual functioning in terms of the precise cognitive process involved. Recent research has also suggested that in DAT and other neurodegenerative conditions such as PD, the neuropsychological sequelae of pharmacological intervention may be closely monitored using computerized tests of cognitive function. The success of this approach has obvious implications for the assessment of potential treatment strategies in dementia and related disorders.

A number of different approaches have also been used to demonstrate how computerized neuropsychological methods may be important in increasing our understanding of the specific neural and neurochemical basis of cognitive dysfunction in dementia. Comparisons between groups of patients with dementia and related neurodegenerative conditions and nondemented groups of patients with well-defined, neurosurgical excisions have proved to be particularly useful in this regard. Recent imaging studies have also suggested that in future the neural substrates responsible for specific neuropsychological deficits in dementia might be more clearly defined by combining advanced computerized assessment of cognitive function with both dynamic (SPET, PET) and structural (CT, MRI) imaging techniques.

The results of all of these studies suggest that computerized assessment may have an important role to play in many areas of neuropsychological assessment. In particular, computerized tests appear to be most useful where small changes are espected which may not be detected using more conventional 'paper and pencil' tests. However, it is important to emphasize that few direct comparisons have been made between these novel, computerized techniques and the more traditional methods of assessment. Such comparisons may be essential before the future role of computerized assessment of cognitive function in dementia and ageing can be fully evaluated.

AN ILLUSTRATIVE EXAMPLE: COMPUTERIZED ASSESSMENT OF SET-SHIFTING ABILITY

In the previous sections of this chapter the benefits of computerized neuropsychological tests have been described together with a number of studies that have exploited this advanced technology.

In order to illustrate how these advantages might be applied to a specific neuropsychological question, one particular test designed to assess attentional set-shifting ability will now be described in detail. The task, from the CANTAB attention battery, has recently been used to assess set-shifting impairments in patients with dementia, and to draw comparisons between patients with related neurodegenerative conditions, patients with localized neurosurgical excisions and monkeys with specific neurochemical lesions.

Test rationale and design
Clinically, 'frontal lobe dysfunction' is often assessed using tests assumed to depend on set-shifting ability such as the Wisconsin Card Sorting Test. (WCST; Grant and Berg, 1948; Milner, 1964; Nelson, 1976). Deficits on the this test have also been reported in a number of neurodegenerative diseases including PD (Lees and Smith, 1983), progressive supranuclear palsy (PSP; Pillon et al., 1986) and Huntington's disease (Josiassen et al., 1983). In DAT, significant deficits have not been reported for the WCST (Pillon et al., 1986) although an

impairment has been observed in a related test of tactile reversal learning (Freedman and Oscar-Bermann, 1987).

However, in addition to set shifting, successful performance on the WCST requires a number of other distinct cognitive abilities including matching to sample and the identification of stimulus attributes. These factors may not depend on frontal lobe mechanisms and may independently contribute to some of the deficits described. Thus, across these patient groups, similar impairments may actually reflect deficits in quite different cognitive mechanisms.

Several computerized analogues of the WCST have also been produced (e.g. Acker and Acker, 1982), although in general, these suffer from the same drawbacks as the standard form of the test. Accordingly, a 'purer' computerized test of attentional set shifting has recently been developed that can be related to the WCST but which is derived from the animal learning literature and is based on the concepts of 'intradimensional' and 'extradimensional' shifts. An intradimensional shift (IDS) occurs when a subject is required to cease responding to one member of a particular stimulus dimension (e.g. 'blue' from the dimension 'colour') and begin responding to a new member of that same dimension (e.g. 'red'). An extradimensional shift (EDS) occurs when the subject is required to switch responding to a novel member of a previously irrelevant dimension (e.g. to 'squares' from the dimension 'shape').

The computerized attentional set-shifting test was specifically designed to improve the comparative assessment of cognition from animals to humans. Therefore, formally identical versions have been developed for use with human subjects and experimentally lesioned monkeys (Roberts *et al.*, 1987). The test was designed and programmed to run on an Acorn BBC Master microcomputer and more recently on an IBM personal computer. In both cases, the programs employ high-resolution colour graphics and responses are made via a touch sensitive screen.

Test description
The subject is required to learn a series of discriminations in which one of two stimuli are correct and the other is not, using feedback provided automatically by the computer. The test is composed of nine stages presented in the same fixed order, beginning with a simple discrimination (SD) and reversal (SDR) for stimuli varying in only one dimension (i.e. two white line configurations). In Fig. 5.2, example stimuli from various stages of the test are presented. A second, alternative dimension is then introduced (purple-filled shapes) and compound discrimination (CD) and reversal (CDR) are tested (Fig. 5.2). To succeed, subjects must continue to respond to the previously relevant stimuli (white lines), ignoring the presence of the new, irrelevant dimension (shapes). At the intradimensional shift (IDS) stage new exemplars are introduced from each of the two dimensions (new lines and new shapes) and subjects are required to transfer the previously learnt rule to a novel set of exemplars of the same stimulus dimension. To succeed, they must continue to respond to one of the two exemplars from the relevant dimension (lines). Following another reversal of contingencies (IDR) the extradimensional shift (EDS) and reversal (EDR) occurs and again novel exemplars from each of the two dimensions are introduced. The subject is required to shift 'response set' to the alternative (previously irrelevant) stimulus dimensions (see Fig. 5.2).

At each stage a change in contingencies occurs once the subject has learnt the current rule to a criterion of six consecutive correct responses. Failure to achieve this criterion within 50 trials results in the premature discontinuation of the test.

Simple discrimination and reversal (initial dimension, white lines)

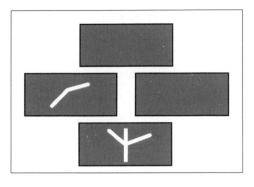 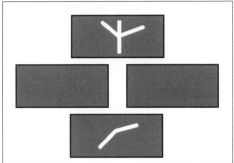

Compound discrimination and reversal (introduce second dimension, filled shapes)

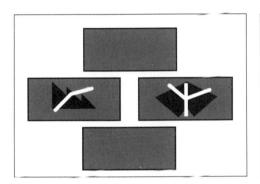 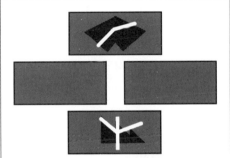

Intra-dimensional or Extra-dimensional shift and reversal (new lines and shapes)

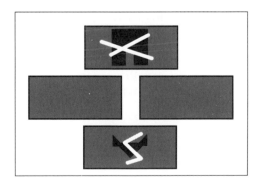 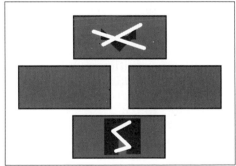

Fig. 5.2 Example stimuli from various stages of the intradimensional and extradimensional set-shifting task. The white line and purple-filled stimuli (shown here in black and white) are presented exactly as they appear on the screen and at each stage, two *typical* trials are given (left box = trial 1, right box = trial 2).

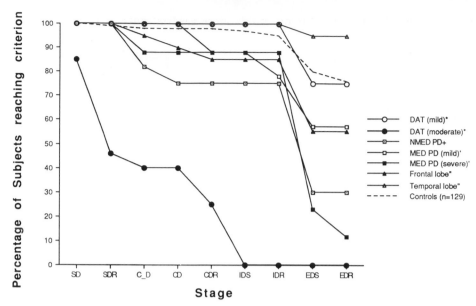

Fig. 5.3 The proportion of subjects reaching criterion at each of the nine stages of the discrimination learning paradigm. *Sahakian *et al.* (1990). +Downes *et al.* (1989). 'Owen *et al.* (1992). "Owen *et al.* (1991). DAT = dementia of Alzheimer type. NMED = non-medicated Parkinson's disease. MEDPD = medicated Parkinson's disease. SD = simple discrimination. SDR = SD reversal. CD = compound discrimination. CDR = CD reversal. IDS = intradimensional shift. IDR = IDS reversal. EDS = extradimensional shift. EDR = EDS reversal.

Comparative studies of dementia of the Alzheimer type, Parkinson's disease and normal ageing
This paradigm has now been used to compare shifting ability directly in patients suffering from neurodegenerative disorders including DAT, PD, PSP and MSA as well as neurosurgical patients with localized excisions of the frontal and temporal lobes.

The combined results of these investigations have shown that impairments on this computerized set-shifting task are both psychologically and pathologically specific (see Fig. 5.3). For example, both medicated and particularly nonmedicated patients with PD are selectively impaired in their ability to perform an extradimensional shift but not an intradimensional shift (Downes *et al.*, 1989). In addition, whilst medicated patients with PD are specifically impaired at the EDS stage of the test, compared to age-matched controls, this deficit is somewhat worse in patients with very severe clinical symptons (Owen *et al.*, 1992).

In contrast, a subgroup of elderly patients in the mild stages of DAT are not impaired on this test of visual discrimination learning despite having significant deficits in short-term visual recognition memory (Sahakian *et al.*, 1990). However, compared to age-matched controls, patients with more severe DAT (unlike severe PD patients) are impaired *throughout* the test, even at the simplest reversal stage. This may reflect a more global deterioration of cognition in this group.

Thus the psychological specificity of the set-shifting deficit is shown by the patients with PD who are selectively impaired on the EDS but not the IDS stage of the test. The neural specificity is shown by the fact that mild DAT patients are far better than even the nonmedicated PD patients with mild clinical symptoms.

The EDS stage of this test is also sensitive to the effects of normal ageing. In a recent study, a group of healthy control subjects of 70+ years with no known neurological condition were significantly impaired at the EDS stage of the test when compared to younger, IQ-matched controls (Owen et al., 1991).

Clearly, in assessing set-shifting ability, this computerized paradigm can distinguish between the patterns of impairment observed in specific neurological populations as well as reliably differentiate between groups of patients at different stages of the disease process.

Comparisons with neurosurgical populations

Comparative studies of neurosurgical patients with localized neurosurgical excisions suggests that impairments at the EDS stage of this test may be related to a disruption of frontal lobe function. Whilst patients who have undergone unilateral temporal lobe resection or unilateral amygdalo hippocampectomy reach criterion at every stage of the test, patients with excisions restricted to the frontal lobes are specifically impaired at the EDS (Owen et al., 1991). This suggests that whilst the severe deficits exhibited by patients late in the course of DAT may reflect a global deterioration of cognition, the specific EDS impairment observed in patients with medicated and nonmedicated PD may follow disruption of frontal or frontostriatal mechanisms.

Lesion studies with nonhuman primates

In order to investigate the neuropathological substrates of the set-shifting impairments described above, comparative studies are also being conducted in nonhuman primates, with selective lesions of defined neurochemical systems. Since this computerized test of set-shifting ability employs nonverbal stimuli and requires nonverbal responses, only slight modifications to the basic design were necessary to make the test suitable for primate studies.

Experimental marmosets with damage to the cholinergic projection to frontal cortex, similar in extent to that seen in PD, are unimpaired on this task (Roberts et al., 1992). In contrast, attentional set-shifting ability is altered following damage to the dopaminergic projection to the frontal cortex (Roberts et al., 1991). This suggests that in PD at least, the deficits in set-shifting ability seen early in the course of the disease may reflect disruption of dopaminergic rather than cholinergic neurotransmitter systems.

The studies described above illustrate how carefully designed computerized tests can be used to establish the neural and neurochemical causes of specific neuropsychological impairments in human patient populations. In this case, a test of attentional set-shifting ability has been used to distinguish groups of patients with different, though related, neurodegenerative conditions and to differentiate between patients at different stages of the disease process. In addition, comparative studies with human neurosurgical patients and primates with selective neurochemical lesions can help to address the question of whether specific neuronal changes are causal to or correlates of these cognitive deficits.

CONCLUSIONS

This chapter has described how recent developments in computing technology can be exploited for the neuropsychological assessment of cognitive function in ageing and dementia. The advantages of computer-based systems over more traditional methods of neuropsychological assessment have been described in the context of several recent studies that have adopted this technology. The sensitivity of computerized tests to cognitive changes during the course of dementia and other neurodegenerative disease and to the effects of pharmacological intervention has been discussed. In addition, a role for computerized neuropsychological testing in other rapidly advancing fields of technology such as neuroimaging has been suggested. A number of comparative human and animal studies which have used analogous computerized tests have also been described. Such comparisons are helping to define the specificity of cognitive impairments in dementia and other neuropsychiatric conditions and the underlying neural substrates responsible.

In future, parallel computerized tests in comparative neuropsychology may guide the direction of research into appropriate treatments for the alleviation of various neurological conditions including dementia and, in addition, may have some diagnostic value. For example, they may provide a means of assessing the probable loci of neuropathology in the early stages of a neurodegenerative disease when other methods are unavailable or insufficiently sensitive to do so.

REFERENCES

Abas, M.A., Sahakian, B.J. and Levy, R. (1990). Neuropsychological deficits and CT scan changes in elderly depressives. *Psychological Medicine*, **20**, 507–20.

Acker, W. and Acker, C.F. (1982). *Bexley–Maudsley Automated Psychological Screening*. NFER-Nelson Publishing Company, London.

Baddley, A.D., Bressi, S., Logie, R. *et al.* (1986). Dementia in working memory. *Quarterly Journal of Experimental Psychology*, **38a**, 603–18.

Carr, A.C., Woods, R.T. and Moore, B.J. (1986). Automated cognitive assessment of elderly patients: a comparison of two types of response device. *British Journal of Clinical Psychology*, **25**, 305–6.

Downes, J.J., Roberts, A.C., Sahakian, B.J. *et al.* (1989). Impaired extra-dimensional shift performance in medicated and unmedicated Parkinson's disease: evidence for a specific attentional dysfunction. *Neuropsychologia*, **27**, 1329–43.

Eagger, S.A., Levy, R. and Sahakian, B.J. (1991a). Tacrine in Alzheimer's disease. *Lancet*, **337**, 989–92.

Eagger, S.A., Morant, N.J. and Levy, L. (1991b). Parallel group analysis of the effects of Tacrine versus placebo in Alzheimer's disease. *Dementia*, **2**, 207–11.

Folstein, M.F., Folstein, S.E. and McHugh, P.R. (1975). 'Mini-Mental State': A practical method for grading the cognitive state of patients for the clinician. *Journal of Psychiatric Research*, **12**, 189–98.

Freedman, M. and Oscar-Bermann, M. (1987). Tactile discrimination learning deficits in Alzheimer's and Parkinson's disease. *Archives of Neurology*, **44**, 394–8.

Gaffan, D. (1992). The role of the hippocampus-fornix-mammillary system in episodic memory. In *Neuropsychology of Memory*, pp. 336–85, Squire, L.R. and Butters, N. (Eds). Guildford Press, New York.

Grant, D.A. and Berg, E.A. (1948). A behavioural analysis of degree of reinforcement and ease of shifting to new responses in a Weigl-type card sorting problem. *Journal of Experimental Psychology*, **38**, 404–11.

Hodkinson, H.M. (1972). Evaluation of a mental test score for the assessment of mental impairment in the elderly. *Age and Ageing*, **1**, 233–9.

Jacoby, R.J. and Levy, R. (1980). Computed tomography in the elderly: 3. Affective disorder. *British Journal of Psychiatry*, **136**, 270–5.

Josiassen, R.C., Curry, L.M. and Mancall, E.L. (1983). Development of neuropsychological deficits in Huntington's disease. *Archives of Neurology*, **40**, 791–6.

Joyce, E.M. and Robbins, T.W. (1991). Frontal lobe function in Korsakoff and non-Korsakoff alcoholics: Planning and spatial working memory. *Neuropsychologia*, **29**, 709–23.

Kendrick, D.C. (1985). *Kendrick Cognitive Tests For The Elderly*. NFER-Nelson Publishing Company Ltd, Windsor.

Lange, K.W., Robbins, T.W., Marsden, C.D. *et al.* (1992). L-Dopa withdrawal in Parkinson's disease selectively impairs cognitive performance in tests sensitive to frontal lobe dysfunction. *Psychopharmacology*, **107**, 394–404.

Lees, A.J. and Smith, E. (1983). Cognitive deficits in the early stages of Parkinson's disease. *Brain*, **106**, 257–70.

Milner, B. (1964). Some effects of frontal lobectomy in man. In *The Frontal Granular Cortex and Behaviour*, Warren, J.M. and Akert, K. (Eds), pp. 313–31. McGraw-Hill, New York.

Mishkin, M. (1982). A memory system in the monkey. *Philosophical Transactions of the Royal Society of London B*, **298**, 85–95.

Morris, R.G. (1986). Short term forgetting in senile dementia of the Alzheimer type. *Cognitive Neuropsychology*, **3**, 77–97.

Morris, R.G., Downes, J.J., Evenden, J.L. *et al.* (1988). Planning and spatial working memory in Parkinson's disease. *Journal of Neurology, Neurosurgery and Psychiatry*, **51**, 757–66.

Morris, R.G., Evenden, J.L., Sahakian, B.J. and Robbins, T.W. (1987). Computer aided assessment of dementia: comparative studies of neuropsychological deficits in Alzheimer type dementia and Parkinson's disease. In *Cognitive Neurochemistry*, Stahl, S.M., Iverson, S.D. and Goodman, E.C. (Eds). Oxford University Press, Oxford.

Nelson, H.E. (1976). A modified card sorting test sensitive to frontal lobe defects. *Cortex*, **12**, 313–24.

O'Brien, J.T., Eagger, S.A., Syed, G.M.S. *et al.* (1992). A study of cerebral blood flow and cognitive performance in Alzheimer's disease. *Journal of Neurology, Neurosurgery and Psychiatry*, **55**, 1182–7.

Olton, D.S. (1982). Spatially organised behaviours of animals. In *Spatial Abilities*, Potegal, M. (Ed.). Pergamon, London.

Owen, A.M., Downes, J.D., Sahakian, B.J. *et al.* (1990). Planning and spatial working memory following frontal lobe lesions in man. *Neuropsychologia*, **28**, 1021–34.

Owen, A.M., James, M., Leigh, P.N. *et al.* (1992). Fronto-striatal cognitive deficits at different stages of Parkinson's disease. *Brain*, **115**, 1727–51.

Owen, A.M., Roberts, A.C., Polkey, C.E. *et al.* (1991). Extra-dimensional versus intra-dimensional set shifting performance following frontal lobe excisions, temporal lobe excisions of amygdalohippocampectomy in man. *Neuropsychologia*, **29**, 993–1006.

Passingham, R.E. (1985). Memory of monkeys (Macaca Mulatta) with lesions in prefrontal cortex. *Behavioural Neurology*, **99**, 3–21.

Pillon, B., Dubois, B., Lhermitte, F. and Agid, Y. (1986). Heterogeneity of cognitive impairment in progressive supranuclear palsy, Parkinson's disease and Alzheimer's disease. *Neurology*, **36**, 1179–85.

Roberts, A.C., Robbins, T.W. and Everitt, B.J. (1987). The effects of intra-dimensional and extra-dimensional shifts on visual discrimination learning in humans and non-human primates. *Quarterly Journal of Experimental Psychology*, **40B**, 321–41.

Roberts, A.C., Robbins, T.W., Everitt, B.J. and Muir, J.L. (1990). A specific form of cognitive rigidity following excitotoxic lesions in the basal forebrain in marmosets. *Neuroscience*, **47**, 251–64.

Roberts, A.C., De Salvia, M., Muir, J.L. *et al.* (1991). The effects of selective prefrontal dopamine lesions on cognitive tests of frontal function in primates. *Society for Neuroscience Abstracts*, **17**, 501.

Robbins, T.W., James, M., Lange, K.W. *et al.* (1992). Cognitive performance in multiple system atrophy. *Brain*, **115**, 271–91.

Roth, M., Tym, E., Mountjoy, C. *et al.* (1986). CAMDEX: a standardised instrument for the diagnosis of mental disorder in the elderly with special reference to the early detection of dementia. *British Journal of Psychiatry*, **149**, 698–709.

Sahakian, B.J., Downes, J.J., Eagger, S. *et al.* (1990). Sparing of attentional relative to mnemonic function in a subgroup of patients with dementia of the Alzheimer type. *Neuropsychologia*, **28**, 1197–213.

Sahakian, B.J., Jones, G., Levy, R. *et al.* (1989). The effects of nicotine on attention, information processing, and short-term memory in patients with dementia of the Alzheimer type. *British Journal of Psychiatry*, **154**, 797–800.

Sahakian, B.J., Levy, R.L. and Eagger, S.A. (1991). The effect of tetrahydroaminoacridine on attention and memory in Alzheimer's disease. *Society for Neuroscience Abstracts*, **17**, 423.25, p. 1074.

Sahakian, B.J., Morris, R.G., Evenden, J.L. *et al.* (1988). A comparative study of visuospatial memory and learning in Alzheimer-type dementia and Parkinson's disease. *Brain*, **111**, 695–718.

Sahgal, A. and Iverson, S.D. (1978). Categorization and retrieval after selective inferotemporal lesion in monkeys. *Brain Research*, **146**, 341–50.

Sahgal, A., Lloyd, S., Wray, C.J. *et al.* (1992). Does visuospatial memory in Alzheimer's disease depend on severity of the disorder? *International Journal of Geriatric Psychiatry*, **7**, 427–36.

Sahgal, A., Sahakian, B.J., Robbins, T.W. *et al.* (1991). Detection of visual memory and learning deficits in Alzheimer's disease using the Cambridge Neuropsychological Test Automated Battery. *Dementia*, **2**, 150–8.

Squire, L.R. and Zola-Morgan, S. (1991). The medial temporal lobe system. *Science*, **253**, 1380–6.

Tomlinson, B.E. (1984). The pathology of Alzheimer's disease and senile dementia of Alzheimer type. In *Handbook of Studies on Psychiatry and Old Age*, Kay, D.W.K. and Burrows, G. (Eds), pp. 89–117. Elsevier, Amsterdam.

Mony J. de Leon

Department of Psychiatry
New York University Medical Center

6 HIPPOCAMPAL FORMATION ATROPHY IN AGEING AND THE PREDICTION OF ALZHEIMER'S DISEASE

INTRODUCTION

Studies of animals and humans have revealed numerous behavioural changes indicative of age-related brain dysfunction. Foremost among the behavioural changes are declines in memory functioning. While animal studies have specifically linked many of these ageing changes to hippocampal alterations, very little direct evidence is available for the human (Zola-Morgan *et al.*, 1986).

Hippocampal pathology in Alzheimer's disease

In Alzheimer's disease (AD) many age-related behavioural changes are markedly exacerbated and there is clear evidence for extensive neuropathological involvement of the hippocampus. However, in AD many other brain regions also show pathological changes and therefore, until recently, the role of hippocampal changes had not been defined.

Alzheimer's disease has been characterized as 'a hippocampal dementia' (Ball *et al.*, 1985). There are many structural hippocampal abnormalities documented in AD. They include neuronal loss, granulovacuolar degeneration, neurofibrillary tangles and neuritic plaques (Kemper, 1984). The important observation of extensive pathology in the hippocampal formation in AD (Hyman *et al.*, 1984) and the documentation of early cases in which histopathological markers of AD are restricted to the hippocampus and the parahippocampal gyrus (Price *et al.*, 1991) have directed researchers towards examining these structures as the site of the earliest neurodegenerative changes associated with AD.

The typical pattern of neuropathological degeneration documented in AD is consistent with the connectivity of the pathways linking the hippocampal

This chapter was co-authored by: J. Golomb, A.E. George, A. Convit, H. Rusinek, J. Morys, M. Bobinski, S. De Santi, C. Tarshish, O. Narkiewicz and H. Wisnicwski from the Departments of Psychiatry, Neurology and Radiology New York University Medical Centre, New York, New York, Nathan S. Kline, Psychiatric Research Centre, Orangesburg, New York and The Institute for Basic Research, Staten Island, New York. This work was made possible with grants from the National Institute on Aging Alzheimer Disease Core Centre, Grants P30 AG08051 and PO1 AG04220; National Institute of Mental Health RO1 43965; New York State Office Of Mental Retardation and Developmental Disabilities; the Orentreich Foundation for the Advancement of Science and Betty Wold Johnson. I am especially indebted to Mr Ken Anderson's excellent technical support with the MRI scanning and the photographic contributions of Ms Martha Helmers and Mr Anthony Jalondoni.

formation and amygdala to the neocortex and also correlates with the neuro-psychological impairments observed. The pyramidal cells of the entorhinal cortex are severely and consistently involved. These are the neurons of the perforant pathway, which possess reciprocal connections with the cortical association areas and project to the hippocampal formation (Hyman *et al.*, 1984, 1987; Van Hoesen *et al.*, 1991). In AD these sites are notable for their excessive deposition of neurofibrillary tangles and senile plaques. More specifically, the major output regions from the hippocampus, the subiculum and the CA1, are sites of perhaps the most extensive pathology. The observed pattern of degeneration results in the 'isolation' of the hippocampal formation from the neocortical association areas (Hyman *et al.*, 1984).

In some normal ageing cases, AD-type histopathologic changes limited to the hippocampus have been observed. From the seventh to the tenth decades, age-related hippocampal neuronal loss, neurofibrillary tangles, granulovacuo-lar degeneration and senile plaques have been documented (Ball, 1978; Terry *et al.*, 1981; Kemper, 1984; Hyman and Van Hoesen, 1988). De la Monte (1989) reported that hippocampi (cornu ammonis) both from AD patients and clinical-ly normal elderly with neuropathological evidence of AD showed volume reductions from 'pure' elderly control values (no histologic evidence for AD). Neocortical changes were found only in the demented AD group, suggesting the primacy of the hippocampal changes. Similarly, Price *et al.* (1991) found, in minimally impaired elderly, evidence for the neuropathologic changes of AD to be restricted to the medial temporal lobe. In addition, some younger Down's syndrome patients show AD pathology restricted to hippocampus, amygdala and entorhinal cortex (Mann and Esiri, 1988). It is unknown how prevalent the hippocampal formation changes are in ageing populations or if these brain changes are related to the mild memory impairments so often reported in clinical studies of nondemented elderly. It is also unknown if long-lived normal elderly individuals with AD-like hippocampal changes will develop neocortical changes and AD-like clinical symptoms.

The severity of hippocampal pathology in AD and the observation of pathology limited to the hippocampal formation in early AD cases, Down's syndrome and elderly normals indicates that the hippocampal formation may be among the earliest regions involved in AD. However, given that the majority of AD patients survive until the latter stages of the illness, when there are diffuse degenerative changes, the location of the early changes in AD cannot be ascertained with confidence at *post-mortem* examination. Therefore, the iden-tification of the early sites of brain involvement in AD and in individuals 'at risk' for AD is dependent upon the application of *in vivo* neuroimaging studies.

A study population of critical research importance is, in our view, the minimally impaired elderly. In clinical practice, the minimally impaired show some objective evidence of cognitive deficits but they cannot be classified as demented or given a diagnosis of probable AD. We have defined this group as having Mini-Mental State Examination scores (MMSE) OF >23 (Folstein *et al.*, 1975) and Global Deterioration Scores (GDS) of <4 (Reisberg *et al.*, 1982). Other groups have characterized the degree of cognitive impairment of this group and their likelihood of dementia as 'very mild', 'borderline', 'questionable', 'mini-mally impaired' and 'incipient' (Hughes *et al.*, 1982; Reisberg *et al.*, 1982; Rubin *et al.*, 1989).

Only a few *in vivo* neuroimaging studies of the hippocampus have been reported in the AD literature. For the most part, these magnetic resonance imaging (MRI) studies have described volume losses in the AD hippocampus relative to controls (Seab *et al.*, 1988; Kesslak *et al.*, 1991; Jack *et al.*, 1992). At present, only our group (de Leon *et al.*, 1989; George *et al.*, 1990; de Leon *et al.*, 1993) has demonstrated, in cross-sectional and longitudinal studies, the early hippocampal changes in AD and the use of this measure to predict future dementia from minimally impaired elderly accurately. It is the goal of this paper to provide further evidence for early hippocampal involvement in the natural history of AD.

Neuropsychology

Minimally impaired subject (GDS = 3), as a group, exhibit a neuropsychological profile that is clearly discriminable from that of the unimpaired elderly. Mild cognitive deficits have been reliably demonstrated on tests of recent memory, remote memory, language function, concept formation and visuospatial praxis (Storandt and Hill, 1989; Flicker *et al.*, 1991). The word-finding difficulty observed in these subjects, on tests of confrontation, naming for example, is particularly notable in that normal ageing is not usually associated with a decline in language abilities (Flicker *et al.*, 1987). However, most of their other language abilities are intact, and they commonly perform as well as the normal elderly on tests of visuoperceptual function, immediate memory and psychomotor speed (Storandt and Hill, 1989; Flicker *et al.*, 1991).

In a 3-year longitudinal study with a group of 32 minimally impaired (GDS = 3) elderly subjects, tests of verbal, visuospatial recall and language were the best predictors of decline to AD levels of performance (Flicker *et al.*, 1991). This is consistent with previous observations that recent memory impairment is the most reliable clinical symptom of AD (Sim and Sussman, 1962; Neary *et al.*, 1986). The language tasks were particularly useful in distinguishing nondeclining from declining patients (Flicker *et al.*, 1991). The results showed that some nondecliners presented with memory deficits, but the minimally impaired subjects who also had language impairments were accurately predicted to deteriorate.

TRANSVERSE FISSURE ANATOMY

In a series of computed tomographic (CT) and MRI studies we have described that enlargement of the cerebrospinal fluid (CSF) spaces in the perihippocampal region are indicative of atrophy and volume losses in the hippocampus and the parahippocampal gyrus. The precise anatomical location of these CSF changes involves the transverse fissure of Bichat and its related extensions: the choroidal and hippocampal recesses or fissures. The transverse fissure curves around the thalamus and in its lateral aspect separates the thalamus from the parahippocampal gyrus (Duvernoy, 1988). On the horizontal or axial view, the transverse fissure is bordered anteriorly by the uncus (see Fig. 6.1). The lateral boundary is the dentate gyrus and the fimbria and medially it communicates with the ambient cistern and cerebral peduncles. The coronal view best permits separation of the choroidal and hippocampal fissure extensions of the transverse fissure (see Fig. 6.2). Both the coronal and sagittal planes of section permit identification of the ventral surface of the transverse fissure (the parahippocampal gyrus, i.e. subiculum), as well as the identification of thalamic structures on the dorsal surface (the lateral geniculate and the pulvinar, see Fig. 6.3).

Due to partial volume averaging, in the axial view the choroidal and hippocampal fissures cannot be easily distinguished from the larger CSF pool. However, the partial volume averaging may actually increase the viewer's

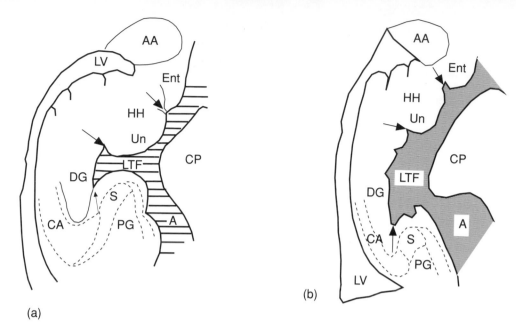

Fig. 6.1 Schematic representation of the axial view of the perihippocampal region. (a) Normal anatomy. (b) Typical changes caused by Alzheimer's disease. LTF = lateral transverse fissure. CR = choroid fissure recess. HR = hippocampal sulcus recess. LV = lateral ventricle. CA = cornu ammonis. PG = parahippocampal gyrus. A = ambient cistern. AA = amygdaloid body. CP = cerebral peduncle. DG = dentate gyrus. Ent = entorhinal cortex. HH = head of hippocampus. S = subiculum. PS = presubiculum. Un = uncus. TC = tela choroidea. Fi = fimbria. LGB = lateral geniculate body. Pul = pulvinar.

sensitivity to slight increases in fissure size. In our previous axial studies, we have referred to this region as the choroidal–hippocampal fissure complex.

Our results, reported below, document: a large cross-sectional and longitudinal axial plane study, coronal MRI validations and anatomical studies. The *in vivo* studies with the axial protocol are designed to cut parallel to the anterior–posterior plane of the hippocampus in order to reveal any enlargement of the transverse fissure and the choroidal–hippocampal fissure complex. A major objective of these studies is to examine the hypothesis that changes in the region of the hippocampus occur relatively early in the natural history of AD and may be of predictive significance. Data supporting this hypothesis will be presented that will contribute to the understanding of the early stages of AD and of the normal ageing process. *In vivo* and *post-mortem* validation studies have established relationships between changes in the fissures and volume losses in the hippocampus and parahippocampal gyrus. Moreover, evidence has been found for the anatomic specificity of the hippocampal formation changes in the minimally impaired.

Cross-sectional hippocampal studies, *n* = 405
Imaging the long axis of the hippocampus, as is done in our modified axial

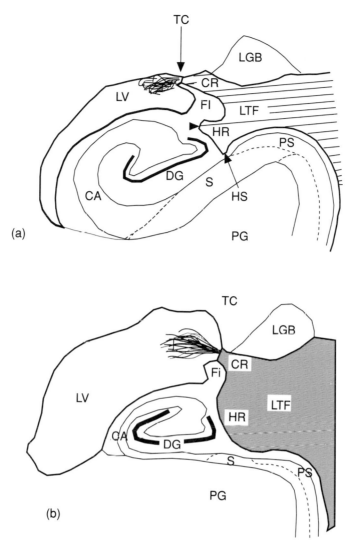

Fig. 6.2 Schematic representation of the coronal view of the perihippocampal region. (a) Normal anatomy. (b) Typical changes caused by Alzheimer's disease. See Fig. 6.1 for abbreviations.

study (See Fig 6.4), makes it possible to evaluate as a single CSF space the dilatation of the transverse fissure and the associated choroidal–hippocampal fissure complex (see Fig. 6.1). Images taken in this plane allow a determination of fissure enlargement to be made from one or two slices. Images not taken in this plane require the reader to integrate the CSF across several slices (see Fig. 6.5).

To estimate the prevalence of hippocampal atrophy (HA) in normal ageing and across severity levels of AD originally the CT scans were examined of a group of 175 AD patients, controls and minimally impaired patients (subjects with mild memory changes but who did not meet criteria for AD; de Leon *et al.*, 1989). This study also included a longitudinal follow-up. The results pointed to the utility of the radiologic examination in evaluating the risk for dementia.

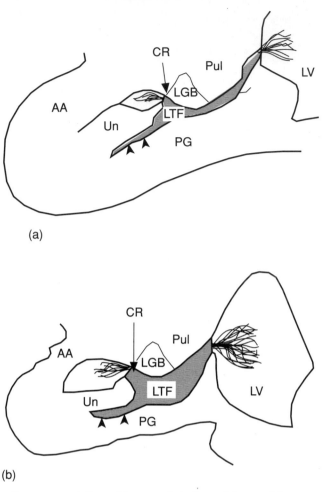

(a)

(b)

Fig. 6.3 Schematic representation of the saggital view of the perihippocampal region. (a) Normal anatomy. (b) Typical changes caused by Alzheimer's disease. See Fig. 6.1 for abbreviations.

Recently, the sample was expanded to include 209 CT studies (GE 9800) and 196 MRI studies (Phillips 1.5T) for a total of 405 patients. As with the earlier study, all patients received an extensive research protocol of medical, neurologic, psychiatric and neuropsychologic examinations. These examinations allowed exclusion from the study of those individuals who showed evidence of changes that could affect brain functioning or structure, other than normal ageing or AD. Subsequently, subjects were divided into four groups. The clinical groups were defined using NINCDS–ADRDA criteria and the GDS. The groups included normal elderly (GDS 1 and 2, $n = 130$), minimal impairment (GDS 3, $n = 72$) mild AD (GDS 4, $n = 73$) and moderate to severe AD (GDS 5 and 6, $n = 130$). For both CT and MRI, all subjects were evaluated using the same subjective assessment scale to rate the extent of HA using the modified axial protocol (see Fig. 6.6). The perihippocampal CSF was separately rated for each study and for each hemisphere using a four-point scale (0 = none, 1 = questionable, 2 = mild and 3 = moderate to severe).

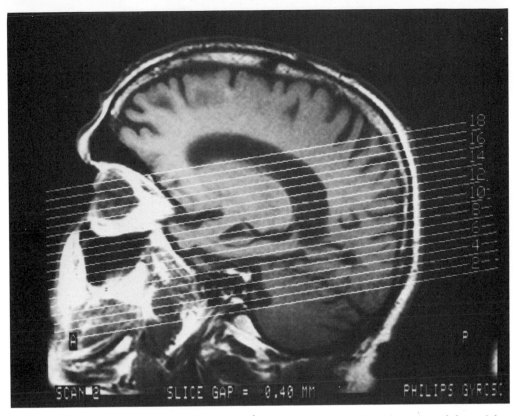

Fig. 6.4 Magnetic resonance images. Sagittal view depicting the orientation of the axial slices. Axial images run parallel to the plane of the hippocampus.

In order to compare the sensitivities of the CT and MRI machines for the clinical detection of HA, a group of 56 individuals who received both CT and MRI studies within a few months ($x = 2.9 \pm 3.0$ months) were compared. Correlation of HA scores between the two machines ranged between $r = 0.87$ for the right hippocampus and $r = 0.89$ for the left hippocampus. Grouping the cases for the presence of HA (score ≥ 2 for either hemisphere) resulted in a high between machine agreement, $\kappa = 0.96$ and $P < 0.0001$. Only 1/56 cases was grouped differently between the CT and MRI machines. Inter-rater reliability was also found to be very high. For a group of 25 CT scans randomly selected from this project, right and left ratings were correlated between two observers at $r = 0.92$ and 0.91, respectively ($P < 0.001$). Grouping the cases for the presence of HA resulted in all cases being correctly classified ($\kappa = 1.0$).

Prior to combining the CT and MRI samples, further analyses were conducted to examine the relationship between type of machine, HA and other clinical variables. An analysis was designed that permitted examination of any machine-related interactions. Using the large cross-sectional samples, ANOVA values were used to examine the effects of machine (CT or MRI) and of HA group on the dependent variables age and cognitive level of functioning (MMSE score). Since the results indicated that the two machine samples were equivalent, the two samples were combined.

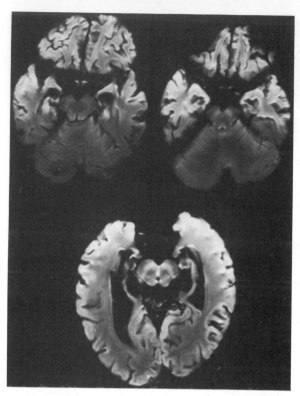

Fig. 6.5 *Post-mortem* magnetic resonance image depicting the hippocampal region. The conventional transaxial canthomeatal plane study is shown in the top two images and the negative angulation from the same patient is below.

For the combined sample, using the HA cut-off rating of ≥ 2 to define the presence of HA, HA was significantly more prevalent in all clinical groups compared with controls. Seventy-eight per cent of the minimally impaired (GDS = 3), 84% of the mild AD (GDS = 4) and 96% of the moderate to severe AD (GDS ≥ 5) groups showed HA. Controls showed HA in 29% of subjects. The prevalence of HA as a function of clinical severity is depicted in Fig. 6.7. Normal controls showed a striking age dependence for HA while the AD groups showed prevalences independent of age (see Fig. 6.8).

Consistent with the neuropathological literature, our normal controls with HA ($n = 37$) were significantly older than those without evidence of atrophy ($n = 93$) [76 ± 6 years versus 70 ± 7 years, $t(128) = 4.9$, $P < 0.001$]. The high prevalence of HA in the patient groups and the relatively low prevalence of HA in controls under the age of 75 years suggest the potential use of this measure as a diagnostic tool. Figure 6.9 graphically depicts the accuracy of the HA measure to differentiate the normal and the AD groups as a function of 5-year age groups. Note the high diagnostic accuracy between the ages of 60 and 75 years. After 75 years of age the accuracy declines for the normals and the utility of the measure is decreased.

The symmetry of the HA was examined in the four study groups. As shown above, with increasing clinical deterioration, there were increased numbers of cases with HA. However, when controlling for the cases with HA, the relationship between unilateral and bilateral changes was found to be proportionately similar across all groups. Approximately one in three cases of HA

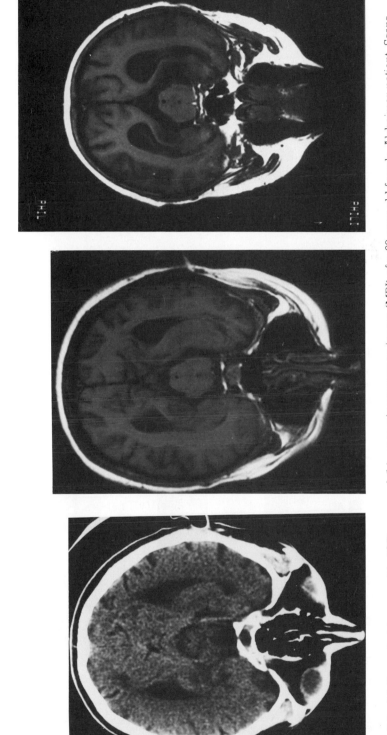
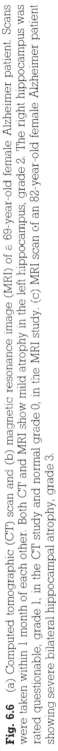

Fig. 6.6 (a) Computed tomographic (CT) scan and (b) magnetic resonance image (MRI) of a 69-year-old female Alzheimer patient. Scans were taken within 1 month of each other. Both CT and MRI show mild atrophy in the left hippocampus, grade 2. The right hippocampus was rated questionable, grade 1, in the CT study and normal grade 0, in the MRI study. (c) MRI scan of an 82-year-old female Alzheimer patient showing severe bilateral hippocampal atrophy, grade 3.

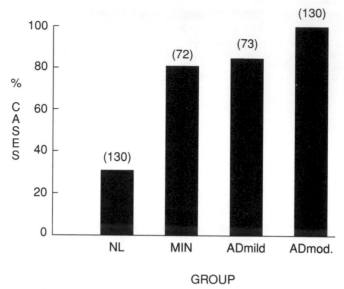

Fig. 6.7 The prevalence of hippocampal atrophy in four groups: normal elderly (NL), minimally impaired elderly (MIN) and Alzheimer patients with two different severity levels of cognitive impairment: ADmild = mild Alzheimer's disease (AD). ADmod. = moderate AD. $n = 405$. Numbers in parentheses = number in study.

were unilateral across groups. Interestingly, for all four of the study groups the left side was most likely to be affected. For each group, when an asymmetry did occur, on approximately 64% of the occasions it was on the left and on 36% occasions on the right side.

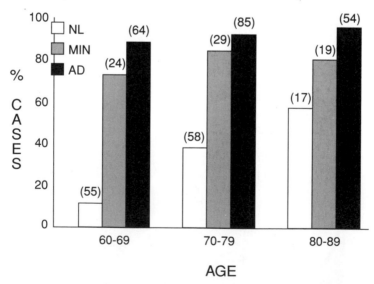

Fig. 6.8 The prevalence of hippocampal atrophy for normal (NL), minimal (MIN) and Alzheimer (AD) groups as a function of age in years. $n = 405$. Numbers in parentheses = number in study.

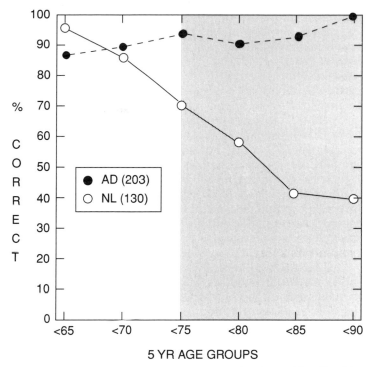

Fig. 6.9 Diagnostic accuracy of the hippocampal evaluation to identify either Alzheimer (AD) patients or normal (NL) controls as a function of 5-year age groups.

Longitudinal studies predicting the development of dementia

The results of our cross-sectional studies suggest that hippocampal changes occur with a high frequency in minimally affected patients and thereby may be predictive of deterioration to symptoms consistent with the course of AD. In order to assess the early diagnostic value of hippocampal changes, de Leon *et al.*, 1993 carried out a 4-year follow-up CT study (*n* = 86) in a normal elderly group (*n* = 54, aged 70 ± 8 s.d. years) and a minimally impaired group (*n* = 32, aged 71 ± 9 s.d. years). A preliminary report of this work based on a smaller sample has been published (de Leon *et al.*, 1989). Over the interval, 23 (72%) of the minimally impaired group and two (4%) of the controls deteriorated to receive the diagnosis of AD (GDS ⩾ 4). Baseline hippocampal ratings ⩾ 2 were present in 91% of the decliners and absent in 89% of the nondecliners. The results also showed that the prediction of decline was not related to age as 31% of the decliners came from the group 75 years of age and greater and 27% came from the group aged 60 to 74 years. Nonsignificant differences were found in the percentages of males and females that declined of 33 and 24% respectively. Both cortical sulcal prominence and ventricular enlargement were related at baseline to the observation of decline. However, compared with the overall prediction accuracies of 88% for HA, these global measures of brain atrophy yielded overall accuracy scores of 70 and 69%, respectively. The relative high accuracies for the prediction of decline in the group showing HA and the high rate of preservation in the group not showing HA suggest the unique potential of this measure as an early and predictive test for AD.

The results of these studies point to the need for the continued longitudinal study of the temporal relation between hippocampal change, neocortical pathology and the development of intellectual dysfunction. Longitudinal study is essential to understand the effects of normal ageing on these measures, to differentiate normal ageing from the early stages of AD and finally to elucidate the progression of AD. As only 2/54 of the normal elderly with HA deteriorated while 6/54 had baseline HA and did not decline, it is felt that the period of observation must be extended beyond the 4 years used in order to evaluate carefully the predictive risk of the hippocampal change and to identify the potentially protective benefit of other factors in describing the risk for cognitive deterioration. It is of great potential interest that data derived from the larger cross-sectional study, shows that normals with HA ($n = 40$), had significantly lower psychometric test performances than normals without HA ($n = 95$) (Golomb *et al.*, 1993). Specifically, differences were found on composite measures of delayed recall derived from eight psychometric tests spanning verbal memory, visuospatial praxis and recall of abstract designs ($t(122) = 2.99$, $P<0.01$). The two groups had identical average MMSE scores of 29.

Magnetic resonance imaging

Using MRI (Phillips 1.5 tesla), the objective was to validate the anatomic and pathologic significance of the observed dilated transverse fissure. In the *first validation* procedure contiguous 4 mm-thick T_1 weighted coronal MRI slices perpendicular to the long axis of the hippocampus were used to determine the volume of CSF in the region of the perihippocampal fissures (see Fig. 6.10). The purpose of this study was to determine the relationship between the subjective estimates of CSF in the perihippocampal fissures, and the actual volume of CSF for the same region. In all studies, the CSF volume was determined from consecutive slices through the length of the hippocampus with the most anterior slice just posterior to the head of the hippocampus. The MRI procedure required drawing a region of interest on an enlarged computer-displayed image and subsequently using an individualized threshold procedure based on pixel intensity to identify the CSF. For all MRI evaluations, estimates of head size (intracranial volumes derived using the inner table as the boundary) were made in order to correct the measures of interest. The results across comparable age groups consisting of 15 AD patients, 17 minimally impaired subjects and 18 controls indicated that CSF volume was significantly associated with the subjective ratings of dilated transverse fissures derived from 4-mm thick (negative angulation) transaxial T_1 studies (Fright [1,48] = 20.8 and Fleft [1,48] = 15.9 with p<0.0001).

In the *second validation study* the above 50 study cases and MRI image data were used to derive the tissue volumes of several structures adjacent to the region of the transverse fissure. This study was designed to assess whether specific parenchymal volume reductions could explain the subjective CSF accumulations. In addition, the hypothesis was investigated that the parenchymal volume reductions like the CSF changes occurred early during the course of AD. The volumes investigated included the hippocampus, the parahippocampal gyrus, and the fusiform gyrus and the perihippocampal CSF.

As shown in Fig. 6.11, the most consistent parenchymal volume losses for the two patient groups compared with controls occur in the hippocampus. Importantly, as compared with controls, the minimally impaired subjects show only significant hippocampal volume reductions that average about 12%. These data, therefore, lend support to the CT and MRI findings of perihippocampal changes appearing consistently and early in the course of AD. With

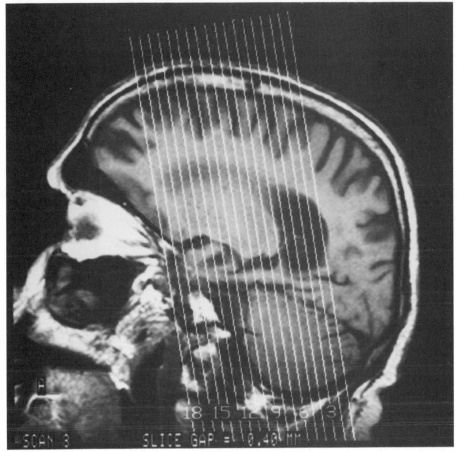

Fig. 6.10 Magnetic resonance images. (a) Sagittal view depicting the orientation of the coronal study. Images are taken perpendicular to the long axis of the hippocampus.

respect to the specificity of early anatomical changes, the hippocampal measures show significant reductions in the minimally impaired group, but this relationship is not found for the parahippocampals and the fusiform gyrus (Convit *et al.*, 1993)

The appearance of the medial temporal lobe on the negative angle axial scan results from the average of the perihippocampal CSF with the hippocampal and the parahippocampal parenchyma. Out of these three volumes, the CSF and the hippocompal volumes were the best combination correctly classifying 80% of the cases by subjective rating of hippocampal atrophy, ($\chi^2 = 23.7$, df = 2, p<0.0001). The parahippocampal volume did not add to the ability to classify the patients by the subjective atrophy assessment.

In the *third validation study*, it was hypothesized that dorsal-ventral dilation of the transverse fissure is largely responsible for its increased volume (Golomb *et al.*, 1992). Consequently, its height was directly measured using a 4× magnified screen projection of the coronal images. Scans from 27 normal elderly controls, 19 minimally impaired subjects, 26 patients with mild and 17 patients with moderate to severe AD were studied. The mean age for the entire sample was 72 years and there were no significant age differences between the

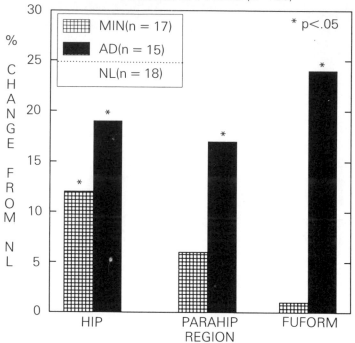

Fig. 6.11 Regional magnetic resonance imaging (MRI) volume changes (%) relative to controls (NL) for the minimally impaired (MIN) and the Alzheimer (AD) groups. Results are depicted for the hippocampus (HIP), parahippocampal gyrus (PARAHIP), fusiform gyrus (FUFORM) and transverse fissure cerebrospinal fluid (CSF-TF).

groups ($F = 2.01$, $P > 0.1$). A ruler was used to find the right and left subicular–thalamic distance of the medial and lateral aspects of the transverse fissure. The measures were taken from immediately posterior to the pes hippocampus extending caudad to the pulvinar of the thalamus approximately at the level of the splenium of the corpus callosum. A mean of all measures was taken as an estimation of fissure height for each case. The results showed that compared with the cognitively normal subjects, the minimally impaired, mild AD and moderate to severe AD patients had significant transverse fissure dilatations of 51.8, 56.9 and 71.8%, respectively ($F = 13.32$, $P < 0.0001$).

Positron emission tomography and fluorodeoxyglucose
Limitations in spatial resolution for the first generations of positron emission tomography (PET) camera technology only permitted the imaging of brain structures greater than 2 cm in all planes. Consequently, the relatively small hippocampus could not be imaged accurately and early PET focussed on relatively large neocortical and subcortical samples (Alavi and de Leon, 1985). In some studies, in the interest of obtaining estimates of homogeneous tissue samples, large areas potentially contributing to partially volumed CSF, such as the Sylvanian fissures were avoided. Other studies have estimated the CSF

using CT or MRI scans and statistically corrected the data on a lobar or whole brain basis. Only recently have coregistration systems become available to map the structural anatomy on to the PET scan thereby permitting precise sampling.

Spatial resolution limitations aside, there is a large literature describing the diagnostic utility of PET in studies of AD (Ferris *et al.*, 1980; Benson *et al.*, 1983; de Leon *et al.*, 1983; Foster *et al.*, 1984; Cutler *et al.*, 1985; Friedland *et al.*, 1985; Duara *et al.*, 1986; Haxby *et al.*, 1986). There is a consensus that temporal lobe and temporoparietal reductions in glucose utilization are typically salient among the global changes seen in AD. Unfortunately, except for a few longitudinal studies (Frackowiak *et al.*, 1981; Duara *et al.*, 1986; Jagust *et al.*, 1988; Smith *et al.*, 1992) very little is known about the inter-relation of the stage of AD and the subsequent progression of the metabolic patterns of brain deficit. The data that are available point to progressive reductions in glucose metabolism in affected regions, for example, temporal and parietal lobes, and the involvement of new regions. Virtually nothing is known about either early features or predictors of dementia, or the relationship between hippocampal changes and neocortical changes.

In earlier studies, prior to coregistration, we examined whether the structural hippocampal lesion as determined by CT is observed before the neocortical temporal lobe metabolic reduction as determined by PET. Normal controls were compared with the minimally impaired group for the following variables: temporal lobe glucose metabolism, the prevalence of hippocampal atrophy and the extent of ventricular enlargement. In this study, hippocampal atrophy differentiated the groups as it was found in 1/21 normal and 7/9 minimally impaired patients. Neither temporal lobe glucose metabolism nor ventricular enlargement revealed any group differentiation. Therefore, with respect to the hypothesized sequence of change, our data suggested that hippocampal atrophy may precede temporoparietal glucose utilization reductions and ventricular enlargement in the minimally affected patients. The observation that structural hippocampal change may predece neocortical involvement further suggests that hippocampal involvement occurs early in the course of AD.

Using current PET hardware, imaging the hippocampus directly is now possible. However, to perform an affective metabolic image analysis of brain substructures one needs the context of specific anatomical location provided by a high-resolution MRI or CT scan. For structures of the size of the hippocampus, image correlation within 2 mm accuracy is required. In dealing with aged and demented patients, such a level of accuracy is not achievable by even the most rigorous positioning of the patient in the respective scanners.

The software system we have implemented for retrospective image correlation performs the tasks of: (a) extracting common surfaces in coronally oriented MR images and transaxial PET images of the same subject, (b) computing coordinate transformation that relates PET and MR image sets, and (c) reformatting PET images along the coronal planes. The registration method is based on a large number of points extracted from brain surfaces in the two scans as described by Pelizzari *et al.* (1989). The method we developed, extends the earlier surface fitting strategy in that it permits us to assign relative weights to individual surface elements (such as planes of sylvanian fissures). Preferential weighting of surfaces that exhibit considerable variation over a small distance improves the accuracy of the registration. From computer simultations and phantoms we have determined the error in translation to be less than 1.7 mm and the error in rotation to be less than $3.8°$.

Using the CTI 931 PET camera with fluorodeoxyglucose (FDG) as the tracer for glucose metabolism, seven normal controls and seven minimally affected patients were studied. Positron emission tomographic scans were obtained using a negative angulation protocol and interleaved such that two sets of 15 slices were obtained. The entire set of 30 PET slices, with midpoints every 3.4 mm, was coregistered to contiguous coronal T_1 weighted MRI scans of 4 mm thickness. The close spacing of the axial study improved the accuracy of the reformatted coronal data. A less than 4% differences was observed in regional glucose metabolism due to coronal reformatting of the functional PET image. The strategy of analysing metabolic images in a coronal orientation presents the hippocampal anatomy with minimum partial volume artefacts.

The age and sex distribution of these groups were comparable. The results show that the metabolic rates for the hippocampus and parahippocampal gyrus are significantly different between the two groups. The minimally impaired patients show metabolic reductions in the magnitude of 20%, that do not overlap with the control values. Importantly other sampled sites such as the fusiform gyrus and the superior temporal gyrus do not distinguish between the groups. These data together with the CT and MRI data described above, show that there is both anatomic and metabolic specificity to the early brain changes in cases at risk for the development of dementia.

Hippocampal atrophy in normal pressure hydrocephalus

Normal pressure hydrocephalus (NPH) is a recognized cause of motoric dysfunction and memory impairment in the elderly (Adams *et al.*, 1965). Symptoms are generally ascribed to the enlarging ventricular volume and the consequent brain compression and damage. The condition is classically diagnosed by the clinical triad of gait dyspraxia, dementia and urinary incontinence in patients exhibiting severe ventriculomegaly on CT or MRI. Such patients typically have CSF flow abnormalities demonstratable by radiosotope lumbar cisternography (Banister *et al.*, 1967; Heinz *et al.*, 1970). In most cases the gait impairment precedes both the cognitive decline as well as the incontinence and it is felt that patients who can be diagnosed at this early stage are most likely to improve with neurosurgical intervention (Fisher, 1977; Graff-Radford *et al.*, 1989). Given the central role of the hippocampus in memory function, it was hypothesized that NPH patients with mild or no cognitive impairment might have structurally preserved hippocampi and smaller transverse fissures than NPH cases with dementia.

Transverse fissure heights were measured in 14 elderly patients with enlarged ventricles, lumbar cisternograms suggestive of NPH and varying degrees of gait and cognitive impairment. Seven patients had severely impaired gaits and six patients were demented (MMSE score <23). Using a two-factor ANOVA with gait severity group and dementia classification as independent variables, significantly increased transverse fissures were found in the demented NPH patients compared to the nondemented NPH patients ($F = 11.08$, $P < 0.01$) and no significant differences in fissure size in patients with severe gait impairment compared with those manifesting minimal gait change ($F = 14$, $P > 0.7$). Fissure height was found to correlate significantly with MMSE scores ($R = 0.58$, $P < 0.05$). This result suggests that dementia in NPH is associated with hippocampal damage. While the mechanism for the dementia is unknown, hypothetically, it could arise either from the mechanical effects of chronic ventricular expansion or from an accompanying AD. Nevertheless, severe ventriculomegaly *per se* is not a sufficient cause of fissure dilatation or dementia. Moreover, these results suggest that HA evaluation may be of potential value in the early differentiation of NPH and AD (Golomb *et al.*, 1992).

Post-mortem studies

Seven confirmed AD cases and five controls were studied. The normal and AD groups were 70.0 ± 3.6 s.d. and 80.8 ± 9.7 s.d. years of age, respectively. The neuropathology protocol included uniform coronal 5-mm thick slabs taken through the entire brain. Following embedding in paraffin, coronal 8-μm thick serial sections were cut and stained with cresyl violet, haematoxylin–eosin, Bielschowsky silver, Loyez methods and immunocytochemical methods for amyloid (MAB 4G8 against amino acids 17–24 of the β-amyloid peptide) and for tangles (MAB tau-1 against tau protein). Consistent with NINCDS–ADRDA criteria, the AD patients showed extensive neurofibrillary tangles, amyloid deposition and neuronal loss in the hippocampal formation and neocortex. Magnetic resonance imaging scans were obtained after 3 weeks formalin fixation. The scan protocol included contiguous 3 mm T_1 weighted coronal images through the hippocampal formation.

All AD cases demonstrated neuropathologic and neuroimaging evidence of dilated transverse fissures. With respect to the interpretation of changes in the transverse fissure, neuropathologic examination of the AD material showed volume losses in the hippocampus and parahippocampal gyrus with relative preservation of the lateral geniculate body and pulvinar (see Fig. 6.12).

For a subgroup of four AD patients and three controls actual volumes were determined and losses found in AD of approximately 40% in the cornu ammonis, 20% in both entorhinal cortex and subicular complex and 12% in the dentate gyrus (Bobinski *et al.*, 1992). As with the visual inspection, the actual volumes of the lateral geniculate body and pulvinar were not changed relative to control. More specific examination of the AD cases for the numbers of plaques, neurofibrillary tangles and neuronal losses further confirmed the hippocampal and entorhinal cortex vulnerability. Among the regions studied, both the cornu ammonis and the entorhinal cortex showed the greatest accumulations of tangles, approximately 20 and 15%, respectively, of neurons were affected (see Fig. 6.13) and the highest numbers of neurons lost (approximately 27 and 17%, respectively). Plaque counts were highest in the entorhinal cortex (26/mm^2) and more or less uniform in the other regions studied (approximately 15/mm^2).

For the quantitative MRI analysis, six of the confirmed AD cases and three of the age-matched normal controls were studied. The *post-mortem* MRI results showed a 40% reduction of the volume of the hippocampal formation (hippocampus and parahippocampal gyrus) in the AD group. Comparable anatomical *in vivo* sampling on 14 AD cases and 16 normal controls yielded a 20% reduction.

These data support the hypothesis that transverse fissure dilatation in AD is directly related to pathologic alterations of the hippocampal formation. The combination of the clinical and the neuropathological data suggests that damage to the hippocampal region begins early in the course of AD and is progressive throughout its course.

CONCLUSIONS

In vivo examination of the hippocampal region appears to be of potential diagnostic and predictive value in the clinical study of AD. Hippocampal changes appear early in the natural history of AD. When such changes are present in the absence of large neocortical metabolic lesions, they appear to be associated with the mild memory and cognitive deficits so often ascribed to the normal ageing process. Early HA appears to be related to the AD process, a

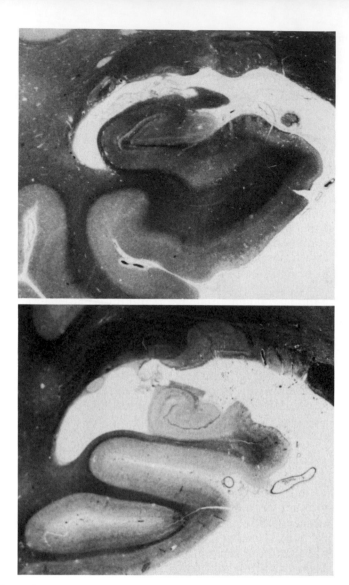

Fig. 6.12 Coronal sections through the hippocampal formation at the lateral geniculate level. (a) Normal control. (b) Alzheimer patient. Loyez stain.

conclusion supported by the *post-mortem* studies of Price *et al.* (1991). It is universally observed that HA occurs in AD at *post-mortem* examination, and these observations have been extended to show a remarkably consistent *in vivo* involvement of the hippocampus in AD. Furthermore, the CT imaged CSF changes are directly related to degenerative parenchymal changes detected with MRI volume studies and identified at *post-mortem*. Our longitudinal data indicate that hippocampal atrophy is predictive of the clinical deterioration to dementia associated with AD, consequently highlighting the clinical significance of this atrophic change. These findings now permit, for the first time, the identification of early patients at risk for AD and therefore provide a marker which may be of value for subject selection in therapeutic trials and in the development of other biological markers.

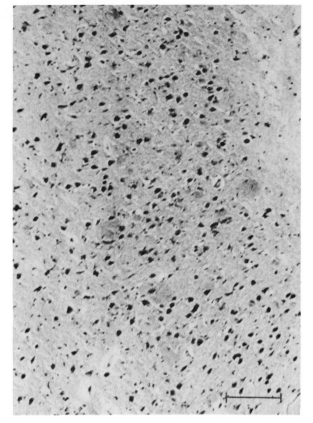

Fig. 6.13 Representative numbers of neurofibrillary tangles in the stratum pyramidale of the CA1 sector in an Alzheimer patient. Scale bar = 170 μm.

Our cross-sectional results also show that the hippocampal volume reductions specifically separate normal elderly subjects from those with minimal cognitive impairment. Other candidate temporal lobe regions were examined and only the hippocampal volume sigificantly separated the groups.

Histopathological evidence suggests that the earliest sites of medial temporal lobe tissue loss in AD, in addition to the hippocampus, consistently include the subiculum and the entorhinal cortex. These later regions in part form the floor of the transverse fissure. Atrophy in these regions, even if very small, may result in conformational changes affecting the orientation of the hippocampal formation and may result in an increase in fissure size. These considerations in part explain why measures of transverse fissure CSF in addition to the hippocampal volume can be used to explain the subjective appearance of the perihippocampal region on the negative angle axial scan.

Hippocampal atrophy as an early marker for AD now provides an opportunity to investigate the emergence of pathophysiologic phenomena and to evaluate their clinical significance. In particular, neuroendocrine dysregulations are related to hippocampal degeneration and cognitive impairment in both animal models (Sapolsky *et al.*, 1986) and in AD (de Leon *et al.*, 1988). In the case of AD, hypothesized relationships over time, between hippocampal and neocortical integrity, dementia and status of the neuroendocrine axis are under investigation. In conclusion, we have renewed optimism that with earlier diagnosis the search for relevant mechanisms of disease and effective treatment will be facilitated.

REFERENCES

Adams, R.D., Fisher, C.M., Hakim, S. *et al.* (1965). Symptomatic occult hydrocephalus with 'normal' cerebrospinal fluid pressure. *New England Journal of Medicine*, **273**, 117–26.

Alavi, A. and de Leon, M.J. (1985). Studies of the brain in aging and dementia with positron emission tomography and x-ray computed tomography. In *Positron Emission Tomography*, Reivich, M. and Alavi, A. (Eds), pp. 273–90. Alan R. Liss, Inc., New York.

Ball, M.J. (1978). Topographic distribution of neurofibrillary tangles and granulovacuolar degeneration in hippocampal cortex of aging and demented patients. A quantitative study. *Neuropathologica*, **42**, 73–80.

Ball, M.J., Hachinski, V., Fox, A. *et al.* (1985). A new definition of Alzheimer's disease: A hippocampal dementia. *Lancet*, **i**, 14–16.

Bannister, R., Gilford, E. and Kocen, R. (1967). Isotope encephalography in the diagnosis of dementia due to communicating hydrocephalus. *Lancet*, **ii**, 1014–17.

Benson, D.F., Kuhl, D.E., Hawkins, R.A. *et al.* (1983). The fluorodeoxyglucose 18F in Alzheimer's disease and multi-infarct dementia. *Archives of Neurology*, **40**, 711–14.

Bobinski, M., Morys, J., Wegiel, J. *et al.* (1992). Topography of pathological changes in the hippocampal formation in AD. *Journal of Neuropathology and Experimental Neurology*, **51**, 318 (abs.).

Convit, A., de Leon, M.J., Golomb, J. *et al.* (1993). Hippocampal atrophy in early Alzheimer's disease: anatomic specificity and validation. *Psychiatric Quarterly* (in press)

Cutler, N.R., Haxby, J.V., Duara, R. *et al.* (1985). Clinical history, brain metabolism, and neuropsychological function in Alzheimer's disease. *Annals of Neurology*, **18**, 298–309.

de la Monte, S.M. (1989). Quantitation of cerebral atrophy in preclinical and end-stage Alzheimer's disease. *Annals of Neurology*, **25**, 450–9.

de Leon, M.J., Ferris, S.H., George, A.E. *et al.* (1983). Positron emission tomography studies of aging and Alzheimer's disease. *American Journal of Neuroradiology*, **4**, 568–71.

de Leon, M.J., George, A.E., Stylopoulos, L.A. *et al.* (1989). Early marker for Alzheimer's disease: The atrophic hippocampus. *Lancet*, **ii**, 672–3.

de Leon, M.J., Golomb, J., George, A.E. *et al.* (1993). The radiologic prediction of Alzheimer's disease: the atrophic hippocampal formation. *American Journal of Neuroradiology* (in press).

de Leon, M.J., McRae, T., Tsai, J.R. *et al.* (1988). Abnormal hypercortisolemic response in Alzheimer's disease linked to hippocampal atrophy. *Lancet*, **ii**, 391–2.

Duara, R., Grady, C., Haxby, J. *et al.* (1986). Positron emission tomography in Alzheimer's disease. *Neurology*, **36**, 879–87.

Duvernoy, H.M. (1988). *The Human Hippocampus. An Atlas of Applied Anatomy.* J.F. Bergmann Verlag, Munchen.

Ferris, S.H., de Leon, M.J., Wolf, A.P. *et al.* (1980). Positron emission tomography in the study of aging and senile dementia. *Neurobiology of Aging*, **1**, 127–31.

Fisher, C.M. (1977). The clinical picture in occult hydrocephalus. *Clinical Neurosurgery*, **24**, 270–315.

Flicker, C., Ferris, S.H., Crook, T. and Bartus, R.T. (1987). Implications of memory and language dysfunction in the naming deficit of senile dementia. *Brain and Language*, **31**, 187–200.

Flicker, C., Ferris, S.H. and Reisberg, B. (1991). Mild cognitive impairment in the elderly: Predictors of dementia. *Neurology*, **41**, 1006–9.

Folstein, M.F., Folstein, S.E., McHugh, P.R. (1975). Mini-Mental State: A practical method for grading the cognitive state of patients for the clinician. *Journal of Psychiatry Research*, **12**, 189–98.

Foster, N.L., Chase, T.N., Mansi, L. *et al.* (1984). Cortical abnormalities in Alzheimer's disease. *Annals of Neurology*, **16**, 649–54.

Frackowiak, R.S.J., Pozzilli, C., Legg, N.J. *et al.* (1981). Regional cerebral oxygen supply and utilization in dementia – a clinical and physiological study with oxygen-15 and positron tomography. *Brain*, **104**, 753–78.

Friedland, R.P., Budinger, T.F., Koss, E. and Ober, B.A. (1985). Alzheimer's disease: Anterior–posterior and lateral hemisphere alterations in cortical glucose utilization. *Neuroscience Letters*, **53**, 235–40.

George, A.E., de Leon, M.J., Stylopoulos, L.A. *et al.* (1990). CT diagnostic features of Alzheimer's disease: Importance of the choroidal/hippocampal fissure complex. *American Journal of Neuroradiology*, **11**, 101–7.

Golomb, J., de Leon, M.J., George, A.E. *et al.* (1992). Medial temporal lobe atrophy in Alzheimer's disease. Presented at the *30th Annual Meeting of the American Society of Neuroradiology*, St Louis, Missouri.

Golomb, J., de Leon, M.J., Kluger, A. *et al.* (1993). Hippocampal atrophy in normal aging: an association with recent memory impairment. *Archives of Neurology* (in press).

Graff-Radford, N.R., Godersky, J.C. and Jones, M.P. (1989). Variables predicting surgical outcome in symptomatic hydrocephalus in the elderly. *Neurology*, **39**, 1601–4.

Haxby, J.V., Grady, C.L., Duara, R. *et al.* (1986). Neocortical metabolic abnormalities precede nonmemory cognitive defects in early Alzheimer's-type dementia. *Archives of Neurology*, **43**, 882–5.

Heinz, E.R., Davis, D.O. and Karp, H.R. (1970). Abnormal isotope cisternography in symptomatic occult hydrocephalus. *Radiology*, **95**, 109–20.

Hughes, C.P., Berg, L., Danziger, W.L. *et al.* (1982). A new clinical scale for the staging of dementia. *British Journal of Psychiatry*, **140**, 566–72.

Hyman, B.T., Van Hoesen, G.W., Damasio, A.R. and Barnes, C.L. (1984). Alzheimer's disease: Cell-specific pathology isolates the hippocampal formation. *Science*, **225**, 1168–70.

Hyman, B.T., Van Hoesen, G.W. and Damasio, A.R. (1987). Alzheimer's disease: glutamate depletion in the hippocampal perforant pathway zone. *Annals of Neurology*, **22**, 37–40.

Hyman, B.T. and Van Hoesen, G.W. (1988). Sites of earliest Alzheimer-type pathological changes in entorhinal cortex and hippocampus visualized by ATZ-50 immunocytochemistry. *Society for Neuroscience Abstracts*, **14** (Part 2), 1084.

Jack Jr, C.R., Petersen, R.C., O'Brien, P.C. and Tangalos, E.G. (1992). MR-based hippocampal volumetry in the diagnosis of Alzheimer's disease. *Neurology*, **42**, 183–8.

Jagust, W.J., Friedland, R.P., Budinger, T.F. *et al.* (1988). Longitudinal studies of regional cerebral metabolism in Alzheimer's disease. *Neurology*, **38**, 909–12.

Kemper, T. (1984). Neuroanatomical and neuropathological changes in normal aging and in dementia. In *Clinical Neurology of Aging*, Albert, M.L. (Ed.). Oxford University Press, New York, Oxford.

Kesslak, J.P., Nalcioglu, O. and Cotman, C.W. (1991). Quantification of magnetic resonance scans for hippocampal and parahippocampal atrophy in Alzheimer's disease. *Neurology*, **41**, 51–4.

Mann, D.M.A. and Esiri, M.M. (1988). The site of the earliest lesions of Alzheimer's disease. *New England Journal of Medicine*, **318**, 789–90.

Neary, D., Snowden, J.S., Bowen, D.M. *et al.* (1986). Neuropsychological syndromes in presenile dementia due to cerebral atrophy. *Journal of Neurology, Neurosurgery and Psychiatry*, **49**, 163–74.

Pelizzari, C.A., Chen, G.T.Y., Spelbring, D.R. *et al.* (1989). Accurate three-dimensional registration of CT, PET, and/or MR images of the brain. *Journal of Computer Assisted Tomography*, **13**, 20–6.

Price, J.L., Davis, P.B. and Morris, J.C. (1991). The distribution of tangles, plaques and related immunohistochemical markers in healthy aging and Alzheimer's disease. *Neurobiology of Aging*, **12**, 295–312.

Reisberg, B., Ferris, S.H., de Leon, M.J. and Crook, T. (1982). The global deterioration scale for assessment of primary degenerative dementia. *American Journal of Psychiatry*, **139**, 1136–9.

Rubin, E.H., Morris, J.C., Grant, E.A. and Vendegna, T. (1989). Very mild senile dementia of the Alzheimer type. I. Clinical assessment. *Archives of Neurology*, **46**, 379–82.

Sapolsky, R., Krey, L.C. and McEwen, B.S. (1986). The neuroendocrinology of stress and aging: The glucocorticoid cascade hypothesis. *Endocrine Review*, **7**, 284–301.

Seab, J.P., Jagust, W.S., Wong, S.F.S. *et al.* (1988). Quantitative NMR measurements of hippocampal atrophy in Alzheimer's disease. *Magnetic Resonance*, **8**, 200–28.

Sim, A. and Sussman, I. (1962). Alzheimer's disease: Its natural history and differential diagnosis. *Journal of Nervous and Mental Disease*, **135**, 489–99.

Smith, G.S., de Leon, M.J., George, A.E. *et al.* (1992). Topography of cross-sectional and longitudinal glucose metabolic deficits in Alzheimers Disease: Pathophysiologic implications. *Archives of Neurology*, **49**, 1142–50.

Storandt, M. and Hill, R.D. (1989). Very mild senile dementia of the Alzheimer type. II. Psychometric test performance. *Archives of Neurology*, **46**, 383–6.

Terry, R.D., Peck, A., De Teresa, R. *et al.* (1981). Some morphometric aspects of the brain in senile dementia of the Alzheimer type. *Annals of Neurology*, **10**, 184–92.

Van Hoesen, G.W. and Damasio, A.R. (1989).

Van Hoesen, G.W., Hyman, B.T. and Damasio, A.R. (1991). Entorhinal cortex pathology in Alzheimer's disease. *Hippocampus*, **1**, 1–8.

Zola-Morgan, S., Squire, L. and Amaral, D. (1986). Human amnesia and the medial temporal region: enduring memory impairment following a bilateral lesion limited to the field CA1 of the hippocampus. *Journal of Neuroscience*, **6**, 2950–67.

Alistair Burns

Department of Old Age Psychiatry
University of Manchester
Withington Hospital
and

Glyn Lewis

Section of Epidemiology and General Practice
Institute of Psychiatry

7 SURVIVAL IN DEMENTIA

INTRODUCTION

The study of survival in dementia is important for a number of reasons:

1. Knowledge of factors affecting survival may facilitate predictions of longevity in individual patients.
2. Details of survival patterns allow for more accurate planning of services.
3. Survival analysis has implications for subtypes of dementia in general and Alzheimer's disease in particular.
4. It is important to know whether the prognosis of dementia is improving over time as this has implications for service provision.
5. It allows, in companion studies, analysis to be made of cause of death in dementia.

An analysis of survival studies in the field reveals several identifiable components. Some work documents the differences in survival in groups of elderly subjects, generally showing that those with organic brain syndromes have a higher mortality. Others attempt to assess differences in survival between different types of dementia and within dementia, usually Alzheimer's disease. This chapter will begin with consideration of methods of investigating survival followed by a review of relevant studies.

The main studies assessing survival/mortality rates are summarized in Table 7.1, comparisons of survival in Alzheimer-type dementia and arteriosclerotic dementia are summarized in Table 7.2 and those studies detailing predictors of mortality are summarized in Table 7.3. The reader is also referred to three reviews by Christie (1985, 1987) and Van Dijk *et al.* (1991) on aspects of survival.

Methodological issues

There are a number of methodological issues surrounding analysis of survival data in dementia. The following summarizes some of the issues involved and, as examples, takes data from the study by Burns *et al.* (1991).

Calculating death rates

Studies of death in dementia will need to calculate a rate. A rate is defined as:

$$\text{Rate} = \frac{\text{Number of events}}{\text{Population at risk}} \tag{1}$$

It is the number of events, for example, deaths or new cases of disease, divided by the population at risk. If rates are not calculated it becomes extremely difficult to draw conclusions or compare the results of different

Table 7.1 Mortality in dementia of the Alzheimer type.

Study	Years examined	Population	Place	Lower age of limit (years)	Number of subjects	Mortality (%)						
						6 months	1 year	2 years	3 years	4 years	5 years	6 years
Camargo and Preston (1945)	1938, 1939, 1940	HA	Maryland (USA)	65	683	—	—	—	70.3	—	—	—
Post (1951)	1946	HA	London	60	158	—	—	—	—	60	—	—
Roth and Morrissey (1952)	1948	HA	Graylingwell (W. Sussex)	60	36	53	—	73	—	—	—	—
Roth (1955)	1934, 1936, 1948, 1949	HA	Graylingwell	60	450	58	—	82	—	—	—	—
Kay (1962)	1931–1937	HA	Stockholm	60	41	—	—	68	—	—	—	—
Kay and Bergmann (1966)	1960	Community	Newcastle-upon-Tyne	65	29	—	—	—	—	69	—	—
Goldfarb (1969)	1957, 1958	HI and NH	New York	64	355 mod. 305 sev.	— —	23 37	44 60	57 75	70 84	78 90	84 93
Shah et al. (1969)	1955–1960	HA	Saxondale (Notts)	60	38	42	53	71	95	85	—	—
Varsamis et al. (1972)	1964	HA	Winnipeg	>765	130	35	49	60	80	79	90	90
Gruenberg (1978)	1947–1957	Community	Lundby Study (Sweden)	N/S	14	—	—	50	—	66	—	100
Gruenberg (1978)	1957–1967	Community	Lundby Study (Sweden)	N/S	27	—	—	33	—	—	—	78
Kasznak et al. (1978)	1970s	HA	Chicago	50	47	—	46	—	—	75	—	—
Thompson and Eastwood (1981)	1969, 1978	HA	Toronto	N/S	24 (1969)	25	—	54	—	84	100	—
Blessed and Wilson (1982)	1969, 1978	HA	Newcastle	65	37 (1978)	43	—	62	—	84	100	—
Christie (1982)	1976	HA	Crichton (Dumfries)	70	320	31	—	68	—	—	—	—
Whitehead and Hunt (1982)	1974–1976	HA	Oxford	60	265	15	—	50	—	—	—	—
Naguib and Levy (1982a)	1975	*	London	—	199	—	35	—	—	—	—	—
Molsa et al. (1986)	1980	Community	Finland	N/S	40	25	—	—	69	—	—	—
Heyman et al. (1987)	1976	HI	N. Carolina	N/S	218	—	—	—	—	—	—	79

Study	Years		Location								
Robinson (1989)	1979–1984	HR	Oxford	49†	92	—	—	—	—	24	—
Neilsen et al. (1991)	1973–1988	HR	Denmark	48	59	36	53	66	78	81	85
Vitaliano et al. (1981)	1984–1985	NH	New York	N/S	51	—	—	25	—	—	—
Martin et al. (1987)	1970s	HR	Pittsburgh	N/S	212	—	—	—	—	66	—
Duckworth et al. 1979	1981–1983	HA	Toronto	>765	202	—	—	301	—	—	—
Burns et al. (1991)	1970s	HR	London	>765	23	13	48	—	—	—	—
Knopman et al. (1988)	1986–1988	HR	Minneapolis	56	178	—	—	47	—	—	—
Walsh et al. (1990)	1982–1984	HR	Washington	N/S	1C1 mild	98	94	92	—	—	—
	1980–1982				adv.	91	77	69	25	—	—
					126		13				46

HA = hospital admissions. HI = hospital inpatients. HR = hospital referrals. NH = nursing home. mod. = moderate dementia. sev. = severe dementia. adv. = advanced. N/S = not stated.
* Patients followed up from computed tomographic study 18–36 months previously.
† Service included organic cases under the age of 65 years.

Table 7.2 Differential survival in patients with Alzheimer-type and vascular dementia.

Study	Number	Year examined	Mortality index	Alzheimer	Vascular	Comparison	Comment
Camargo and Preston (1945)	683	1938–1940	% dead at 3 years	71%	66%	AD = MID	Diagnostic criteria not stated
Roth (1955)	318	1948–1949	% dead at 2 years	82%	73%	AD = MID	Operationally defined cases
Corsellis (1962)	81	1953–1957	Duration from onset to death	4.6 years	4.0 years	A = MID	Neuropathologically confirmed cases
Kay (1962)	686	1931–1937	Survival as fraction of normal population	M = 0.33 F = 0.23	0.16 0.39	MID > AD	Prognosis worse in men with vascular disease
Shah et al. (1969)	75	1955–1960	% dead at 2 years	M = 80% F = 68%	80% 35%	AD > MID	Only study to show better prognosis in AD
Varsamis et al. (1972)	130	1964	% dead at 2 years	60%	80%	AD = MID	Four-year follow-up revealed a similar pattern
Duckworth et al. (1979)	28	1964	% dead at 2 years	48%	60%	AD = MID	Same diagnostic criteria as Roth (1955)
Christie (1982)	132	1974–1976	% dead at 2 years	50%	66%	AD = MID	Same diagnostic criteria as Roth (1955)
Barclay et al. (1985a)	268	N/S	50% survival since onset	8.1 years	6.7 years	MID > AD	Prognosis for mixed cases same as MID
Molsa et al. (1986)	333	1976	% dead at 2 years	20%	30%	MID > AD	Difference continued until 6-year follow-up
Martin et al. (1987)	202	1982–1983	% dead at 2 years	18%	28%	AD = MID	
Hier et al. (1989)	95	1981–1988	Survival from diagnosis till death	4.3 years	4.5 years	AD = MID	
Nielsen et al. (1991)	87	1984–1985	% dead at 3 years	25%	45%	MID > AD	Chi-squared analysis showed significant difference

M = male. F = female. AD = Alzheimer's disease. MID = multi-infarct dementia. N/S = not stated.

Table 7.3 Predictors of death in Alzheimer-type dementia.

Study	Population	Number	Age (years) (mean of range)	Features predictive of death	Follow-up (months)	Comment
McDonald (1969)	HI	57	80.3	Young age Parietal lobe signs	6	Parietal lobe signs and survival established in different samples
Kaszniak et al. (1978)	HA	47	52–88	Expressive language dysfunction EEG abnormalities	12	Possible bias – of 60, 13 excluded and 12 lost to follow-up
Vitaliano et al. (1981)	NH	693	72.9 (median)	Male (Age >80)	60	Interesting cross-cultural study (New York and Tokyo)
Barclay et al. (1985b)	HR	199	73.3	Male (Age <65) Behavioural disturbance	up to 1300 days	Cognition not related to survival
Diesfeldt et al. (1986)	NH	297	53–97 (onset)	Behavioural disturbance onset (Age <75)	12	No effect on survival of age in those with onset at age >75
Heyman et al. (1987)	HA	92	62.4	Language dysfunction Poor cognitive function	60	Young patients with severe cognitive impairment had shorter survival than elderly patients with some degree of impairment
Knopman et al. (1988)	HR	101	70.6	Poor cognitive function Behavioural disturbance Activity of daily living impairment	36	Age not implicated in reduced survival

Table 7.3 Continued

Study	Population	Number	Age (years) (mean of range)	Features predictive of death	Follow-up (months)	Comment
Christie et al. (1988)	HA	83	Two separate groups: age 65–74 and 85 and over	Age	1–96	Elderly patients spent less time in hospital and had a more benign course
Ballinger et al. (1988)	HI	100	65–94	Impaired mobility	12	Geriatric and psychiatric populations. Cognitive function not implicated. Psychotic symptoms protected
Hier et al. (1989)	HR	61	71 (onset)	Hypertension Visuoconstructive and language dysfunction	64 (mean)	Race, age and sex not predictive
Walsh et al. (1990)	HR	126	77.6	Poor cognition Behavioural problems	72	Duration and age not predictive
Nielsen et al. (1991)	Community	51	54–85	High ischaemic score Low body mass index Low verbal fluency Wide pulse pressure (men only)	36	Combination of vascular and Alzheimer dementia
Burns et al. (1991)	HR	178	80.4	Increasing age Long duration of illness Male Physical illness Apraxia Depression Absence of misidentification	36	Rigorously defined population based Alzheimer cases

HA = hospital admissions. HI = hospital inpatients. HR = hospital referrals. NH = nursing home. EEG = electroencephalography.

studies. Although this point seems blindingly obvious, it is a fundamental principle which is occasionally ignored. There are also circumstances when the population at risk needs to be carefully defined.

In studies examining survival in dementia, death rates will therefore need to be calculated. Death rates are a special case of an incidence rate.

Incidence rate is defined as:

$$\text{Incidence rate} = \frac{\text{Number of new events}}{\text{Person–years at risk}} \qquad (2)$$

Death rate is defined as:

$$\text{Incidence rate} = \frac{\text{Number of deaths}}{\text{Person–years at risk}} \qquad (3)$$

In calculating an incidence rate the population at risk is most accurately defined as the person–years at risk. For example, in Fig. 7.1 a hypothetical longitudinal study is outlined in which six subjects are followed up for the period of the study. Three of the subjects die and two are lost to follow-up. Only one person is followed up to the end of the study. The population at risk in this 'study' is the total time that all six subjects spent in the study, before death or loss to follow-up. Subjects are still 'at risk' until they actually die.

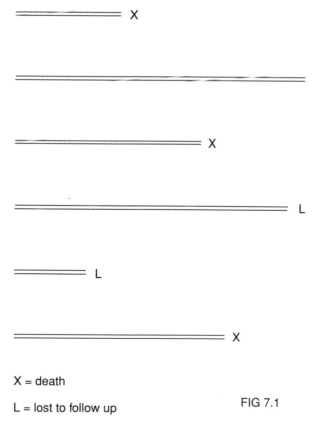

X = death

L = lost to follow up

FIG 7.1

Fig. 7.1 Calculating a death rate requires knowledge of the person-years at risk.

Likewise, those subjects who were lost to follow-up were still at risk while they were in the study. Once the subject has left the study the researcher does not know if the subject is alive or dead therefore the subject is no longer 'at risk' of death. In many circumstances, the exact person–years is not known. In that case one can usually assume that, on average, all the people who died did so half-way through the follow-up period.

Some studies have tended to calculate the proportion of the sample that has died rather than calculate death rates (see Table 7.1). The proportion who have died is not a very useful statistic. In the long run we all die as the follow-up period becomes longer, so one would expect the proportion who have died to increase – eventually it will reach 100%. It is then very difficult to compare studies as the proportion who have died will depend upon the follow-up period.

Selection of cases
In studying the survival of those with dementia, the source of the cases studied will affect the validity of the conclusions that can be drawn. There are two important issues to be considered.

Prevalent or incident cases
It is tempting to use the current cases in a clinical service for study. They are readily accessible and this method of selecting cases will reduce costs and thereby increase sample size. However, subjects who are prevalent within the category of those with dementia will tend to be those who have survived for a longer period. This is because subjects who died rapidly would have less of a chance of being included in the sample. Therefore, a study which uses prevalent cases will not be able to conclude in a general way about subjects with dementia. However, if one is concerned with the survival of those patients with dementia who are within a clinical service, then cases that are prevalent are the correct ones to choose. In a clinical service, the more long-lived patients will tend to be rather overrepresented, therefore, conclusions about the mortality of the patients in a clinical service should use a sample of prevalent cases. If one wishes to make conclusions about people with dementia or Alzheimer's disease then an incident sample of cases is needed.

From a defined catchment area
Referral to a specialist service occurs for a variety of reasons. Many of these may have something to do with the clinical characteristics, but the evidence from the referral of patients with depression (Goldberg and Huxley, 1980) suggests that a number of other factors tend to bias referral patterns. It is therefore important to take these into account in any epidemiological study. One of the simplest strategies is to ensure that the subjects all come from a defined catchment area. However, only a few of the potential subjects with dementia will be referred to a specialist psychiatric service. Evidence also exists that suggests that general practitioners do not know of all the patients with dementia on their list (Williamson, 1964; O'Connor, 1988). Therefore it is possible that the mortality experience of patients with dementia in a specialist service is different from that of all people with dementia. For example, it is possible that those with coexistent physical problems are referred to psychiatrists. Alternatively, perhaps patients with more disturbed behaviour are more likely to be referred, but they also have an increased likelihood of death.

The only approach that will avoid this potential bias is to screen the general population, and establish the incident cases of dementia by repeating the screen after an interval. This is the methodology being adopted by the Medical Research Council Cognitive Function and Ageing Study (Copeland *et al.*, 1992).

Comparison with the general population

To establish the mortality of patients with dementia requires reference to the general population. The death rates of demented subjects are less meaningful if they cannot be compared to members of the general population of the same sex and age as the patients. The standard method for this is to use the Standardized Mortality Ratio (SMR). This is a statistic which compares the death rate in patients with dementia with the death rate in the general population. Since mortality varies considerably by age and sex and it is necessary to adjust for these. The SMR uses a method of indirect standardization, relying upon calculating standard rates from the reference population and applying this to the age and sex stratified sample population. An SMR of 100 indicates that the mortality of the sample is that expected of the general population, given the age and sex structure of the sample.

A number of studies have calculated SMRs for their populations (e.g. Kay, 1962; Burns *et al.*, 1991). Burns *et al.* (1991) were the only ones to use standard death rates from the catchment area from which the patients originated. There are considerable geographical variations in mortality. Using national figures would have overestimated the SMRs in the study of Burns *et al.* as Camberwell, a deprived inner city area, has itself a high all cause SMR. However, the size of the increase in mortality seen in dementia could not be entirely explained by this bias.

The Burns *et al.* study gave the following results. The SMR for men was 3.00 [95% confidence interval (CI) 1.75–4.83%] and for women it was 3.86 (95% CI 3.02–4.94). There is a markedly elevated SMR for both men and women. There is no evidence that the SMR for men and women is different. This was established by conducting a test for heterogeneity ($P = 0.34$; Breslow and Day, 1987) which determines whether there is a statistically significant difference between the two SMRs. That is not the same as saying that women and men have the same death rates. Women have lower death rates than men. However, the ratio of death rates in patients with dementia in relation to the general population is the same for men and women. Overall the SMR of the whole cohort studied by Burns *et al.* was 3.64 (95% CI 2.92–4.53). The authors also found a trend for younger subjects to have a higher SMR than older patients. Again, this is not suggesting that younger demented subjects have an increased rate of death, but that the relative rate of death is higher in this group.

Examining clinical heterogeneity

An important question concerns whether different clinical groups have the same prognosis. This information is useful in its own right, allowing clinicians to advise relatives on the likely prognosis more accurately. There is also the hope that such methods can define groups who differ in other respects as well. Therefore, studies of pathophysiology and aetiology could be informed by such observations and in turn lead to other distinctions of clinical usefulness.

An approach to this question can be made by comparisons within a cohort of subjects with dementia. Again death rates need to be considered. The main univariate method of analysing death rates is by using the method of Kaplan–Meier. In effect the outcome of interest is the survival time. The method can accommodate subjects who are lost to follow-up or who do not die (i.e. censored data). This is an approach similar to that of life tables. The probability of dying during successive time periods is calculated. The cumulative probability of death can therefore be plotted and two or more groups compared.

The main limitation of this method is that of all univariate methods. When potential factors of prognostic importance are correlated with each other, all may show a strong univariate relationship. With multivariate methods, it is possible to take account of these and therefore determine which factors are important in their own right in determining prognosis. This is the standard confounding problem and readers are referred to textbooks of epidemiology to have this fully explained.

The most commonly used method of analysis for survival times is the proportional hazards model of Cox. It is a multivariate technique. It assumes that the hazard or risk of death for all individuals is proportional throughout the period of study. It also assumes that the effect of explanatory variables is multiplicative. The coefficients generated by the proportional hazards model can be exponentiated and the resulting 'hazard ratios' can be interpreted as relative risks. A hazard ratio of greater than one then indicates an increased death rate while a value below one indicates a reduced death rate.

Previously published results from the cohort of Burns *et al.* (1991) are given in Table 7.4. The aim of this analysis was to discover whether clinical and computed tomographic (CT) scan features were related to survival in dementia. The first analytic step was therefore to examine each variable of interest in turn in a univariate fashion. This could have been done using the Kaplan–Meier

Table 7.4 Univariate models for the effect of various factors on survival in Alzheimer's disease.

Variables comparison	Hazard ratio	Significance P
Increase in age by 1 year	1.06	0.002
Female *v.* male	0.76	0.32
Increase in duration of illness by 1 month	1.005	0.06
Incident *v.* prevalent cases	0.82	0.38
Probable *v.* possible AD	0.80	0.41
Hallucinations: present *v.* absent	1.47	0.17
Thought disorder: present *v.* absent	0.94	0.80
Misidentification: present *v.* absent	0.55	0.02
Depression: present *v.* absent	1.70	0.04
Family history: present *v.* absent	0.64	0.08
Increase in MMSE score by one point	0.95	0.001
Increase in CAMDEX praxis score by one point	0.90	0.001
Increase in CAMDEX language score by one point	0.96	0.005
Increase in CAMDEX memory score by one point	0.93	0.03
Increase in VBR by 1	0.91	0.58
Cortical atrophy (1) *v.* 0	0.72	0.36
Marked cortical atrophy (2) *v.* 0	1.98	0.03

A hazard ratio of >1 means that the first normal variable causes more rapid death and <1 means the variable causes less rapid death, on comparison with the baseline. The size of the hazard ratio is not directly associated with the degree of significance because of the different units of measurement in the variables.
AD = Alzheimer's disease. CAMDEX = Cambridge Mental Disorders of the Elderly schedule.
MMSE = Mini-Mental State Examination. VBR = ventricular–brain ratio.
Reproduced from Burns *et al.* (1991) with permission.

Table 7.5 Multivariate model for predicting survival in Alzheimer's disease.

Variables	Hazard ratio	Significance P
Increase in MMSE score by 1	0.93 (0.90, 0.97)	0.001
Increase in age by 1 year	1.06 (1.02, 1.10)	0.008
Depression: present v. absent	1.80 (1.11, 2.89)	0.02
Female v. male	0.55 (0.32, 0.95)	0.03
Probable v. possible AD	0.56 (0.32, 0.97)	0.04
Misidentification: present v. absent	0.55 (0.33, 1.02)	0.06

95% confidence intervals in parentheses.
Reproduced with permission from Burns et al. (1991. MMSE = Mini-Mental State Examination.
AD = Alzheimer's disease.

model but it was decided to use the Cox proportional hazards model in order to be able to compare with the multivariate analyses.

The advantages of a multivariate approach can be illustrated with these data. Women have a lower death rate in this cohort (hazard ratio 0.76) but this was not statistically significant. However, after the important variables (i.e. significantly related to survival at the 5% level) were added to the model (Table 7.5), the women in the cohort had a hazard ratio of 0.55 ($P = 0.03$). This is because women also had other characteristics, including lower scores on the Mini-Mental State Examination (MMSE) in this cohort. Therefore, such other features confounded the relationship between survival and gender.

In general multivariate methods are most useful when testing specific hypotheses. It has been suggested that poor survival is associated with low scores on visuospatial tasks (McDonald, 1969). This could be tested by including all three scales (praxis, language and memory) from the Cambridge Mental Disorders of the Elderly schedule (CAMDEX) (Roth et al., 1986) in the same model (Table 7.6). The results show that the praxis scale is a better predictor than the other two scales. However, this was not statistically significant.

THE INFLUENCE OF ORGANIC BRAIN DISEASE ON SURVIVAL

The influence of organic factors on the survival of patients has been documented for some time. Much of the current nosology in old age psychiatry results from the pioneering work of Roth (1955) who, for the first time, established a satisfactory classification of psychiatric disorders in the elderly. This was achieved by a study of 450 patients admitted to Graylingwell Hospital in Essex in the years 1934, 1936, 1948 and 1949 and who were followed up for

Table 7.6 A multivariate model including the three CAMDEX subscales.

	Hazard ratio	Significance P
Increase in praxis score by 1	0.90 (0.79, 1.03)	0.13
Increase in language score by 1	1.00 (0.95, 1.06)	0.98
Increase in memory score by 1	1.00 (0.91, 1.10)	0.93

95% confidence intervals in parentheses.
Reproduced with permission from Burns et al. (1991). CAMDEX = Cambridge Mental Disorders of the Elderly.

2 years. The five categories were affective psychosis, senile psychosis, late paraphrenia, arteriosclerotic psychosis and acute confusion. Senile psychosis was defined as '. . . a condition with a history of gradual and continually progressive failure in the common activities of everyday life and the clinical picture dominated by failure of memory and intellect and disorganization of a personality, where these were not attributable to specific causes such as infection, neoplasm, chronic intoxication or cerebrovascular disease known to have produced cerebral infarction'. Arteriosclerotic psychosis was diagnosed in patients in whom there were focal signs and symptoms of vascular disease and who had a fluctuating course and any one of emotional incontinence, preservation of insight or seizures.

The survival patterns at 2 years of 318 patients admitted in 1948 and 1949 showed clear differences between the groups. Those patients with dementia did worse – 82% with Alzheimer's disease and 73% with arteriosclerotic psychosis had died. This compared to just below 20% of those with affective psychosis and just above 20% of those with late paraphrenia. Fifty per cent of patients with acute confusion had died, the other 50% had been discharged home. Thus, it was confirmed that individuals with dementia had a significantly shorter survival time than those with functional illness. The high death rate of those with confusional states presumably reflected the presence of physical disease in these individuals. This is substantiated by another report on the same population (Kay and Roth, 1955) which specifically documented the presence of physical illness in the population. Those with defined physical disorder in the five categories were: affective disorder (48%), late paraphrenia (50%), arteriosclerotic psychosis (66%), senile psychosis (39%) and acute confusion (89%). These authors found, however, that the most important determinant of mortality was the psychiatric diagnosis and not the accompanying physical illness.

Ten years earlier, Camargo and Preston (1945) had shown that in patients admitted to state mental hospitals in the years 1938 to 1940, two-thirds of those with cerebral-arteriosclerosis had died compared with 71% of those with senile psychosis. However, no information is provided with regard to the diagnostic practices employed and, as such, it is reasonable to consider Roth's work as the starting point for the investigation of mortality in operationally defined cases of dementia.

The poor prognosis associated with organic disorders has been confirmed in a number of studies (Kay, 1962; Larsson et al., 1963; Goldfarb, 1969; Versamis et al., 1972; Peck et al., 1978; Duckworth et al., 1979; Whitehead and Hunt, 1982; Robinson, 1989; Eagles et al., 1990).

Kay (1962) looked at all admissions to the psychiatric hospital in Stockholm. He found the death rates of subjects with dementia to be one-quarter and one-third those of the Stockholm population for women and men, respectively. Standard mortality rates of those with other psychiatric disorders was 0.88 for women and 0.80 for men compared to the population. Kay used the same operationally defined criteria as Roth (1955). While one of the original intentions of the study was to assess the role of vascular brain pathology in the genesis of depression, the study revealed much useful information about the prognosis of psychiatric disorders in the elderly. Varsamis et al. (1972) found that subjects with either vascular or primary degenerative dementia had higher death rates than those with other psychiatric disorders in patients admitted to the Winnipeg Psychiatric Institute.

Duckworth et al. (1979) found that 48% of those with senile dementia were dead 2 years after admission compared to 60% of those with arteriosclerotic dementia. Just over 10% of those with paraphrenia and affective psychoses had died. Goldfarb (1969) found that four characteristics were associated with high mortality within 1 year of admission to long-term care institutions (state hospitals, voluntary and nursing homes), two of which were clearly associated with dementia – the presence of chronic brain syndrome, poor cognitive impairment, physical dependence and incontinence. Whitehead and Hunt (1982) examined 200 consecutive referrals to a psychiatric unit over the age of 60 years and followed them for 5 years. The diagnosis of 'chronic brain syndrome' (the diagnosis made on admission – no operational criteria were given) was associated with an increased death rate compared to the normal population only in patients aged 60–74 years and not in those aged 75 years or over. This accords with the general view that early onset cases of Alzheimer's disease are associated with poorer survival.

The study by Whitehead and Hunt (1982) confirmed the findings of the classic work by Larsson *et al.* (1963) who found an excess mortality in dementia to be much greater in younger subjects and to be significantly associated with increasing age. Peck *et al.* (1978) found no difference in mortality in men in patients with or without chronic brain syndrome but found *women* with chronic brain syndrome to have excess mortality, in particularly if they had poor physical health. The presence of chronic brain syndrome outweighed the presence of physical illness (as it did in the study by Kay and Roth, 1955) as women admitted with chronic brain syndrome who were physically well had a poorer prognosis than women with purely physical problems.

Go *et al.* (1978) calculated life expectancy times for patients with dementia and compared these to the normal population of Geneva. Subjects with dementia had one-third the life expectancy of controls and, when they were admitted to hospital, the life expectancy was only 10%. Neuropathological examination revealed that subjects with neurofibrillary tangles in the neocortex had the *longest* survival times.

Two recent studies have addressed similar questions and have essentially confirmed earlier work. Robinson (1989) is a long-term study over 15 years of new referrals to a psychogeriatric service found distinct survival patterns for Alzheimer's disease and depression. The 2, 5, 10 and 15 year mortality rates for Alzheimer's disease and depression were 53, 81, 98 and 100% and 35, 57, 78 and 93%, respectively. Eagles *et al.* (1990) performed a case control study of 410 elderly subjects over the age of 65 years and divided them into cognitively impaired or not cognitively impaired depending on the results of a mental test score. Those with cognitive impairment were 3.5 times more likely to die than those without cognitive impairment (there was no difference in mortality in those with severe or moderate impairment). While this is helpful in emphasizing the association of cognitive impairment with poor survival, it does not show a specific association between dementia and increased mortality (a disadvantage noted by the authors). Thus, many conditions where cognitive impairmant may be detected or may be the end point (i.e. depression, confusion, physical illness) may all contribute to the findings. It may be applicable to general practice where an exact diagnosis of dementia is often eschewed but where a finding of cognitive impairment may signal early death. There did not appear to be a linear relationship between degree of impairment and risk of death.

SURVIVAL IN DIFFERENT TYPES OF DEMENTIA

Many studies have assessed differential survival in dementia. Most have compared Alzheimer's disease and multi-infarct dementia. These are summarized in Table 7.2. The majority show either no difference in survival between the two types of dementia or a worse prognosis for vascular dementia. Studies with the former pattern of mortality sometimes demonstrated a trend in favour of a better prognosis in Alzheimer's disease but this failed to reach statistical significance (e.g. Duckworth *et al.*, 1979; Martin *et al.*, 1987). Differences for men and women have been noted with men generally having a poorer prognosis than women, particularly in vascular dementia. The only study to show a poorer prognosis in Alzheimer's disease was that of Shah *et al.* (1969). This increased mortality was sustained from 3 months to 4 years of follow-up after admission showing that it was not merely a transient phenomenon noted in the months following admission to hospital. The reasons for the findings of Shah *et al.* are not immediately apparent. The methodology is sound and the study was obviously carefully performed using psychiatric case records. The numbers involved were comparatively small compared to others ($n = 75$) and the authors state that 'patients ... were not likely to be admitted unless the illness was already severe ...'. It may be that there was some differential mortality prior to admission, because of the shortage of beds, resulting in the more acutely ill subjects with vascular disease dying before they got to hospital. Shah *et al.* (1969) state that conventional thinking is that subjects with vascular dementia live longer than those with Alzheimer's disease and their study showed that Van Dijk *et al.* (1991) highlight this and suggest that prior to the 1970s, subjects with vascular dementia presented early in their illness, and hence apparently had a longer survival. More recent appreciation of the significance of dementia with an insidious onset has led to these disorders being referred earlier and hence longer survival being found. This argument is partly borne out by the data in this chapter as only one of the four studies prior to that of Shah *et al.* showed vascular dementia having a worse prognosis while this finding has been documented in three of the eight subsequent reports.

With regard to 'other types' of dementia, scant attention has been paid to this and presumably the prognosis is directly related to the underlying cause. The only study to mention specifically their comparative rates of survival is that of Varsamis *et al.* (1972). Twelve out of 72 patients with dementia were placed in this category and included dementia secondary to alcoholism and neurosyphilis. This group had better survival than either the Alzheimer or vascular subjects.

FACTORS ASSOCIATED WITH DEATH

There have been many investigations of factors which are predictive of death in Alzheimer's disease. These were summarized in Table 7.3. The results suggest that male sex, poor cognitive function and behavioural difficulties are consistently associated with increased mortality. Specific cognitive deficits are particularly predictive of poor prognosis: visuoconstructive performance (Burns *et al.*, 1991; Hier *et al.*, 1989; Macdonald, 1969) and aphasia (Kaszniak *et al.*, 1978; Hier *et al.*, 1989). The presence of behaviours may reflect a global increase in dementia and are associated with premature death (Burns *et al.*, 1990) but specific problems such as wandering and falling (Walsh *et al.*, 1990) and incontinence are strongly predictive of poor survival (Burns *et al.*, 1990). Misidentification is protective (Drevets and Rubin, 1989; Burns *et al.*, 1991).

The reasons for this are unclear especially as misidentifications are generally associated with a younger age of onset (Burns et al., 1990). Depression is said to be protective in some studies (e.g. Naguib et al., 1982) but recently was found to signify an increased mortality (Burns et al., 1991). It may be that there was some diagnostic inaccuracy in the earlier study leading to cases of pseudodementia being included as dementia and having a better prognosis.

Age is implicated in a number of studies. Young age is said to be associated with poor prognosis (Mcdonald, 1969; Seltzer and Sherwin, 1983). Burns et al. (1991) showed *relative* mortality (i.e. SMR) to be higher in the younger age group, *absolute* mortality being greater in the elderly. There is a complex interaction between age and degree of cognitive impairment. Heyman et al. (1987) showed that young patients with severe cognitive impairment had a shorter survival time compared to elderly patients and Christie and Wood (1988) separated patients with dementia into two groups – those under the age of 75 years on admission and those aged 85 years and over. Generally, the elderly patients spent less time in hospital and had a more benign course than the younger group but overall there was no difference in mortality. Hier et al. (1989), Walsh et al. (1990) and Knopman et al. (1988) showed that age had no influence on survival.

CHANGES IN SURVIVAL OVER TIME

Several studies have addressed the issue of whether the prognosis of Alzheimer's disease has changed with time. Many of the comparisons have been with Roth's 1955 work, often using the same diagnostic criteria based on case note evaluation. Roth (1955) studied the years 1934, 1936, 1948 and 1949. Studies comparing mortality to Roth's work will be considered first.

Shah et al. (1969) found that survival rates for patients admitted between 1955 to 1960 to Saxondale Hospital in Nottingham with both vascular and senile dementia had lower mortality than Roth's study at 6 months and 2 years after admission (with the exception of vascular dementia at 6 months follow-up where the prognosis was the same). However these results did not reach statistical significance.

Duckworth et al. (1979) compared subjects admitted to psychiatric hospitals in Toronto with those of Roth (the latter being recalculated to include only those over the age of 65 years). Significantly lower rates of mortality were seen in those dying at 6 months and 2 years after admission in senile dementia (Roth's figures: 61% and 86% mortality; Duckworth's figures: 13% and 48% mortality at 6 months and 2 years, respectively). Vascular dementia had a slightly decreased mortality but this did not reach statistical significance. However, the diagnostic categories were not identical (Duckworth used ICD8), referral policies may differ and the populations were in different countries which makes the comparison open to question.

Christie (1982) used the same criteria as Roth (1955) to assess admissions to Crichton Royal Hospital in Dumfries. He presented evidence that admissions to Graylingwell and Crichton Royal were very similar and so the direct comparison between the two was valid. Christie (1982) found that the mortality, 25 years later (1948/9 compared to 1974/6) had improved. At 2 years, the mortality rate for senile dementia was 50% (compared to 88%) and 69% for vascular dementia (compared to 82%). Blessed and Wilson (1982) performed a similar study in Newcastle and found a similar improvement in mortality: 32% difference at 6 months' outcome and 14% difference at 2 years. This was particularly marked in elderly female patients. The difference was confined to

Alzheimer's disease, there being no difference in prognosis for vascular dementia. These data suggest, convincingly, that the prognosis for senile dementia has improved over time.

Other work has not concentrated on a comparison with Roth's data but has involved internal comparisons over time in a number of settings. Wood et al. (1991) assessed survival time in dementia over a 30-year period (seven on-year cohorts, 5 years apart) at Crichton Royal Hospital in Dumfries from 1957 to 1987. In males, later cohorts survived three times as long as earlier admissions, a difference not accountable by variation within the populations. In females, the survival time approximately doubled in later years. The authors considered at length the reasons for the increased survival: alteration in the natural history of Alzheimer's disease, change in age or disability at the time of admission, referral bias and changes in hospital care (treatment and environmental factors). The authors conclude that the changes reflect those occurring in the general population and are not peculiar to those with dementia or those in hospital. Use of SMRs would address this issue.

Three other studies have examined mortality rates over time. Rorsman et al. (1985) followed up the Lundby study and found that over a 25 year follow-up, the mortality of those with 'age psychosis', i.e. dementia of Alzheimer type or vascular dementia, had not changed. Saugstad and Odergard (1979) examined mortality in psychiatric hospitals in Norway over the period 1950 to 1974 and found a decrease in mortality of 20–30% in those with organic psychoses. This appeared to be a greater decline than in the general population in which a decrease of 12% mortality in females and an increase of 12% in mortality in males over the same period, was seen. The decrease in mortality in those with organic psychosis is greater than in that with the functional disorders.

Thompson and Eastwood (1981) examined survival in patients in a nursing home in Toronto over a 10-year period. No change was seen over time. The authors discussed methodological problems in such studies, for example, reliability of death certificate data, representative nature of the population and diagnostic issues. These are shown to have been relatively stable over the time suggesting that the finding of no increased survival is a true one.

In summary, the data concerning the possible improvement in the prognosis of dementia over time are conflicting. Of the studies reported here, five suggest an improvement, three suggest none. No study has shown that the prognosis of dementia has worsened over time. It may that hospitalized patients do have an increased survival due to some of the factors discussed by Wood et al. (1991) but that community patients (e.g. in the Lundby study; Rorsman et al., 1985) or nursing home patients (Thompson and Eastwood, 1981) do not. The study suggesting that there was no improvement in a hospital sample (Shah et al., 1969) did show a trend for improved survival which was not statistically significant. Overall, it would seem that survival for demented patients is improving at a rate which parallels that of the general population (Wood et al., 1991) or may at times outstrip it (Saugstad and Odergard, 1979).

CAUSE OF DEATH

Cause of death is usually considered alongside survival in dementia (Christie, 1985, 1987). Christie (1985) noted that 'remarkably little attention' was paid to cause of death in dementia. The commonest cause of death in dementia is bronchopneumonia (Burns et al., 1990). Burns (1992) has recently reviewed this field.

CONCLUSIONS

There is no shortage of studies looking at various aspects of survival and common themes emerge. Subjects with dementia survive a shorter time than nondemented invididuals, multi-infarct dementia tends to carry a poorer prognosis than dementia of the Alzheimer type, demented patients may be living longer and several features predict prognosis in dementia of the Alzheimer type such as age, specific cognitive deficits, behavioural problems and some psychiatric symptoms. However, there are several factors which make the analysis of survival data difficult to interpret such as choice of subject, choice of population, length of follow-up and the way in which 'drop outs' are dealt with. Using SMRs based on the population from which the sample is drawn is the best method for predicting true estimates of the increased death rate resulting from dementia, but they have rarely been used. When attempting to predict which factors are associated with poor survival, multivariate methods of analysis are preferred (such as the proportional hazards model of Cox). This takes into consideration intercorrelated variables (such as age and apraxia) which using univariate analysis may appear to be related to survival.

It is suggested that these techniques be used in future studies of survival to facilitate accurate identification of the true increased risk of dementia and factors predictive of poor survival.

REFERENCES

Ballinger, B.R., McHarg, A.M., MacLennan, W.J. and Ogston, S. (1988). Dementia psychiatric symptoms and immobility: a one-year follow-up. *International Journal of Geriatric Psychiatry*, **3**, 1125–9.

Barclay, L., Laurie, L., Zcmcov, A., Blass, J.P. and Sansone, J. (1985a). Survival in Alzheimer's disease and vascular dementias. *Neurology*, **35**, 834–40.

Barclay, L., Laurie, L., Zemcov, A., Blass, J.P., McDowell, F.M. and Fletcher, H. (1985b). Factors associated with duration of survival in Alzheimer's disease. *Biological Psychiatry*, **20**, 86–93.

Blessed, G. and Wilson, I.D. (1982). The contemporary natural history of mental disorder in old age. *British Journal of Psychiatry*, **141**, 59–67.

Breslow, N. and Day, N. (1987). *Statistical Methods of Cancer Research*, Vol. 2, *The Design and Analysis of Cohort Studies*. IARC, Lyon.

Burns, A. (1992). Cause of death in dementia. *International Journal of Geriatric Psychiatry*, **7**, 461–4.

Burns, A., Jacoby, R., Luthert, P. and Levy, R. (1990). Cause of death in Alzheimer's disease. *Age and Ageing*, **19**, 341–4.

Burns, A., Lewis, G., Jacoby, R. and Levy, R. (1991). Factors affecting survival in Alzheimer's disease. *Psychological Medicine*, **21**, 363–70.

Camargo, O. and Preston, H. (1945). What happens to patients who are hospitalised for the first time when over sixty-five years of age. *American Journal of Psychiatry*, **102**, 168–73.

Christie, A.B. (1982). Changing patterns in mental illness in the elderly. *British Journal of Psychiatry*, **140**, 154–9.

Christie, A.B. (1985). *Survival in Dementia: A Review. Recent Advances in Psychogeriatrics*, Arie, T. (Ed.). Churchill Livingstone, Edinburgh.

Christie, A.B. (1987). Alzheimer's Disease: The Prognosis: 'Dementia', Pitt, B. (Ed.). Churchill Livingstone, Edinburgh.

Christie, A.B. and Wood, E.R.M. (1988). Age, clinical features and prognosis in S.D.A.T. *International Journal of Geriatric Psychiatry*, **3**, 63–8.

Copeland, J.R.M., Davidson, I.A., Dewey, M.E. *et al.* (1992). Alzheimer's disease, other dementias, depression and pseudo-dementia: prevalence, incidence and three-year outcome in Liverpool. *British Journal of Psychiatry*, **161**, 230–9.

Diesfeldt, L., van Houte, L.R. and Moerkens, R.M. (1986). Duration of survival in senile dementia. *Acta Psychiatrica Scandinavica*, **73**, 366–71.

Drevets, W. and Rubin, E. (1989). Psychotic symptons in the longitudinal course of senile dementia of the Alzheimer type. *Biological Psychiatry*, **25**, 39–43.

Corsellis, J.A.N. (1962). Mental illness and the ageing brain. *Maudsley Monograph* No. 9, Oxford University Press.

Duckworth, G.S., Kedward, H.B. and Bailey, W.F. (1979). Prognosis of mental illness in old age. *Canadian Journal of Psychiatry*, **24** (Review).

Eagles, J.M., Beattie, J.A.G., Restall, D.B. *et al.* (1990). Relation between cognitive impairment and early death in the elderly. *British Medical Journal*, **300**, 239–40.

Go, R., Todorov, A., Elston, R. and Constantinidis, J. The Malignancy of dementias. *Annals of Neurology*, **3**, 559–61.

Gruenberg, E. (1978). Epidemiology of senile dementia. In *Advances in Neurology*, Vol. 19 (Ed.) Schoenberg, B. Raven Press, New York.

Goldfarb, A.I. (1969). Predicting mortality in the institutionalised aged. *Archives of General Psychiatry*, **21**, 172–6.

Goldberg, D.P. and Huxley, P. (1980). *Mental Illness in the Community: The Pathway to Psychiatric Care.* Tavistock, London.

Heyman, A., Wilkinson, W.E., Hurwitz, B.J. *et al.* (1987). Early-onset Alzheimer's disease: clinical predictors of institutionalisation and death. *Neurology*, **37**, 980–4.

Hier, D.B., Warach, J.D., Gorelick, P.B. and Thomas, J. (1989). Predictors of survival in clinically diagnosed Alzheimer's disease and multi-infarct dementia. *Archives of Neurology*, **43**, 1213–16.

Kasczniak, A.W., Fox, J., Gandell, D.L. *et al.* (1978). Predictors of mortality in presenile and senile dementia. *Annals of Neurology*, **31**, 246–52.

Kay, D. and Bergmann, K. (1966). Outcome and cause of death in mental disorders of old age. *Acta Psychiatry Scandinavica*, **38**, 249–76.

Kay, D.W.K. (1962). Outcome and cause of death in mental disorders of old age: a long-term follow-up of functional and organic psychoses. *Acta Psychiatrica Scandinavica*, **38**, 249–76.

Kay, D.W.K. and Roth, M. (1955). Physical accompaniments of mental disorder in old age. *Lancet*, **ii**, 740–45.

Knopman, D.S., Kitto, J., Deinard, S. and Heiring, J. (1988). Longitudinal study of death and institutionalisation in patients with primary degenerative dementia. *Journal of the American Geriatrics Society*, **36**, 108–12.

Larsson, T., Sjogren, T. and Jacobson, G. (1963). Senile dementia. *Acta Psychiatrica Scandinavica*, **167** (Suppl.). 1–259.

Martin, D.C., Miller, J.K., Kapoor, W. *et al.* (1987). A controlled study of survival with dementia. *Archives of Neurology*, **44**, 1122–6.

McDonald, C. (1969). Clinical heterogeneity in senile dementia. *British Journal of Psychiatry*, **115**, 267–71.

Molsa, P.K., Marttila, R.J. and Rinne, U.K. (1986). Survival and cause of death in Alzheimer's disease and multi-infarct dementia. *Acta Neurologica Scandinavica*, **74**, 103–7.

Naguib, M. and Levy, R. (1982). Prediction of outcome in senile dementia – a computed tomography study. *British Journal of Psychiatry*, **140**, 263–7.

Nielsen, H., Lolk, A., Pedersen, I. *et al.* (1991). The accuracy of early diagnosis and predictors of death in Alzheimer's disease and vascular dementia – a follow-up study. *Acta Psychiatrica Scandinavica*, **84**, 277–82.

O'Connor, D.W., Pollitt, P.A. Hydge, J.B. *et al.* (1988). Do general practitioners miss dementia in elderly patients? *British Medical Journal*, **297**, 1107–10.

Peck, A., Wolloch, L. and Rodstein, M. (1978). Mortality of the aged with chronic brain syndrome: further observations in a five-year study. *Journal of the American Geriatrics Society*, **26**, 170–6.

Post, F. (1951). The outcome of mental breakdown in old age. *British Medical Journal*, **1**, 436–40.

Robinson, J.R. (1989). The natural history of mental disorder in old age – a long-term study. *British Journal of Psychiatry*, **154**, 783–9.

Rorsman, B., Hagnell, O. and Lanke, J. (1985). Mortality and age psychosis in the Lundby study: death risk of senile and multi-infarct dementia. *Neuropsychobiology*, **14**, 13–16.

Roth, M. (1955). The natural history of mental disorder in old age. *Journal of Mental Science*, **101**, 281–301.

Roth, M. and Morrissey, J. (1952). Problems in the diagnosis and classification of mental disorder in old age. *Journal of Mental Science*, **98**, 66–80.

Roth, M., Tym, E., Mountjoy, C.Q. *et al.* (1986). CAMDEX: A standardised instrument for the diagnosis of mental disorder in the elderly, with special reference to the early detection of dementia. *British Journal of Psychiatry*, **149**, 698–709.

Saugstad, L.F. and Odegard, O. (1979). Mortality in psychiatric hospitals in Norway 1950–74. *Acta Psychiatrica Scandinavica*, **59**, 431–47.

Seltzer, B. and Sherwin, I. (1983). A comparison of clinical features in early- and late-onset primary degenerative dementia. *Archives of Neurology*, **40**, 143–6.

Shah, K.V., Banks, G.D. and Merskey, H. (1969). Survival in atherosclerotic and senile dementia. *British Journal of Psychiatry*, **115**, 1283–6.

Thompson, E.G. and Eastwood, M.R. (1981). Survivorship and senile dementia. *Age and Ageing*, **10**, 29–32.

van Dijk, P.T.M., Dippel, D.W.J. and Habbema, J.D.F. (1991). Survival of patients with dementia. *Journal of the American Geriatrics Society*, **39**, 603–10.

Varsamis, J., Zuchowski, T. and Maini, K.K. (1972). Survival rates and causes of death in geriatric psychiatric patients. A six-year follow-up study. *Canadian Psychiatric Association Journal*, **17**, 17–22.

Vitaliano, P.P., Peck, A. and Johnson, D.A. *et al.* (1981). Dementia and other competing risks for mortality in the institutionalised aged. *Journal of the American Geriatrics Society*, **29**, 513–19.

Walsh, J.S., Welch, H.G. and Larson, E.B. (1990). Survival of outpatients with Alzheimer-type dementia. *Annals of Internal Medicine*, **113**, 429–34.

Whitehead, A. and Hunt, A. (1982). Elderly psychiatric patients: a five-year prospective study. *Psychological Medicine*, **12**, 149–57.

Williamson, J., Stokoe, I.H., Gray, S. *et al.* (1964). Old people at home: their unreported needs. *Lancet*, **i**, 1117–20.

Wood, E., Whitefield, E. and Christie, A. (1991). Changes in survival in demented hospital in-patients 1957–87. *International Journal of Geriatric Psychiatry*, **6**, 523–8.

Emile H. Franssen

Aging and Dementia Research Center
Department of Psychiatry
New York University Medical Center

8 NEUROLOGIC SIGNS IN AGEING AND DEMENTIA

INTRODUCTION

Several years ago, an editorial in a leading neurology journal asked the startling question, whether the importance of the detailed neurologic examination is becoming obsolete with the emergence of powerful new imaging techniques (Ziegler, 1985). The defence put forward in favour of the neurologic examination made it clear that a careful neurologic examination reveals abnormal findings in a variety of nervous system diseases in which imaging does not disclose abnormality. Conversely, abnormalities, detected in neuroimaging techniques, are not always reflected in physical abnormalities. The importance of a most sophisticated and most meticulous type of neurologic examination on the contrary increases with the emergence of ever more sensitive techniques of measurements because it needs to match the increasing sensitivities of those machines. The neurologic examination looks for neurologic signs. A neurologic sign is an objective evidence of disordered function. A discussion of neurologic signs in ageing needs to ask the question whether ageing itself is accompanied by neurologic dysfunction and, if so, to what extent is that 'normal'. Where lies the border between involution, that part of the human life-cycle that is characterized by a decline in the normal function of the body and its organs, and disease? The normal stages of development in the infant and child, which depend on the maturation and evolution of the brain and which are characterized by the timely acquisition of function and the simultaneous disappearance of earlier movement patterns, have been well described. The disappearance of developmental reflexes for instance, which heralds a new stage in motor system development, occurs within a specific well-documented period of time. The stages of involution have yet to be described. Onset and progression of involutionary changes vary individually. How should normal ageing be defined? Should it simply be regarded as the mean performance on a set of given tests of a given age? Or should it be defined as the average performance of aged individuals free of known disease and functioning independently? Or should it possibly be defined as equivalent to ideal function for all healthy adults? If for instance one accepts that some degree of pyramidal and extrapyramidal dysfunction is common in the elderly, then these elderly are not normal in the sense of being free of dysfunction. It is then not possible to state at the same time that healthy normal adults commonly display primitive reflexes, because these elderly are not normal in the sense of being free of dysfunction.

This study was supported in part by the US Department of Health and Human Services grants AG-03051, MH-35976, P50 MH43486, MH-43486 and AG-08051. The methodology described herein is the subject of a United States patent No. 5,150,716. International patent pending. The author would like to acknowledge gratefully Liduïn Souren for valuable advice and assistance in preparing the manuscript.

During the process of development of the brain functions in the child, brain plasticity is to a considerable extent sacrificed to increasing specialization and stabilization of brain functions. This leads to a long period of equilibrium and stability of brain function. During the process of involution, plasticity of the brain has declined to the extent that even small losses in function can be less well compensated for. This leads to instability of brain function. In a dementing illness such as Alzheimer's disease, brain plasticity is for the greatest part lost; the compensatory mechanisms fall short. A progressively degenerative process resembling an abnormal and accelerated involution of brain function now appears to recapture the evolution of brain function in reverse. In the ageing human being the borderline between the minimum standard for what can still be considered as normal function and disease-induced abnormality becomes indistinct. The clinician must decide, based on the context in which certain signs appear, whether these signs represent a disease or simple involution.

REFLEXES

The testing of the reflexes has been called the most objective procedure of the neurologic examination. To the clinical neurologist the definition of a reflex is 'any action performed involuntarily as the result of an impulse or an impression which is transmitted along afferent fibres, and then calls into action certain cells, muscles and organs (DeJong, 1979). Given that the peripheral afferent and efferent fibres are intact, the reflex is a measure of sensory–motor integration within the central nervous system. Alterations in intensity and character of reflexes may be the earliest and most subtle objective signs of disturbance in neurologic, *in casu*, central nervous system function. It is exactly owing to their assumed involuntariness that reflexes have gained their important status in the practice of clinical neurology. Their evaluation requires a minimum of cooperation from the patient. This quality in particular should make them preeminently suited for tracking the course of a progressive dementia such as Alzheimer's disease. However, when reflexes are not consciously controlled, the inference is that they are therefore not significantly influenced by cortical activity, at least in so far as this activity involves cognitive processes. This would make these signs not very useful as early markers of Alzheimer's disease, an illness which initially involves mainly the hippocampus, entorhinal cortex, temporoparietal cortex and to a lesser extent the frontal association cortex. The possible usefulness of reflexes for diagnosing and staging dementia will be examined for deep tendon reflexes, cutaneous reflexes and primitive reflexes.

DEEP TENDON REFLEXES

The term deep tendon reflexes is actually a misnomer, and its widespread use demonstrates how misconceptions continue to persevere in professional parlance. Around the turn of the century it was believed that these reflexes were elicited by stimulation of receptors in the tendon, hence the term tendon reflexes. Wartenberg in his 1945 classic monograph 'The examination of reflexes: a simplification', proposed the denomination 'deep reflexes' when it had become evident that the receptors for these reflexes were the muscle spindles which are located inside the muscles and which are activated by a short-lasting sudden stretching. The correct name for these reflexes is therefore muscle stretch reflexes. Because of its widespread usage, however, the term deep tendon reflexes will be used here. The character and intensity of these reflexes change with the continuing growth and maturation of the sensorimotor system, and adult responses, which begin to emerge approximately 6 to 8 years after birth, are well developed in the 12-year-old child. However, even in the healthy adult, deep tendon reflexes are not stable entities, but they fluctuate under various conditions in their intensity. Consequently, variability of deep tendon reflexes under special circumstances is a normal physiological phenomenon (Stam and Tan, 1987). It has for instance been demonstrated, that voluntary contraction of muscle in remote parts increases the vigorousness of deep tendon reflexes (Delwaide and Toulouse, 1981). Mental activity such as motor preparation (Brunia and Vuister, 1979) or a voluntary mental effort to alter a reflex response, can also increase the briskness of deep tendon reflexes (Stam and Speelman, 1989). Hence increasing evidence is emerging that deep tendon reflexes are influenced by cortical mechanisms which also govern voluntary activity and cognition. This could have important consequences for the study of deep tendon reflex changes in dementia research.

Because the vigorousness of reflexes shows considerable individual variation, there exists no golden standard for normality with respect to their degree of activity. Nevertheless, very vigorous reflexes suggest central nervous system pathology while very low to absent reflexes are associated with peripheral pathology. Slight asymmetry of reflexes is also not uncommon in normal adults and does not necessarily imply serious pathology. Extension of the stimulus zone over which a reflex can be elicited, or irradiation of a reflex response to a neighbouring joint or even to an opposite extremity do also not necessarily always have an implication of pathology when they occur in a symmetric fashion. These characteristics do however provide measures of excitability by which the activity and vigorousness of a reflex can be rated. As such they are useful as indicators of change in activity over a period of time. Currently there exists no generally accepted scale which measures the activity of deep tendon reflexes. Their evaluation is often based on dichotomous clinical judgment. Neurologists sometimes grade them 0 = absent; + = present but diminished; ++ = normal; +++ = increased but not necessarily to a pathologic degrees, and ++++ = markedly hyperactive, often with associated clonus. Another scale sometimes used is the Mayo Clinic Scale which uses nine points, from −4 (absent) through zero (normal) up to +4 (clonus).

DEEP TENDON REFLEXES AND AGEING

Early reports of a decrease in the activity of deep tendon reflexes in healthy elderly subjects have generally not been substantiated by more recent studies. A decrease in ankle jerk activity with ageing which has been commonly cited, but has recently been refuted (Impallomeni et al., 1984). That deep tendon reflexes do not lose their vigorousness in the healthy aged has also been supported by quantitative measurements; patellar tendon reflexes were, on the contrary, found to be brisker in healthy active older adults compared to young individuals (Kamen and Koceja, 1989).

DEEP TENDON REFLEXES AND DEMENTIA

Prominent reflex asymmetry is a sign of focal neurologic dysfunction. Consequently it is associated more in particular with vascular dementia, especially multi-infarct dementia, where abnormal and asymmetric deep tendon reflexes are also likely to occur at a relatively early stage of cognitive decline. In prensenile dementia, increased deep tendon reflexes have been reported to occur in 20% of patients (Liston, 1979). Huff *et al.* (1987) found increased deep tendon reflexes in 10.5% of patients with Alzheimer's disease, while asymmetric deep tendon reflexes occurred in 3% of Alzheimer patients, an incidence not significantly different from in normal aged controls. Davous *et al.* (1989) reported an absence of ankle jerk reflexes in 33% of Alzheimer patients. Galasko *et al.* (1990) found no significant differences in incidence of abnormal deep tendon reflexes in patients with mild and moderately severe Alzheimer's disease compared to normal controls. Burns *et al.* (1991) reported unequal deep tendon reflexes in 4% of Alzheimer patients during their initial evaluation. These authors observed an increase of 8% in the incidence of asymmetric deep tendon reflexes in the same group of patients over a 12-month follow-up period.

In some of these studies the reflexes were rated on nonstandardized low-grade scales. With the exception of the last study, change of reflex activity over time, or with progression of cognitive or functional deterioration, was not reported. Our own findings will be discussed below.

SUPERFICIAL REFLEXES OR CUTANEOUS REFLEXES

These reflexes are elicited by the application of a stimulus to the skin or mucous membrane. The receptors for this category of reflexes lie in the skin or in the mucous membranes. The response is more slow than in the deep tendon reflexes and tends to fatigue after a relatively small number of repeated stimuli. After a short waiting period they can then again be elicited. The response is dependent on the amount of pressure exerted: too noxious a stimulus may call forth a defence reaction. Dissociation of reflexes, i.e. an absence of superficial reflexes in the presence of hyperactive deep tendon reflexes is often, but not invariably, seen in pyramidal tract disease. Superficial reflexes may sometimes be increased in extrapyramidal system dysfunction and certain superficial reflexes may be increased in states of anxiety and tension. The more commonly tested superficial reflexes are the abdominal reflexes, the cremaster reflex, the gluteal reflex, and the plantar reflex. The palmar reflex, which also is a superficial reflex, consists of flexion of the fingers in response to gentle stroking of the hand palm; it is generally considered as a pathologic response. As such, it is also known as the grasp reflex and will also be discussed with the primitive reflexes. The palmomental reflex also belongs to this category but will be discussed with the primitive reflexes. Little research has been done with regard to an alteration of most of these reflexes with ageing, although a decrease in abdominal reflexes has been reported. The plantar reflex or plantar response is probably the most eminent procedure of the neurologic examination.

THE PLANTAR RESPONSE

Despite its fame there are some misconceptions surrounding this reflex. They have been discussed by van Gijn (1977) and are summarized here. The normal response to the stimulus consists of a fairly rapid plantar flexion of the toes and foot. The abnormal response, the Babinski sign, consists of an extension of the great toe, somewhat confusingly called dorsiflexion. It is essential that the dorsiflexion of the big toe is associated with a noticable contraction of the extensor hallucis longus muscle, which can almost always be seen or palpated along the lateral border of the tibia. It is also essential that the dorsiflexion of the great toe is associated with a contraction of the knee flexors and the hip flexors, which not necessarily needs to lead to a visible movement of the leg. It is important furthermore to distinguish a spinal reaction, which is pathological, from a fright reaction, which is not pathological. In a true spinal reaction, the reflex response is proportional to the strength of the stimulus. In a fright reaction, the response often varies with the same stimulus strength. The fanning of the toes is not a necessary requirement for a positive Babinski reflex. Also, the dorsiflexion of the great toe does not necessarily have to be slow. Elication of the reflex is performed by moving a blunt point such as a broken tongue blade, a key or the stem of the reflex hammer along the lateral border of the sole of the foot, from the heel forward on to the ball of the foot. It may be necessary to continue along the ball of the foot from the little to the great toe. Stimulation of the space in between the ball of the foot and the toes should be avoided, lest a false pathological reflex might occur. The stimulus should be as light as possible so as to avoid a fright reaction, but tickling may cause voluntary withdrawal. Wherever possible, the patient should be warned not to withdraw his or her leg. Slight pressure on the ball of the foot alone may in pathological conditions elicit a foot grasp reflex (see primitive reflexes) and should be avoided. It is also important that during the examination the legs are fully relaxed and to this purpose should rest on a solid underlayer, while the leg is uncovered. In general, reflexes should be tested under uniform circumstances in a quiet environment with comfortable room temperature.

The dorsiflexion of the great toe is actually a part of the flexor reflex. This reflex is stronger and faster in the infant and dorsiflexion of the toes is a normal part of the flexor reflex until approximately 12 to 24 months after birth. Thereafter the dorsiflexion response of the great toe is gradually changed to a plantar flexion. The flexor response of the knee and hip also gradually diminishes and is in most normal adults barely visible.

No significant changes in plantar response have been reported with consistency in normal ageing. A positive Baninski reflex is always pathological. When encountered bilaterally and accompanied by hyperactive symmetric deep tendon reflexes and a normally active jaw jerk reflex, the elderly patient most often has significant cervical spondylosis. Other causes should be suspected when cervical spine roentgenograms are normal (Jenkyn, 1989).

Jenkyn et al. (1977) found an abnormal plantar response not to be significantly associated with mild or moderate diffuse cortical impairment. The presence of an extensor plantar reflex is more commonly associated with vascular dementia, in particular when the dementia is of mild or moderate severity. Huff et al. (1987) found an abnormal plantar response in approximately 5% of mildly demented patients with Alzheimer's disease, a percentage similar to that found in the normal control group. Davous et al. (1989) elicited a definite Babinski sign in 4% of patients with Alzheimer-type senile dementia and Galasko et al. (1990) found a Babinski sign in 9% of patients with mild and moderately severe Alzheimer's disease compared to 6% in control subjects.

Burns et al. (1991) found a frequency of 3.4% in patients with Alzheimer's disease at the time of the initial examination. At 12-months follow up, 5.3% of patients had extensor plantar reflexes. These patients tended to have a significantly greater ventricular–brain ratio. Abnormal plantar responses do not appear to be significantly associated with mild or moderately severe Alzheimer's disease, but there is some evidence that the frequency of extensor plantar response may increase with severity of dementia. Franssen et al. (1991b) found extensor plantar reflexes in 15% of severely demented Alzheimer patients. Recently obtained data by Franssen *et al.* indicate that the prevalence of an extensor plantar sign is much higher in severe stage dementia, where patients are unable to ambulate, probably as high as 45% (Franssen *et al.*, 1993).

PRIMITIVE REFLEXES

Primitive reflexes are stereotype motor responses to specific external stimuli which occur in patients with diffuse cortical dysfunction. Primitive reflexes appear in neurologic conditions such as the diencephalic stage of the central syndrome of rostral–caudal deterioration in the evolution of coma resulting from supratentorial lesions. They occur transitorily in metabolic encephalopathies and in acute psychosis. Their teleology is not clear and most of these signs have eluded attempts to associate them with anatomical localizations. They resemble developmental reflexes, i.e. the typical motor responses which are present in the neonate and the infant during the early stages of brain maturation. Primitive reflexes are also called release signs, because it is assumed that they originate from the activity of subcortical structures which are released from cortical inhibitory influences. The adjective 'frontal', which is sometimes used in conjunction with this latter term, indicates that it is believed that the frontal lobe cortex in particular has an inhibitory influence on the manifestation of these signs. This has actually been demonstrated for the grasp reflex which occurs contralaterally with focal lesions of the frontal lobe. But in general, primitive reflexes are usually considered to be signs of diffuse brain dysfunction. Foetal, neonatal, developmental, archaic or primary reflexes (frontal) release signs, primitive reflexes, cortical disinhibition signs and neurological soft signs are often all bracketed together as one category. The first five designations are used to indicate the age-specific motor responses which occur in the young infant, and which disappear with erect stance and gait. In paediatric neurology those responses serve as undisputed markers of normal development and maturation of the central nervous system. The adjective 'primitive' has a connotation of regression and is a vestige of the days when a strictly hierarchical concept of brain functions was still prevalent (Touwen, 1984). Schaltenbrand was probably the first one to use the term primitive reflexes to denote certain motor phenomena which he observed in infants and which resembled behaviour seen in experimentally brain-damaged mid-brain animals. The implication was that the normal infant's brain, compared to that of the human adult, and even to that of the normal full-grown animal was inferior, primitive and not yet inhibited by the cerebral cortex; i.e. in essence, it was a subcortically functioning structure. Buckley probably introduced the term primitive reflexes first into the English literature 'to designate a mechanism by which a particular type of response is brought about by the activity of either a single nervous arc or several nervous arcs, such reflexes as have been observed in embryonic and later life in lower forms of animals and in human beings' (Buckley, 1927). It had occurred to him that there existed striking similarities between these normal behaviours which could be observed in the embryo, during infancy and early childhood and certain reactions which could be seen in psychosis and advanced dementia. The volitional responses could be entirely absent while there existed no demonstrable paralysis. He stated that with advancement in the functional development of the individual, inhibitory functions gradually emerged; 'neural excitations which were capable of neutralizing or counteracting the effect of an excitation which normally would bring about the response in question' (i.e. the primitive reflex). Buckley mentioned specifically the swallowing and sucking reflexes elicited by the application of tactile stimuli, the sucking response evoked by visual stimuli, the pouting reaction, the grasping reflex of the hand and the 'primitive dominance of the flexor reflex responses'. He concluded that 'in general, it may be stated that the reflexes appearing earliest in the order of functional development are apt to be the last to disappear in the process of functional disintegration. In similar manner, the last reflexes to be acquired are likely to disappear early in the course of the dementia'. Buckley's observations were concerned with responses that could be 'examined without depending upon the patient's statements for any part of the explanation of the symptoms in question'. The cooperation of the patient who needs to comprehend and act upon instructions was thus not a prerequisite. The original assumption that the infant brain is a reflex organism, functioning at the mid-brain or diencephalon level, is not supported any more by modern studies (Touwen, 1984). A healthy infant's brain with its high degree of plasticity can not be compared to a damaged adult's brain. Furthermore, there is now some evidence, for instance, that corticospinal and corticobulbar tracts do already mediate some motor functions in the human newborn (Sarnat, 1989), and that the developmental reflexes are modified by, and possibly in tandem with, myelination of these tracts and with the development of the cerebral cortex in a specific manner. This leads to their integration into volitional behaviour. The primitive reflexes, however, which accompany the involution of brain function and the subsequent loss of volitional behaviour are stereotypic and pathological and only show a phenomenological similarity to the developmental reflexes which occur in the healthy infant. If the developmental reflexes can be utilized as markers of normal brain development, one could hypothesize that primitive reflexes might also be useful as markers of the process of cerebral involution, in particular in those cases where involution appears to recapture evolution in reverse.

The utilization of primitive reflexes as diagnostic markers for dementia gained more prominence in the sixties, after de Ajuriaguerra *et al.* (1963) described the reoccurrence of oral reflexes in dementia and found these to be especially frequent in severe Alzheimer's disease, where their intensity changed with progression of the disease. Paulson and Gottlieb (1968) wrote their now classic paper in an effort to link these special responses as seen in aged demented patients to those seen during normal development. They stated that these signs are best considered as a group of related responses rather than as individual reflexes, and they presumed that these responses are probably repeatedly represented in the central nervous system and might be exposed by imbalances at more than one area and by destruction at more than one site. As such, they believed, it would be unlikely that exact pathological correlates of any of these reflexes may ever be found, and indeed may not be the same, in different patients. In all, they arbitrarily selected seven inter-related reflexes which were present in many senile persons: the sucking reflex, the snout reflex, gegenhalten or paratonia, the palmomental reflex, the hand grasp and foot grasp reflexes, the corneomandibular reflex and inappropriate associated movements. They concluded on the basis of a series of 85 aged patients carrying the diagnosis 'chronic brain syndrome', that the reappearance of these developmental reflexes in these aged patients is almost always attributable to diffuse, bilateral and irreversible central nervous system disease. Since the publication of Paulson and Gottlieb's paper, more than a dozen studies have been published on the occurrence of primitive reflexes in dementia and in particular in Alzheimer's disease. The more recent of these studies have also included mostly small groups of normal aged controls. The results of these studies will be briefly summarized, but first a description of the more commonly examined reflexes will be given:

1. *The hand grasp reflex* is elicited by a distal moving contact in the palm of the hand of the patient from proximal toward distal, while the patient where possible is requested not to do anything. The response is flexion of the fingers with adduction of the thumb and grasping of the stimulus. The reflex is present in the neonate and has disappeared in most children around the twelfth month of age. It should not be confused with a traction response, which occurs secondary to stretching of the fingers of the patient.

2. *The foot grasp reflex or tonic foot response* is elicted by direct mild pressure upon the ball of the foot or the toes. The response is flexion and adduction of the toes and sometimes incurving of the foot. It is present in the neonate and disappears at approximately 12 months of age.

3. *Paratonia or gegenhalten* is an often inconstant, sudden increase in muscle tone of an extremity as a response to passive irregular movement. It does not have a cogwheel quality and is in contrast to lead pipe rigidity not consistently present over the entire range of motion. The hypertonicity occurs in both agonists and antagonists. Paratonia is elicited by rapid irregular passive movements of the extremity by the examiner, while the patient may or may not be urged to 'relax'. Paratonia is usually not elicited when the extremity is moved in a slow, regular and gentle manner.

4. *The sucking reflex* consists of the appearance of sucking mouth movements in response to gentle stroking of the lips with the finger or a tongue blade, which is grasped by the lips. Sometimes the patient may attempt to follow the stimulus with pursed lips, and smacking and chewing movements may occur. Once it has been grasped by the teeth, biting of the stimulus may also occur. In addition to the tactile-elicited sucking reflex, which in the infant lasts until 3 or 4 months of age, there exists also a visual sucking reflex. Here, the tongue blade is moved towards the mouth of the patient and this visual stimulus elicits opening of the mouth and sucking or licking movements with lips and tongue, without the tongue blade actually touching the lips.

5. *The tactile rooting reflex* is elicited by stroking the corners of the mouth or the perioral area with a tongue blade. This results in turning of the head towards the stimulus and grasping it with the lips. It has been said that presence of this reflex suggests more loss of inhibition than does a snout or sucking reflex. The reflex disappears between the fourth and seventh months in the normal infant. A variant elicited by a visual stimulus also exists.

6. *The snout or pouting reflex* consists of a puckering or protrusion of the lips in response to a gentle tap with the finger or reflex hammer to the philtrum, the area above the upper lips, or by applying quick pressure with the knuckle, to the area above the upper lip, below the nose.

7. *The glabellar blink reflex* (syn. orbicularis oculi reflex) consists of the blinking of both eyes in response to a slight quick tap with the finger to the root of the nose between the eyebrows. Care must be taken that the patient is unable to see the approaching finger, because otherwise a menace reflex will result. The complex ontogeny of this reflex has been described in detail (Zametkin *et al.*, 1979). A mature response is reached in the 12-year-old child.

8. *The palmomental reflex or palm-chin reflex* is elicited by a brisk mildly noxious stroke of a key or other blunt instrument on the thenar eminence of the palm of the hand from proximal to distal, and consists of a twitch of the ipsilateral mentalis muscle of the chin which may be accompanied by ipsilateral protrusion and elevation of the lower lip.

9. *The corneomandibular reflex* is elicited by gentle backward pressure of the gloved index finger on the cornea of the eye. The result is slight opening of the jaw with a slight lateral and downward movement of the jaw to the contralateral side.

10. *The nuchocephalic reflex* of Jenkyn *et al.* is elicited by rotating the standing patient by the shoulders, preferentially with his eyes closed. Normally, the head of the patient follows the direction of the shoulders after a brief lag. The reflex is positive when the head does not follow the shoulders or when it turns in block with the shoulders. In the child it disappears around the fourth year.

Some of these reflexes are more complex motor responses and involve the cooperation of several muscles, such as the sucking reflex, the grasp reflexes and the rooting reflex. Other reflexes involve the contraction of one muscle: the orbicularis oris muscle in the snout reflex, the orbicularis oculi muscle on both sides in the glabellar blink reflex and the mentalis muscle in the palmomental reflex. Some reflexes have a 'prehensile' or grasping character such as the grasp reflexes of hand and foot, and, in a sense the sucking reflex of the lips. Some reflexes are considered to be nociceptive in character, such as the glabellar blink reflex, the snout reflex and the palmomental reflex, all of which are elicited by a potentially harmful stimulus. Some reflexes, in addition to their association with diffuse brain damage, are also sometimes associated with dysfunction of a particular system, such as the glabellar blink reflex with dysfunction of the nigrostriatal dopaminergic system in Parkinson's disease and in some forms of parkinsonism. The hand and foot grasp reflexes and paratonia, besides occurring in diffuse brain damage, can also be observed in focal brain lesions of the frontal lobe. The hand grasp reflex, paratonia, the snout reflex and the palmomental reflex have also been observed with pyramidal tract lesions.

One argument brought forward against the usefulness of primitive reflexes in the diagnosis of dementia is their occurrence in normal aged individuals. Few special studies involving large groups of subjects have yet been conducted. The largest study hitherto conducted on the occurrence of primitive reflexes in normal ageing is that of Jenkyn *et al.* (1985) on 2029 elderly volunteers 50 to 93 years of age. The primitive reflexes tested in that study were the nuchocephalic reflex, the glabellar blink reflex, the snout reflex and paratonia. These investigators tested in addition vertical gaze, visual pursuit, reverse spelling and memory recall. They found the rates of abnormal responses to remain constant until the age of 70 years after which there occurred a significant increase of abnormal responses for all the signs examined, while at the same there also occurred an increase in number of abnormal signs per subject. Memory word recall however was an exception; it did not become increasingly more abnormal until the age of 80 years. All subjects were free of psychiatric and neurologic disease, but they did not receive more extensive formal cognitive testing. The authors concluded from the statistical methods employed that several signs frequently occurred in associated pairs which did vary together with increasing age, and that a common factor thus was responsible for the variation. Tweedy *et al.* (1982), who had previously investigated primitive reflexes in patients with dementia, had not found strong pair wise linkages. From this they concluded that individual signs are independent and that it is unlikely that any of these signs is produced by a deeper or more severe version of the lesion that produces some other sign. The interesting finding in the study of Jenkyn *et al.* (1985) is that primitive reflexes and other signs of subtle neurologic dysfunction preceded signs of memory recall by 10 years. When this occurs in normal ageing, the appearance of primitive reflexes and other signs of subtle neurologic dysfunction prior to evidence of cognitive impairment might also occur in abnormal ageing and serve as a predictor and marker of cognitive decline in dementia. More than a dozen papers on the possible usefulness of primitive reflexes as predictors and markers of dementia, in particular Alzheimer's disease, have been published since Paulson and Gottlieb's classic study (Table 8.1). Some but not all of these studies did include a normal control group. No unanimity exists amongst all these investigators with respect to the significance of the individual primitive reflexes as useful diagnostic markers, although the general impression is that these signs are not early markers of Alzheimer's disease. Considerable variance also exists in reported prevalence of primitive reflexes in age-matched control subjects in these studies (Table 8.1). The extent to which neuropsychological evaluation of the studied subjects was performed, as well as the method and the degree of clinical staging of dementia severity varies in many studies. Jenkyn *et al.* (1977) found these signs to be useful predictors of diffuse cerebral dysfunction. Basavaraju *et al.* (1987) found only the palmomental reflex and the grasp reflex to be helpful in discriminating between patients with senile dementia of the Alzheimer type and elderly patients with hemiplegia associated with cerebral vascular accident. Tweedy *et al.* (1982) found that only the snout reflex and the grasp reflex correlated with impaired performance on cognitive testing in patients with dementia of various aetiologies. Sucking and rooting reflexes were associated only with the terminal phase of dementia. In their study, primitive reflexes in general were more strongly correlated with evidence of ventricular dilatation than with cortical atrophy. Koller *et al.* (1983) found an abnormal glabellar blink reflex to be more common in demented patients with presumed Alzheimer's disease than in normal controls, but found no significant difference in prevalence of any primitive reflex and presence of cerebral atrophy on the computed tomographic (CT) scan or of abnormal psychometric tests. Huff and Growdon (1986) assessed suck, snout, grasp and palmomental reflexes in four subgroups of patients with increasingly severe Alzheimer's disease and found these signs, with exemption of the palmomental reflex, to be significantly associated with dementia severity, regardless of age. Huff *et al.* (1987) found primitive reflexes in patients with Alzheimer's disease and in control subjects, with prevalences of 55 and 9% respectively. They examined the glabellar blink, snout, palmomental and grasp reflexes. Their population did not include severely demented patients with Mini-Mental State Examination scores of less than 10 out of 30. Bakchine *et al.* (1989) found the presence of snout, sucking and grasp reflexes to correlate significantly with the severity of cognitive impairment and with presence of extrapyramidal signs. No correlation was found in their study between occurrence of primitive reflexes and age, depression or drug therapy. Davous *et al.* (1989) looked at reflex grasping, the snout reflex, the palmomental reflex and a persistent glabellar blink reflex in a standardized neurological examination of patients with senile dementia of the Alzheimer type (SDAT). They found gait abnormalities in 57%. Only the grasp reflex and rigidity, mainly paratonia, correlated with the gait abnormality. Girling and Berrios (1990) found the grasp reflex, glabellar blink reflex and snout reflex to correlate well with scores for extrapyramidal signs (EPS), whereas scores for EPS correlated well with scores for (impaired) cognitive function in patients with SDAT. Galasko *et al.* (1990) studied snout, sucking, grasp and glabellar blink reflexes in patients with Alzheimer's disease; only the grasp reflex correlated significantly with the degree of cognitive impairment.

Table 8.1 Frequency of primitive reflexes in dementia and normal ageing.

Reference	N	Grasp	Snout	Palmomental	Suck	Glab.	Plantar	Paratonia
Paulson and Gottlieb (1968)	85	18	52	21	53	N.A.	N.A.	29
Villeneuve et al. (1974)	56	25	79	61	39	N.A.	N.A.	50
Jenkyn et al. (1977)	75	(0)	(11)	(6)	(0)	(29)	N.A.	(6)
Kokmen et al. (1977)	51	(7)	(31)	(41)	N.A.	N.A.	N.A.	N.A.
Basavaraju et al. (1981)	50	34	70	60	N.A.	N.A.	N.A.	N.A.
		(0)	(36)	(34)				
Tweedy et al. (1982)	32	17	19	47	3	79	N.A.	57
Koller et al. (1983)	52	2	54	N.A.	N.A.	23	N.A.	N.A.
		(0)	(54)			(8)		
Bakchine et al. (1989)	91	5	33	33	8	19	N.A.	N.A.
Davous et al. (1989)	75	24	31	27	N.A.	23	4	28
Molloy et al. (1991)	207	18	25	28	4	N.A.	N.A.	N.A.
Galasko et al. (1991)	135	17	46	N.A.	21	27	9	N.A.
Burns et al. (1991)	178	7	41	2	N.A.	N.A.	4	N.A.

The numbers in parentheses indicate percentages of primitive reflexes in normal aged subjects.
N.A. = not applicable (no frequency listed for this reflex).

Risse *et al.* (1990) found paratonia in 86% in a group of longitudinally followed Alzheimer patients. Molloy *et al.* (1991) found that Alzheimer patients with snout, sucking, grasp and palmomental reflexes had more severe impairment of the functions of activities of daily living (ADL) and dysfunctional behaviour for an equal level of cognitive function than patients without these signs. Burns *et al.* (1991) found a grasp reflex and EPS to be associated with severe cognitive impairment; EPS were associated with increased third ventricular size and with basal ganglia calcification, while the grasp reflex was associated with frontal lobe atrophy on CT scan. In their study, 7% of patients developed a grasp reflex during a 12-month follow-up. These patients were more cognitively impaired and had greater lateral ventricular size than those patients who did not develop the reflex. In summary, data from these studies show that prevalence of primitive reflexes increases with dementia severity in Alzheimer's disease while the grasp, rooting and sucking reflexes are associated mainly with the more severe stages of the illness, and these particular reflexes are thus definitely not useful as early neurologic markers of dementia in Alzheimer's disease. Increased prevalence of primitive reflexes is also associated with the presence of extrapyramidal symptomatology and with impaired functionality in Alzheimer's disease. No primitive reflexes in particular are specific for Alzheimer's disease or are by themselves useful as early markers of the disease. It should be emphasized that these signs derive their significance from the specific context within which they are placed. The finding of one primitive reflex in a healthy individual is obviously not significant. However, if it could be shown that there is a specific sequential pattern of specific primitive reflexes in specific diseases, such as Alzheimer's disease, these signs may become more interesting, both as diagnostic and as research tools.

In our own laboratory, reflexes are studied as part of a standardized comprehensive neurologic examination in patients with progressive cognitive decline and in normal control subjects. In order to assess possible changes in activity of deep tendon reflexes, plantar responses and primitive reflexes with progressive cognitive impairment, a semiquantitative seven-point scale was developed (Franssen *et al.*, 1991b) for rating the presence and changes in activity of these signs, even when subtle. Points 1, 3, 5 and 7 are well defined; points 2, 4 and 6 are intermediate scores. Increased activity of deep tendon reflexes was measured in terms of increased briskness, amplitude, clonus, extent of the stimulus zone within which a reflex could be elicited and irradiation of the reflex response activity over neighbouring joints. This latter criterion for hyperactivity was especially useful in severe stage Alzheimer patients, in whom classic responses of, for instance, the knee jerk reflex could sometimes no longer be obtained because of contractures of the joints. For elicitation of the deep tendon reflexes, i.e. the right and left biceps, triceps, quadriceps (knee jerk) and gastrocnemius-soleus (ankle jerk) reflexes and for the right and left plantar responses, standard methodology was employed. These reflexes were elicited with the patient in a sitting position. Examination of the plantar reflex was carried out while the exposed leg rested on a supporting underlayer. The sitting position proved to be the easiest way to examine the reflexes in both ambulant and nonambulant patients. Also, more severely demented patients often had difficulty with climbing on an examination table and seemed often more at ease and cooperative when sitting in a comfortable chair. Paratonia, the grasp reflexes of the hand and foot, the tactile and visual sucking reflexes and the palmomental reflex were elicited according to the methodology of Paulson and Gottlieb, described earlier in this chapter. The precise methodology used for the elicitation of the reflexes and for scoring

Table 8.2 Semiquantitative neurologic assessment methods

Seven-point rating scale for the examination of reflexes and release signs*

I. Deep tendon reflexes (muscle stretch reflexes)

biceps,

triceps,

quadriceps (knee jerk),

gastrocnemius-soleus or triceps surae (ankle jerk).

Elicitation: tap with a rubber reflex hammer. The examiner places his index finger firmly over the tendon of the muscle to be examined near the point of its insertion, and firmly taps his finger with a soft rubber reflex hammer. Extension of the stimulus zone over which the reflex can be elicited is tested by placing one's finger over a point which lies 10 to 15 centimeters from the insertion of the tendon of the muscle to be examined.

Response rating*
1. Normal or decreased briskness of contraction; deflection of the extremity, if any, should be less than approximately 20° and there is no extension of the stimulus zone.
3. Notably increased briskness of contraction with deflection of the extremity of approximately 30° to 40° and extension of the stimulus zone.
5. Prominently increased briskness of contraction, with extension of stimulus zone or prominent extension of the stimulus zone alone.
7. Very prominently increased briskness of contraction, with marked extension of the stimulus zone and with irradiation of the reflex response to muscles other than that whose tendon is percussed, resulting in simultaneous contraction of adjacent joints, a multiple reflex and/or non-exhaustible clonus may occur. For contracted joints: marked extension of the stimulus zone and irradiation, of the reflex response resulting in contraction of adjacent joints or occurrence of a multiple reflex.

II. Plantar response

Elicitation: blunt point such as a wooden applicator, moving with as little pressure as needed, over the lateral plantar surface, from the heel towards the ball of the foot, with the knee extended whenever possible and the leg resting on a flat surface. The reflex should be tested at least three times before the response is scored.

Response rating*
1. Plantar flexion of the great toe.
3. No distinct flexion or extension of the great toe; indistinct and inconsistent, rapid dorsiflexion of the great toe, not proportional to the stimulus, may occur.
5. Distinct and consistent dorsiflexion of the great toe which is proportional to the stimulus, with noticeable simultaneous contraction of the flexors of the leg.
7. Prominent dorsiflexion of the great toe proportional to the stimulus, often with fanning of the other toes, and with prominent contraction of the flexors of the leg. A spinal defence reflex may occur.

III. Release signs

A. Paratonia (gegenhalten)

Elicitation: passive alternating flexion and extension of the elbow of the patient in 10

Table 8.2 *Continued*

subsequent trials of increasing rapidity and amplitude. The pattern of movement should be sudden and irregular. The sitting patient is quietly asked not to resist, and several trials should be attempted before scoring the response.

Response: a palpable simultaneous contraction of flexors and extensors of the examined extremity, resulting in an involuntary resistance to the movement and a temporary locking of the joint.

Response rating*
1. absent: no paratonia with 10 trials
3. paratonia occurs in 1 to 4 out of 10 trials
5. paratonia occurs in 5 to 9 out of 10 trials
7. paratonia is present on every attempt of passive limb manipulation.

Note: it is necessary before testing an extremity for presence of paratonia, to move the extremity first in a slow, regular and gentle fashion in order to register presence of plastic (lead pipe) rigidity or cogwheel rigidity, on which paratonia may be superimposed.

B. Prehensile Release Signs

1. Sucking reflex (tactile)

Elicitation: 15 seconds of continuous gentle stroking of the lips with a tongue blade, per trial.
Response: sucking movements of the mouth.

Response rating*
1. Absent: no response at all.
3. Slight parting and protrusion of the lips, but lips do not actually grasp the stimulus.
5. Lips grasp the stimulus, followed by distinct sucking movements, and sometimes with licking, chewing or swallowing.
7. Very prominent and persistent sucking – the protruded lips will follow the stimulus when it is withdrawn – licking, chewing, swallowing, and biting of the stimulus often occurs.

2. Sucking reflex (visual)
Elicitation: a clearly visible object, such as a tongue blade, is slowly moved within the visual field of the subject towards the mouth of the subject for 15 seconds, without actually touching the lips.
Response: sucking movements of the mouth.

Response rating*
1. Absent: no response at all.
3. Slight parting and protrusion of the lips in response to the approaching visual stimulus, but lips do not attempt to grasp the stimulus.
5. The head is moved towards the stimulus and the lips grasp the approaching stimulus, followed by distinct sucking movements, and sometimes with licking, chewing or swallowing.
7. Very prominent and persistent sucking occurs; the head moves towards the stimulus which is grasped by the lips; the protruded lips follow the stimulus

Table 8.2   *Continued*

when it is withdrawn; licking, chewing, swallowing and biting of the stimulus often occur.

3. Hand grasp reflex

Elicitation: 15 seconds gentle stroking with one's finger of the hand palm and palmar surface of the fingers, from proximal towards distal, while the patient is quietly distracted and asked to remain inactive. Care should be taken not to exert traction upon the fingers.
Response: grasping movement of the hand and fingers.

Response rating*

1. Absent: no response at all.
3. Flexion of the fingers, and abduction with or without flexion of the thumb, with occasional brief grasping of the stimulus.
5. Distinct grasping of the stimulus; the grasping increases when an attempt is made to extricate the fingers.
7. Trapping of the stimulus, with or without groping after stimulus; grasping is persistent and may be clonic, extrication of the fingers is possible only with considerable difficulty.

4. Foot grasp reflex (tonic foot response)

Elicitation: 15 seconds of slight to moderate pressure to the ball of the foot or the plantar surface of the toes.
Response: grasping movement of the toes.

Response rating*

1. Absent: no response at all.
3. Slight plantar flexion of the toes in response to stimulus.
5. Distinct plantar flexion and adduction of the toes.
7. Persistent prominent tonic plantar flexion and adduction of the toes with arching of the foot.

5. Rooting reflex

Elicitation: 15 second of gentle stroking of the corner of the mouth or the adjacent cheek with the finger or a tongue blade.
Response: turning of the head towards the stimulus.

Response rating*

1. Absent: no response at all.
3. Slight movement of the lips and slight turning of the head towards the stimulus.
5. Head distinctly turns towards stimulus, the lips may part.
7. Head turns prominently towards the stimulus and the lips grasp the stimulus; sucking may occur.

C. Nociceptive release signs

1. Snout reflex

Elicitation: slight but brisk tapping over the upper lip, with the tip of the flexed finger, with a rate of 1 tap per second and repeated 10 times.
Note: in patients with a positive visual sucking reflex, the eyes are covered before the stimulus is applied.
Response: pursing of the lips.

Table 8.2 *Continued*

Response rating*
1. Absent: no response at all.
3. Slight brief puckering or protrusion of the lips, occurs less than 5 times in response to 10 subsequent stimuli.
5. Distinct puckering or protrusion of the lips which does not habituate with 5 to 10 subsequent stimuli.
7. Prominent and continuous protrusion of the lips in response to each stimulus, with extension of the stimulus zone – no habituation occurs.

2. Glabellar (blink) refex
Elicitation: repeated slight and brief tapping of the glabella, between the eyebrows, with the tip of the flexed finger, with a rate of 1 tap per second, and repeated 20 times.
Note: the examiner's finger approaches the patient from above the forehead, outside the visual field, in order to avoid a menace reflex; several trials are made without actually touching the glabella and no blinking should occur then.
Response: blinking of both eyes.

Response rating*
1. 0 to 5 blinks in response to 20 subsequent stimuli.
3. 5 to 10 blinks in response to 20 subsequent stimuli.
5. 10 to 20 blinks in response to 20 subsequent stimuli.
7. 20 or more blinks, no habituation in response to 20 subsequent stimuli; extension of stimulus zone over the forehead or beyond.

9. Palmomental reflex (palm-chin reflex)
Elicitation: scratching over thenar eminence of the hand with a blunt point, such as a key, from distal towards proximal with a rate of 1 scratch per second, while applying moderate pressure.
Response: contraction of the ipsilateral mentalis muscle.

Response rating*
1. Absent: no response at all.
3. Habituation occurs after 1 to 5 slight contractions of the ipsilateral mentalis muscle in response to 10 subsequent stimuli.
5. Habituation occurs after 5 to 10 distinct contractions of the ipsilateral mentalis muscle in response to 10 subsequent stimuli; some elevation and protrusion of the ipsilateral lower lip occurs.
7. No habituation occurs after 10 subsequent stimuli; distinct elevation of the ipsilateral lower lip occurs; extension of the stimulus zone outside the palm of the hand occurs.

---

* In situations falling between the four well-defined points 1, 3, 5 and 7, intermediate numerical scores 2, 4 and 6 are used.
©Copyright 1993 by Emile H. Franssen, M.D. and Barry Reisberg, M.D.

the responses on the seven-point rating scale is depicted in Table 8.2. For all bilaterally elicited reflexes (i.e. biceps, triceps, quadriceps, gastrocnemius-soleus, plantar response, paratonia, grasp reflexes, rooting reflexes and pal-momental reflexes) the highest of the two scores obtained was always entered.

In addition to these individual reflexes, five measures consisting of combinations of these individual reflexes were studied. These combination or summary measures were: all deep tendon reflexes, plantar responses and primitive reflexes (release signs) as one measure; all deep tendon reflexes combined as one measure; all individual primitive reflexes (release signs) combined as one measure (paratonia, although usually regarded as a release sign, was not included in this measure); all five release signs with either a manual or oral prehensile character combined as one measure and including the hand and foot grasp reflexes, the tactile and visual sucking reflexes and the rooting reflex; and all three release signs whose elicitation has a potentially threatening or disagreeable character, collectively labelled nociceptive release signs, and including the snout reflex, the glabellar blink reflex and the palmomental reflex combined as one measure. A summary measure was given a score of 3 when any of its constituents yielded a score of 3 or greater on the neurologic rating scale. The score of the constituent individual reflex with the highest rating on the neurologic scale was then entered and represented the score of the summary measure. The summary measure was thus given a score of 1, 3, 5 or 7, just like the individual reflexes. The rationale for the summary measures is based upon the observation that there exists considerable variability of scores obtained on individual reflex responses in different subjects, and sometimes even in the same subject on subsequent examinations, and on the general assumption that the pathological process in Alzheimer's disease more or less diffusely but not necessarily homogeneously afflicts the brain. The summary measures may thus provide an early cognition-independent neurologic measure of diffuse brain dysfunction. A computerized analysis of all the scores obtained on the activity rating scale for reflexes and release signs and of the scores of the summary measures was performed employing three different cut-offs, reflecting three levels of conservativeness for defining the registered score as hyperactive. An activity rating of 3 or greater represented the least conservative cut-off, an activity rating of 5 or greater represented a moderately conservative cut-off and an activity rating of 7 represented the most conservative cut-off. A chi-squared analysis of the obtained activity ratings was carried out both from the viewpoint of prevalence of increased activity of reflexes, employing the three above-mentioned cut-off criteria, and from the viewpoint of mean activity rating value, obtained for both the individual reflexes and the summary variables on the neurologic rating scale. Prevalence and mean values for all individual and summary measures were determined for six groups of subjects with different degrees of cognitive impairment and including normal controls, subjects with mild cognitive impairment and subjects with probable Alzheimer's disease in successive stages of clinical severity.

In all, 135 subjects were studied (Franssen et al., 1991b). The demographic characteristics are shown in Table 8.3. Their cognitive and functional status was determined using the Global Deterioration Scale (GDS) of Reisberg et al. (1982). This is a seven-point rating instrument for staging of the magnitude of cognitive and functional capacity in normal ageing, age-associated memory impairment (AAMI) and primary degenerative dementia (PDD). It is designed to reflect the characteristic phenomenology of these conditions, and the progression of PDD. The GDS stages 1 and 2 represent, respectively, subjects with no memory defect on clinical interview and subjects with very mild subjective, but not objectively demonstrable deficit on clinical interview. The following GDS stages represent subjects with mild, objectively demonstrable cognitive impairment on detailed clinical interview (GDS stage 3), subjects with moderate cognitive decline on interview (GDS stage 4), subjects with moderately severe cognitive decline consistent with early dementia (GDS stage 5), subjects with severe cognitive decline or middle dementia (GDS stage 6) and subjects with very severe cognitive decline or late dementia (GDS stage 7). The

Table 8.3 Subject characteristics. *

| GDS stage | Mean age (years) | | | | | | Mean MMSE score |
	n	Men	n	Women	n	Total	
GDS 1 and 2	9	69.7 ± 12.3	18	58.7 ± 7.4	27	68.7 ± 12.1	29.0 ± 1.2
GDS 3	6	70.8 ± 14.1	14	73.6 ± 6.4	20	72.8 ± 9.1	24.9 ± 3.3
GDS 4	8	70.6 ± 8.3	25	72.5 ± 7.0	33	72.1 ± 7.3	20.1 ± 3.4
GDS 5	16	71.6 ± 9.0	15	76.0 ± 8.8	31	73.7 ± 9.0	14.7 ± 3.3
GDS 6	5	77.7 ± 6.7	12	71.5 ± 8.7	17	73.3 ± 8.5	7.3 ± 5.4
GDS 7	1	87.6 ± 0.0	6	81.5 ± 5.5	7	82.4 ± 5.5	0.0 ± 0.0
All subjects	45	72.0 ± 10.1	89	72.9 ± 9.2	135	72.6 ± 9.5	18.8 ± 8.6

* Values are mean ± S.D. GDS = Global Deterioration Scale. MMSE = Mini-Mental State Examination.
From Franssen *et al.* (1991b).

GDS stage 1 and 2 subjects were used as normal age-matched controls. All subjects in GDS stages 4 to 7 were diagnosed as having probable Alzheimer's disease and fulfilled the NINCDS–ADRDA criteria for Alzheimer's disease (McKhann *et al.*, 1984). All subjects underwent comprehensive neuropsychological, psychiatric, neurological and physical examinations, including routine laboratory tests and computed tomographic or magnetic resonance imaging studies of the brain. All patients with evidence of cerebrovascular disease on the brain scan were excluded. None of the subjects had any other condition which could adversely affect cognition or function. All subjects had a Modified Ischaemia Scale (Rosen *et al.*, 1980) score of less than 4.

In using the previously described methodology, a recognizable pattern of reflexes and release signs (primitive reflexes) with regard to their sequence of appearance, prevalence and activity was observed with progression of cognitive impairment and dementia. Figures 8.1 to 8.9 depict the percentages of activity responses for all three levels of conservativeness for some of the reflexes and release signs and some of the summary measures across the GDS stages. Patients with mild cognitive decline (GDS stage 3) and patients with moderate cognitive decline (GDS stage 4) had a significantly higher prevalence of increased activity ratings on the summary measure which combined all 14 individual reflex measures and on the summary measure which combined all deep tendon reflexes, and on the summary measure which combined all nociceptive primitive reflexes, then normal age-matched controls (GDS stages 1 and 2) (Table 8.4), while none of the individual reflexes or release signs showed a significant difference in prevalence between these two groups. The specificity for the summary measure combining all 14 individual measures in differentially diagnosing normal subjects from subjects with mild but objective cognitive deficit was 56%, the sensitivity was 87% and the overall accuracy was 80%. Patients with moderately severe cognitive decline (GDS stage 4), i.e. patients who had clinical manifestations of early dementia, showed in addition to significantly higher prevalence values on these summary measures a significant increase in the mean activity rating of the summary variable combining all primitive reflexes (release signs) compared to normal control subjects (GDS stages 1 and 2) (Table 8.5). Patients with severe cognitive decline (GDS stage 6), i.e. patients in the middle phase of dementia, showed in addition significantly higher prevalence values on the summary measure, combining all prehensile release signs compared to normal controls (Table 8.4) and they also had

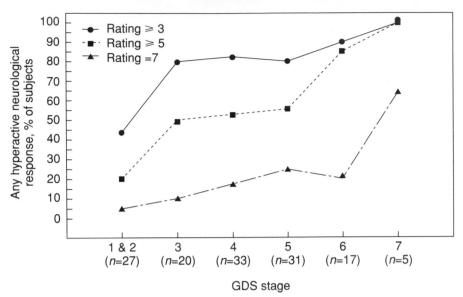

Fig. 8.1 Percentage of subjects showing any hyperactive neurological response studied (i.e. any hyperactive deep tendon reflex, plantar response, muscle tone, or release sign) as a function of the Global Deterioration Scale (GDS) stage using three different ratings of hyperactivity. n = number of patients. Reproduced with permission from Franssen *et al.* (1991b).

significantly higher mean values for paratonia, hand and foot grasp reflexes and the snout reflex than patients in the previous GDS group (Table 8.5). Patients with very severe cognitive impairment (GDS stage 7), i.e. with late dementia, had in addition significantly higher mean values for the

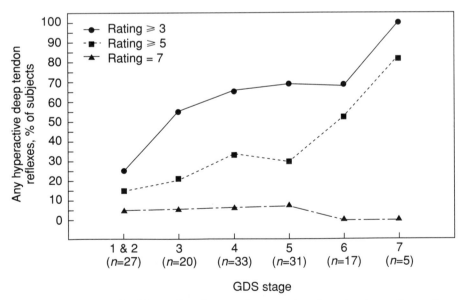

Fig. 8.2 Percentage of subjects showing any hyperactive deep tendon reflexes (i.e. any biceps, triceps, quadriceps, or gastrocnemius-soleus reflex hyperactivity) as a function of the Global Deterioration Scale (GDS) stage using three different ratings of hyperactivity. n = number of patients. Reproduced with permission from Franssen *et al.* (1991b).

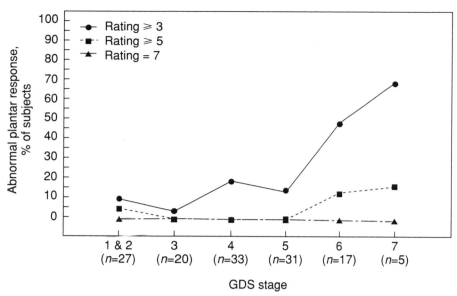

Fig. 8.3 Percentage of subjects showing an abnormal plantar response as a function of the Global Deterioration Scale (GDS) stage using three different ratings of abnormality. *n* = number of patients. Reproduced with permission from Franssen *et al.* (1991b).

summary measure which combined all deep tendon reflexes, for paratonia and for the summary measure for all individual prehensile release signs compared to patients in GDS stage 6 (Table 8.5). The highest mean values (4 or greater) for any reflex in any GDS stage were obtained for deep tendon reflexes, paratonia, sucking reflexes (tactile and visual) and hand grasp reflexes; all occurred in the stage of late dementia (GDS stage 7). The highest mean values for the summary

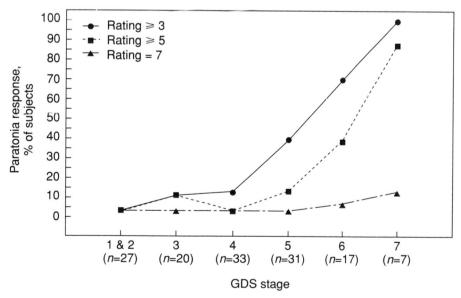

Fig. 8.4 Percentage of subjects showing paratonia as a function of the Global Deterioration Scale (GDS) stage using three different ratings of activity. *n* = number of patients. Reproduced with permission from Franssen *et al.* (1991b).

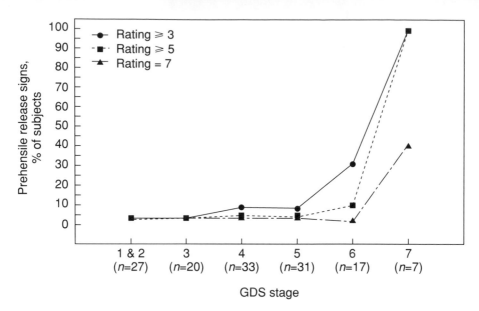

Fig. 8.5 Percentage of subjects showing prehensile release signs as a function of the Global Deterioration Scale (GDS) stage using three different ratings of activity. n = number of patients. Reproduced with permission from Franssen *et al.* (1991b).

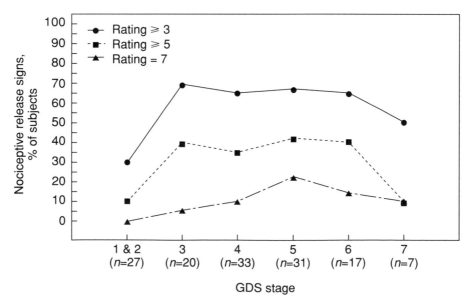

Fig. 8.6 Percentage of subjects showing nociceptive release signs as a function of the Global Deterioration Scale (GDS) stage using three different ratings of activity. n = number of patients. Reproduced with permission from Franssen *et al.* (1991b).

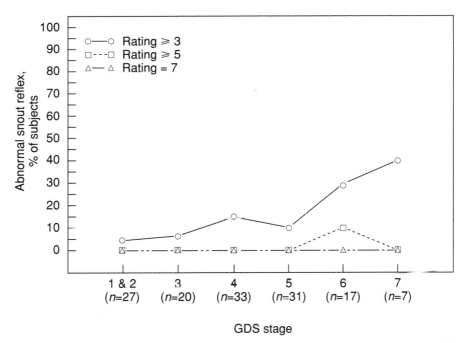

Fig. 8.7 Percentage of subjects showing a snout reflex as a function of the Global Deterioration Scale (GDS) using three different ratings of activity. n = number of patients.

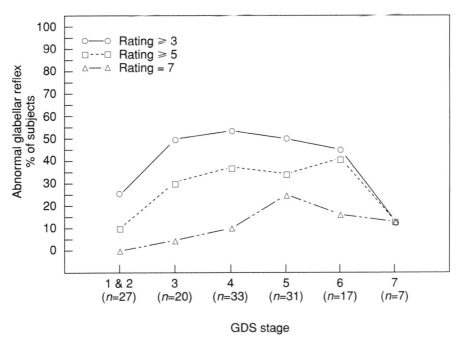

Fig. 8.8 Percentage of subjects showing a glabellar blink reflex as a function of the Global Deterioration Scale (GDS) using three different ratings of activity. n = number of patients.

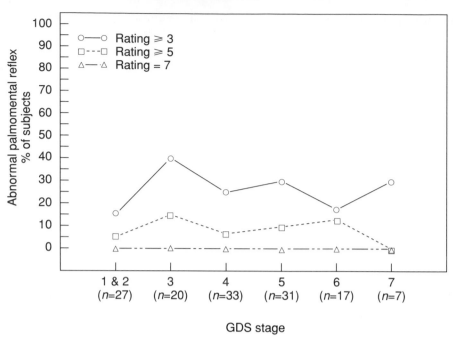

Fig. 8.9 Percentage of subjects showing a palmomental reflex as a function of the Global Deterioration Scale (GDS) using three different ratings of activity. n = number of patients.

measure for noceptive reflexes was observed in GDS stages 4, 5 and 6, i.e. before the stage of late dementia (GDS stage 7); in that stage the mean value for this summary measure was lower than in the preceding stages. In recently obtained new data on a larger population of severely and very severely demented patients, the above observed trends are maintained (Franssen *et al.*, 1993). The use of an activity rating scale for reflexes and release signs (primitive reflexes) as well as the use of summary measures thus provides significant new information on reflex behaviour in Alzheimer's disease. In fact, these methodologies made it possible to observe changes in activity of deep tendon reflexes and primitive reflexes in subjects with only mild but objectively demonstrable cognitive impairment compared to normal age-matched control subjects. This latter finding emphasizes the need for more extensive formal psychometric testing and cognitive evaluation of potential control subjects before they can be considered as normal controls. The use of the above techniques also allowed the demonstration of the continuing progression of neurologic deficit as an indicator of disease progression in severely demented patients at a stage when cognitive tests bottom out. This is possible because the reflexes and release signs are evaluated in patients within each well-defined stage of cognitive and functional impairment decline separately. Particular patterns in the sequence and prevalence of reflexes also did become manifest because the neurological examination was performed on patients who were staged on a cognitive rating scale which measured global dementia severity.

EXTRAPYRAMIDAL SIGNS

Extrapyramidal signs have been reported in Alzheimer's disease patients with a prevalence varying from approximately 12 to 92%. As is the case with

Table 8.4 χ^2 analyses of prevalence of neurological abnormality for cognitively impaired subjects in comparison with normal elderly control subjects using differentially strict ratings for neurological abnormality.*

Neurological variable rating required for abnormality	P value in GDS stages				
	3	4	5	6	7
Any hyperactive neurological response					
≥3	<0.05	<0.001	<0.001	<0.001	<0.05
≥5	<0.05	<0.05	<0.01	<0.001	<0.001
7	N.S.	N.S.	<0.05	<0.05	<0.001
Any hyperactive deep tendon reflexes					
≥3	<0.05	<0.01	<0.001	<0.001	<0.01
≥5	N.S.	N.S.	N.S.	<0.01	<0.01
7	N.S.	N.S.	N.S.	N.S.	N.S.
Abnormal plantar response					
≥3	N.S.	N.S.	N.S.	<0.01	<0.001
≥5	N.S.	N.S.	N.S.	N.S.	N.S.
7	N.S.	N.S.	N.S.	N.S.	N.S.
Paratonia response					
≥3	N.S.	N.S.	<0.001	<0.001	<0.001
≥5	N.S.	N.S.	N.S.	<0.001	0.001
7	N.S.	N.S.	N.S.	N.S.	N.S.
Prehensile release signs					
≥3	N.S.	N.S.	N.S.	<0.001	<0.001
≥5	N.S.	N.S.	N.S.	N.S.	<0.001
7	N.S.	N.S.	N.S.	N.S.	<0.001
Nociceptive release signs					
≥3	<0.01	<0.01	<0.01	<0.05	N.S.
≥5	<0.05	<0.05	<0.01	<0.05	N.S.
7	N.S.	N.S.	<0.01	<0.05	<0.05

* GDS = Global Deterioration Scale. N.S. = not significant ($P < 0.05$). GDS stages 3 to 7 refer to cognitively impaired subjects in comparison with control subjects (GDS stages 1 and 2). From Franssen et al. (1991b).

primitive reflexes, this wide range in prevalence probably reflects different patient populations, different scoring methodologies and differences in the inclusion or exclusion of particular signs (depending on the rating scale used) that are considered indicators of extrapyramidal dysfunction. Several studies have found extrapyramidal signs to be more prevalent in the cognitively and functionally more impaired patients (Pierce, 1974; Pomara et al., 1981; Mölsa et al., 1984; Mayeux et al., 1985). Other studies have found a relation between these signs and the occurence of snout, sucking and grasp reflexes, signs which are also more prevalent in the advanced stages of the illness (Bakchine et al., 1989; Burns et al., 1991). Recent observations generally indicate that extrapyramidal signs are more prevalent in moderately severe and severe Alzheimer's disease and less common in the early stages of the illness (Drachman et al., 1990; Chen et al., 1991; Soininen et al., 1992; Fransen et al. 1993).

Some studies have assessed only very specific signs of parkinsonism, such as

Table 8.5 Activity rating of all neurological variables and all combinations of variables as a function of severity of cognitive and functional impairment by GDS.*

Neurological variable	GDS stage						
	1 and 2 ($n = 27$)	3 ($n = 20$)	4 ($n = 33$)	5 ($n = 31$)	6 ($n = 17$)	7 ($n = 5-7$)	P†
Four deep tendon reflexes, plantar response, muscle tone, and all release sign variables combined (i.e. 14 individual variables combined)							
$\bar{X}$	1.25	1.60‡§	1.68‡	1.79‡	2.21‡§	3.84‡§	
S.D.	0.38	0.51	0.51	0.57	0.71	0.18	<0.0001
Four deep tendon reflexes combined							
$\bar{X}$	1.51	2.20	2.38‡	2.52‡	2.91‡	4.30‡§	
S.D.	1.05	1.25	1.31	1.50	1.58	0.65	<0.001
Biceps							
$\bar{X}$	1.48	2.15	2.27	2.58‡	3.18†	4.00‡	
S.D.	1.22	1.27	1.59	1.73	1.81	1.55	<0.01
Triceps							
$\bar{X}$	1.22	2.00	2.15‡	2.42‡	3.12‡	4.33‡	
S.D.	0.85	1.26	1.42	1.75	1.80	1.03	<0.0001
Quadriceps							
$\bar{X}$	1.81	2.40	2.58	2.68	3.18	4.14‡	
S.D.	1.47	1.57	1.68	1.78	1.94	1.46	<0.05
Gastrocnemius-soleus							
$\bar{X}$	1.52	2.25	2.51	2.42	2.18	3.3	
S.D.	1.42	1.62	1.91	1.80	1.59	1.86	N.S.
Plantar response							
$\bar{X}$	1.22	1.10	1.39	1.29	2.29‡§	2.71‡	
S.D.	0.85	0.45	0.86	0.69	1.53	1.38	<0.0001
Muscle tone (paratonia)							
$\bar{X}$	1.00	1.40	1.24	2.10‡§	3.47‡§	5.42‡§	
S.D.	0.00	1.23	.66	1.45	1.96	0.48	<0.0001
All release sign variables combined							
$\bar{X}$	1.15	1.38	1.42‡	1.44‡	1.68‡	3.56‡§	
S.D.	0.27	0.32	0.42	0.39	0.69	0.48	<0.0001
All five prehensile release sign variables combined (sucking, grasping, and rooting)							
$\bar{X}$	1.00	1.00	1.04	1.03	1.35‡§	4.43‡§	
S.D.	0.00	0.00	0.12	0.10	0.67	1.27	<0.0001
Sucking tactile							
$\bar{X}$	1.00	1.00	1.09	1.13	1.41	6.00‡§	
S.D.	0.00	0.00	0.38	0.50	1.18	1.00	<0.0001
Sucking visual							
$\bar{X}$	1.00	1.00	1.03	1.00	1.18	5.43‡§	
S.D.	0.00	0.00	0.17	0.00	0.73	1.40	<0.0001
Hand grasp							
$\bar{X}$	1.00	1.00	1.00	1.00	1.53‡§	4.43‡§	
S.D.	0.00	0.00	0.00	0.00	0.87	1.62	<0.0001
Foot grasp							
$\bar{X}$	1.00	1.00	1.06	1.00	1.65‡§	3.71‡§	
S.D.	0.00	0.00	0.35	0.00	1.27	1.50	<0.0001

Rooting							
$\bar{X}$	1.00	1.00	1.00	1.00	1.00	2.58‡§	
S.D.	0.00	0.00	0.00	0.00	0.00	2.15	<0.0001

All nociceptive release sign variables combined
(snout, glabellar blink and palmomental reflexes)

$\bar{X}$	1.41	2.02	2.05	2.13	2.24	1.89	
S.D.	0.72	0.85	1.03	0.97	1.23	1.31	N.S.
Snout							
$\bar{X}$	1.11	1.10	1.30	1.23	1.88‡§	1.86	
S.D.	0.42	0.45	0.73	0.72	1.50	1.07	<0.05
Glabellar blink							
$\bar{X}$	1.74	2.75	3.15	3.29	3.18	2.00	
S.D.	1.38	2.05	2.25	2.57	2.55	2.45	N.S.
Palmomental							
$\bar{X}$	1.37	2.20	1.70	1.87	1.65	1.57	
S.D.	0.97	1.61	1.31	1.45	1.36	0.98	N.S.

* Values are mean ($\pm$s.d.). GDS = Global Deterioration Scale; N.S. = not significant ($P > 0.05$).
+P values show significance of change in neurologic variable with GDS (F probability).
‡Significantly different from control subjects (GDS stages 1 and 2) at $P < 0.05$ (one-way analysis of variance using Newman-Keuls follow-up procedure).
§Significantly different from preceding GDS category at $P < 0.05$ (one-way analysis of variance using Newman-Keuls follow-up procedure).
From Franssen *et al.*, Archives of Neurology Vol. 48 (1991).

rigidity and tremor, while other studies have included assessments of brady-kinesia, measures of gait and posture, activities of daily living, speech, rapid alternating movements and the glabellar blink reflex among others. It is common practice to assess extrapyramidal signs in patients with Alzheimer's disease by scales that were developed for assessing patients with Parkinson's disease or with drug-induced parkinsonism. A recent study found, in general, good inter-rater reliability for the presence or absence of extrapyramidal signs in patients with Alzheimer's disease, assessed on a widely used Parkinson's disease rating scale (Richards *et al.*, 1991). It has been pointed out that assessing extrapyramidal signs in demented patients on scales originally developed for Parkinson's disease may sometimes lead to difficulties in interpretation of the results obtained (Tyrrell and Rossor, 1989). This is especially true for patients in the advanced stages of dementia. Severely demented patients are often unable to cooperate with the examination. Spatial disorientation, apraxia and loss of purposeful movements, all common in advanced stage Alzheimer's disease, may be difficult to differentiate from true parkinsonian bradykinesia. Rigidity and bradykinesia in late-stage Alzheimer's disease may be different, both in their character and aetiology from Parkinson's disease. The evaluation of extrapyramidal features in many patients with Alzheimer's disease, in particular in the advanced stages, is also confounded by the use of neuroleptics in this group. The possible effect of these drugs on the presence of those signs in patients with Alzheimer's disease deserves more attention. In a recent study, 75 to 100% of neuroleptic-treated patients showed bradykinesia, rigidity or orofacial dyskinesia (Soininen *et al.*, 1992).

The denomination 'extrapyramidal' often implies striatonigral or basal ganglia pathology. Although decrease in cerebrospinal fluid (CSF) monoamine markers has been reported in Alzheimer's disease with extrapyramidal features

(Kaye *et al.*, 1988). Levodopa does not appear to have an effect on dementia-related rigidity (Duret *et al.*, 1989). Levels of monoamine markers in severe stage Alzheimer's disease have been reported to be consistently lower compared to levels in less severe stage Alzheimer's disease regardless the presence of extrapyramidal symptoms (Blennow *et al.*, 1991). This suggests that a decrease in CSF homovanillic acid and, presumably, the occurrence of extrapyramidal symptoms in severe stage Alzheimer's disease are related to the pathologic process of Alzheimer's disease rather than to concomitant parkinsonian pathology. Recent positron emission tomographic (PET) studies with fluor-18-dopa in Alzheimer's disease patients with an extrapyramidal syndrome have shown a normal uptake in the caudate nucleus and the putamen, in contrast to patients with Parkinson's disease who showed a marked reduction of uptake in the putamen (Tyrrell *et al.*, 1990). The most common extrapyramidal symptoms which have been observed in patients with Alzheimer's disease are rigidity, often with a paratonic quality, and bradykinesia, whereas tremor is uncommon (Koller *et al.*, 1983; Huff and Growdon, 1986; Bakchine *et al.*, 1989; Franssen *et al.*, 1993). Slowing of gait and small stepped gait are also common accompaniments of more advanced Alzheimer's disease (Visser, 1983; Galasko *et al.*, 1990; Franssen *et al.*, 1993). The suggestion that the extrapyramidal syndrome in Alzheimer's disease probably results from other mechanisms than concurrent parkinsonian type striatonigral pathology alone is also supported by autopsy studies (Morris *et al.*, 1989). There is some suggestion that the presence of periventricular white matter changes, visible as hypodense areas on CT scans or as hyperintensities on magnetic resonance imaging (MRI) brain scans, and observed in Alzheimer's disease patients with a frequency twice that of normal aged subjects, may contribute to some of the observed gait abnormalities in Alzheimer's disease patients, whereas in cognitively normal subjects they may have no clinical significance (George *et al.*, 1986). The importance of extrapyramidal features in Lewy body dementia have been emphasized (McKeith *et al.*, 1992).

FUTURE STUDIES

The study of neurologic signs is beginning to provide significant information about central nervous system function in ageing and dementia. The study of reflexes in ageing and dementia is beginning to show how these indicators of motor function and sensorimotor integration are related to the cognitive and other integrating functions of the brain and possibly also to behaviour and its pathology. Many intriguing problems are awaiting further studies. Does involution, the decline of the normal functions of the central nervous system that occurs with age, also occur in a patterned fashion, just like the evolution and maturation of the brain in infancy and childhood? If this is the case, what are the accompanying neurologic signs? Does the pattern of functional loss as it occurs in uncomplicated Alzheimer's disease indeed follow the pattern of the normal development of these functions in reverse? If that were the case, is the functional loss in Alzheimer's disease a matter of an accelerated process of involution? Are some clinical signs of neurologic dysfunction as they are observed in advanced Alzheimer's disease due to degenerative lesions in the cerebral white matter and brain stem, and are they then manifestations of a process that proceeds independently of the disorder that results in dementia, as has been hypothesized (Tweedy *et al.*, 1982)? Or are they the result of the pathologic process that causes Alzheimer's disease? If they result from that process, do these signs then proceed according to a disease-specific pattern?

Assuming again that this is the case, neurologic signs could then be utilized as noncognitive, independent markers of disease progression and as indicators of excess pathology. One area for which this would have immediate consequences is that of the psychopharmacological treatment of behavioural symptomatology, which often accompanies Alzheimer's disease. Patients in the late stages of this disease appear exquisitely sensitive to the side effects. The examination of deep tendon reflexes and primitive reflexes may also provide a reliable differential diagnostic methology for differentiating dementia of various aetiologies. It has been reported that certain primitive reflexes predominate in vascular dementia with lacunas (Ishi *et al.*, 1986). If the neurologic symptoms which accompany Alzheimer's disease represent an independent pathologic process, which does not necessarily closely follow cognitive decline, reflexes are still important as markers of the progression of that process. It is however necessary in future studies of reflexes that the methods of elucidation and scoring become more standardized and refined. The search for pair wise linkages of these signs and the use of combination (summary) measures deserves further attention in future research. This is of particular importance if these signs are to have any usefulness as early indicators of abnormal brain function and dementia. Reflexes and release signs are not quick, cheap and easy measures for cognitive behaviour. They are very helpful clinical tools in addition to and in combination with cognitive testing, neuropsychological evaluation and neuroimaging studies, provided that they are more standardized. With this reservation, the question whether the examination of these signs still has any place in the study of ageing and dementia can be answered affirmatively.

REFERENCES

Bakchine, S., Lacomblez, L., Palisson, E. *et al.* (1989). Relationship between primitive reflexes, extrapyramidal signs, reflective apraxia and severity of cognitive impairment in dementia of the Alzheimer type. *Acta Neurologica Scandinavica*, **79**, 38–46.

Basavaraju, N.G., Silverstone, F., Libow, L. and Paraskeros, K. (1987). Primitive reflexes and perceptual sensory tests in the elderly: their usefulness in dementia. *Journal of Chronic Diseases*, **34**, 367–77.

Blennow, K., Wallin, A., Gottfries, C.G. *et al.* (1991). Significance of decreased lumbar CSF levels of HVA and SHIAA in Alzheimer's disease. *Neurobiology and Aging*, **13**, 103–13.

Brunia, C.H.M. and Vuister, F.M. (1979). Spinal reflexes as indicator of motor preparation in man. *Physiology and Psychology*, **7**, 377–80.

Buckley, A.C. (1927). Observations concerning primitive reflexes as revealed in reactions in abnormal mental states. *Brain*, **50**, 573–8.

Burns, A., Jacoby, R. and Levy, R. (1991). Neurological signs in Alzheimer's disease. *Age and Ageing*, **20**, 45–51.

Chen, J.Y., Stern, Y., Sano, M. and Mayeux, R. (1991). Cumulative risks of developing extrapyramidal signs, psychosis or myoclonus in the course of Alzheimer's disease. *Archives of Neurology*, **48**, 1141–4.

Davous, P., Lamour, Y. and Roudier, M. (1989). Etude neurologique standardisee dans la demence senile de type Alzheimer. *L'Encephale*, **XV**, 387–96.

de Ajuriaguerra, J., Rego, A. and Tissot, R. (1963). Le reflexe oral et quelques activites orales dans les syndromes dementiels du grand age. Leur signification dans la disintegration psycho-motrice. *L'Encephale*, **52**, 179–219.

DeJong, R.N. (1979). *The reflexes, in The Neurologic Examination, Part V.* Harper & Row, Philadelphia.

Dewaide, P.J. and Toulouse, P. (1987). Facilitation of monosynaptic reflexes by voluntary contractions of muscle in remote parts of the body. Mechanisms involved in the Jendrassik manoevre. *Brain,* **104,** 701–19.

Drachman, D.A., O'Donnell, B.F., Lew, R.A. and Swearer, J.M. (1990). The prognosis in Alzheimer's disease. 'How far' rather than 'how fast' best predicts the course. *Archives of Neurology,* **47,** 851–6.

Duret, M., Goldman, S., Messina, D. and Hildebrand, J. (1989). Effects of L-dopa on dementia-related rigidity. *Acta Neurologica Scandinavica,* **80,** 64–7.

Franssen, E.H., Reisberg, B. and Kluger, A. (1991a). Utility of cognition-independent neurologic signs as markers of mild cognitive impairment and as measures of dementia severity in patients with Alzheimer's disease. Fifth Congress of the International Psychogeriatric Association (IPA) Abstracts, p. 79.

Franssen, E.H., Reisberg, B., Kluger, A. *et al.* (1991b). Cognition independent neurologic symptoms in normal aging and probable Alzheimer's disease. *Archives of Neurology,* **48,** 148–54.

Franssen, E.H., Kluger, A., Torossiani, C.L. and Reisberg, B. (1993). The neurologic syndrome of severe Alzheimer's disease: relationship to functional decline. *Archives of Neurology* (in press).

Galasko, D., Kwo-on-Yuen, P.E., Klauber, M.R. and Thal, L.J. (1990). Neurological findings in Alzheimer's disease and normal aging. *Archives of Neurology,* **47,** 625–7.

George, A.E., de Leon, M.J., Gentes, C.I. *et al.* (1986). Leukoencephalopathy in normal and pathologic aging: 1: CT of brain lucencies. *American Journal of Neuroradiology,* **7,** 561–6.

Gijn, J. van (1977). The plantar reflex; a historical, clinical and electromyographic study. Dissertation. Erasmus University, Rotterdam.

Girling, D.M. and Berrios, G.E. (1990). Extrapyramidal signs, primitive reflexes and frontal lobe function in senile dementia of the Alzheimer type. *British Journal of Psychiatry,* **157,** 888–93.

Huff, F.J. and Growdon, J.H. (1986). Neurological abnormalities associated with severity of dementia in Alzheimer's disease. *Canadian Journal of Neurological Science,* **13,** 403–5.

Huff, F.J., Boller, F., Luchelli, F. *et al.* (1987). The neurologic examination in patients with probable Alzheimer's disease. *Archives of Neurology,* **44,** 929–32.

Impallomeni, M., Flynn, M.D., Kenny, R.A. *et al.* (1984). The elderly and their ankle jerks. *Lancet,* **i,** 670–2.

Ishi, N., Nishihara, Y. and Imamura, T. (1986). Why do frontal lone symptoms predominate in vascular dementia with lacunas? *Neurology,* **36,** 340–5.

Jenkyn, L.R. (1989). Examining the aging nervous system. *Seminars in Neurology,* **9,** 82–7.

Jenkyn, L.R., Reeves, A.G., Warren, T. *et al.* (1985). Neurologic signs in senescence. *Archives of Neurology,* **42,** 154–7.

Jenkyn, L.R., Walsh, D.B., Culver, C.M. and Reeves, A.G. (1977). Clinical signs in diffuse cerebral dysfunction. *Journal of Neurology, Neurosurgery and Psychiatry,* **40,** 956–66.

Kamen, G. and Koceja, D.M. (1989). Contralateral influences on patellar tendon reflexes in young and old adults. *Neurobiology of aging,* **10,** 311–15.

Kaye, J.A., May, C., Daley, E. *et al.* (1988). Cerebrospinal fluid monoamine markers are deceased in dementia of the Alzheimer type with extrapyramidal features. *Neurology*, **38**, 554–7.

Kokmen, E., Bossemeyer, R.W., Barney, J. *et al.* (1977). Neurological manifestations of ageing. *Journal of Gerontology*, **32**, 411–19.

Koller, W.C., Glatt, S., Wilson, R.S. and Fox, J.H. (1983). Primitive reflexes and cognitive function in the elderly. *Annals of Neurology*, **12**, 302–4.

Liston, E.H. (1979). Clinical findings in presenile dementia. A report of 50 cases. *Journal of Nervous and Mental Diseases*, **167**, 337–42.

Mayeux, R., Stern, Y. and Spanton, S. (1985). Heterogeneity in dementia of the Alzheimer type: Evidence of subgroups. *Neurology*, **35**, 453–61.

McKeith, I., Fairbairn, A., Perry, R., Thompson, P. and Perry, E. (1992). Neuroleptic sensitivity in patients with senile dementia of Lewy body type. *British Medical Journal*, **305**, 673–8.

McKhann, G., Drachman, D., Folstein, M. *et al.* (1984). Clinical diagnosis of Alzheimer's disease: Report of the NINCDS–ADRAD work group under the auspices of the Department of Health and Human Services Task Force on Alzheimer's disease. *Neurology*, **34**, 939–44.

Molloy, D.W., Clarnette, R.M., Mullroy, W.E. *et al.* (1991). Clinical significance of primitive reflexes in Alzheimer's disease. *Journal of the American Geriatric Society*, **39**, 1160–3.

Mölsa, P.K., Martila, R.J. and Rinne, U.K. Extrapyramidal signs in Alzheimer's disease. *Neurology*, **34**, 1116–16.

Morris, J.C., Drazner, M., Fulling, K. *et al.* (1989). Clinical and pathological aspects of parkinsonism in Alzheimer's disease. A role for extranigral factors? *Archives of Neurology*, **46**, 651–7.

Paulson, G. and Gottlieb, G. (1968). Developmental reflexes: the reappearance of foetal and neonatal reflexes in aged patients. *Brain*, **91**, 37–52.

Pierce, J. (1974). The extrapyramidal disorder of Alzheimer's disease. *European Neurology*, **12**, 94–103.

Pomara, N., Reisberg, B., Albers, S. *et al.* (1981). Extrapyramidal symptoms in patients with primary degenerative dementia. *Journal Clinical Psychopharmacology*, **1**, 398–400.

Reisberg, B., Ferris, S.H., de Leon, M.J. and Crook, T. (1982). The global deterioration scale for assessment of primary degenerative dementia. *American Journal of Psychiatry*, **139**, 1136–9.

Richards, M., Marder, K., Bell, D.G. *et al.* (1991). Interrater reliability of extrapyramidal signs in a group assessed for dementia. *Archives of Neurology*, **48**, 1147–9.

Risse, S.C., Lampe, T.H., Bird, T.D. *et al.* (1990). Myoclonus, seizures and paratonia in Alzheimer's disease. *Alzheimer Disease and Associated Disorders*, **4**, 217–25.

Rosen, W.G., Terry, R.D., Fuld, P.A. *et al.* (1980). Pathological verification of ischemia score in differentiation of dementias. *Annals of Neurology*, **7**, 486–8.

Sarnat, H.B. (1989). Do the corticospinal and corticobulbar tracts mediate functions in the human newborn? *Canadian Journal of Neurological Science*, **16**, 157–60.

Schaltenbrand, G. (1925). Normale Bewegungs-und Lagereactionen bei ei Kindern. *Deutsche Zeitschrift für Nervenheilkunde*, **87**, 23–95.

Soininen, H., Laulumaa, V., Helkala, *et al.* (1992). Extrapyramidal signs in Alzheimer's disease: a 3-year follow-up study. *Journal of Neurological Transmitters*, **4**, 107–19.

Stam, J. and Tan, K.M. (1987). Tendon reflex variability and method of stimulation. *Electroencephalography and Clinical Neurophysiology*, **67**, 463–7.

Stam, J., Speelman, H.D. and Crevel H. van (1989). Tendon reflex asymmetry by voluntary mental effort in healthy subjects. *Archives of Neurology*, **46**, 70–3.

Touwen, B.C.L. (1984). Primitive reflexes. Conceptual or semantic problem. In *Continuity of Neural Functions from Prenatal to Postnatal Life*, Prechtl, H.F.R., (Ed.). *Clinics in Developmental Medicine*, Vol. 94, pp. 115–25. Spastics International Medical Publications with Blackwell Scientific Publications Ltd, Oxford and J.B. Lippincott Co., Philadelphia.

Tweedy, J., Reding, M., Garcia, G. *et al.* (1982). Significance of clinical disinhibition signs. *Neurology*, **32**, 169.

Tyrrell, P.J. and Rossor, M.N. (1989). Extrapyramidal signs in dementia of Alzheimer type. *Lancet*, **ii**, 920.

Tyrrell, P., Sawle, G., Ibanez, V. *et al.* Clinical and PET studies of the extrapyramidal syndrome of dementia of the Alzheimer type. *Archives of Neurology*, **47**, 1318–23.

Villeneuve, A., Turcotte, J., Bouchard, M. *et al.* (1984). Release phenomena and iterative activities in geriatric patients. *Canadian Medical Associated Journal*, **110**, 147–53.

Visser, H. (1983). Gait and balance in senile dementia of Alzheimer's type. *Age and Ageing*, **12**, 296–301.

Wartenberg, R. (1945). *The examination of reflexes, a simplification*. The Year Book Publishers, Inc., Chicago.

Zametkin, A.J. Steven, J.R. and Pittman, R. (1979). Ontogeny of spontaneous blinking and of habituation of the blink reflex. *Annals of Neurology*, **5**, 453–7.

Ziegler, B.K. (1985). Is the Neurologic Examination Becoming Obsolete? *Neurology*, **35**, 559.

Philip J. Luthert

Department of Neuropathology
Institute of Psychiatry
London

9 NEUROPATHOLOGY AND NEUROCHEMISTRY OF AGEING AND DEMENTIA

INTRODUCTION

The aim of this chapter is to review the rapidly growing armamentarium of structural and chemical tools available to the investigator of ageing and dementing disorders. The boundaries between neuropathology, neurochemistry and other branches of neuroscience are now much less distinct than previously and the former, for instance, might arguably include the latest in molecular biology on one hand and the sophistication of *in vitro* brain slice technology on another. This chapter, however, will concentrate upon tools that can be applied to *post-mortem* or biopsy tissue in which there is no attempt to maintain cellular viability. In the same way neurochemistry might be taken to include every aspect of neural biochemistry but here transmitter chemistry and 'histological' neurochemistry will provide the focus of attention. Discussion will be restricted to the central nervous system and to methodologies appropriate to human tissue. Clearly these can also be applied to experimental systems but the greater versatility animal models offer in terms of manipulation of genetic and environmental factors, by means of transgenic models and neurotoxicology, will not be addressed specifically.

Aims of neuropathology and neurochemistry in the study of ageing and dementia

In ageing, neuropathological and neurochemical studies have initially been primarily concerned with providing an accurate description of morphological and biochemical changes occurring as part of the ageing process. In parallel with these phenomenological studies, similar tools have been brought to bear to elucidate the mechanisms underlying the documented changes. Given the profound age-dependence of dementing processes, a precise description of ageing-related events is also required as a moving baseline from which to study dementia.

In dementia, again, both phenomena and their associated pathogenesis are the targets of attention. More specifically, however, there is a requirement to assemble coherent sets of phenomena as 'diseases' or, less satisfactorily, 'syndromes' and to provide an integrated view of their pathogenesis; the whole disease being of more interest than the sum of its parts. The interaction between plaque and tangle formation would be an example of this. Another valuable rôle of these disciplines is to provide an insight into the mapping between pathological and clinical phenomena, in other words to play a part in clinicopathological studies. Typical questions would be 'Is it plaques or tangles that relate most closely to cognitive loss?', 'Which neurotransmitter deficit is associated most closely with cognitive decline?' or, at a more fundamental diagnostic level, 'How precisely can clinical criteria be used to predict histological diagnosis?' (Burns *et al.*, 1990). The value or otherwise of these questions, and the interpretation of their answers, is beyond the scope of this chapter.

CHARACTERIZATION OF NEURONAL CHANGES

A priori there are several things that can 'go wrong' with a nerve cell and specific techniques are employed to tackle each of these possible eventualities. Neurons can die, possibly without trace (however, see below) and measures of nerve cell number therefore become of major importance. (Being postmitotic they cannot increase in number.) Remaining cells may suffer loss or alteration of a pre-existing structure or biochemical component and to study this eventuality the anatomical or chemical tools used to define the normal state of affairs can simply be applied to the pathological state. Potentially more demanding is the circumstance where neuronal pathology is characterized by qualitative changes. At worst, the change will not be readily detectable by conventional methodologies and will therefore go unnoticed: It was not until the advent of silver impregnation techniques that tangles and Pick bodies were discovered. Similarly, more recently, ubiquitin immunohistochemistry has revealed cortical structural abnormalities in dementia associated with motor neuron disease that are undetectable by other techniques (Wightman *et al.*, 1992).

Biochemical approaches may also be confounded by the inherent nature of the structures under investigation. Neurofibrillary tangles and extracellular amyloid in Alzheimer's disease and prion disorders probably accumulate because of their resistance to digestion by various enzymes; biochemical analysis has also been hampered by this insolubility.

Determination of nerve cell loss

Loss of neuronal tissue is fundamental to the 'organic' dementias and of fundamental importance in the study of ageing. Macroscopical indices can demonstrate tissue loss but can not distinguish between cell death and cell shrinkage. In some instances, dying neurons leave so-called 'flag-stones', such as extracellular tangles, declaring their prior existence to microscopic examination, but generally, the only rigorous method is to estimate numbers of neurons. Demonstration of the presence or absence of actual nerve cell death in ageing or in a given dementing illness is one of the most critical tasks of contemporary neuropathology as without this knowledge it is not even clear whether we should be looking, in a given context, for causes of neuronal death or neuronal dysfunction.

Macroscopical methods

The simplest approach to assessing loss of neuronal tissue (i.e. cells or their processes) macroscopically is to measure brain weight. There is no doubt that brain weight declines with age (Dekaban and Sadowsky, 1978) and the only realistic explanation for this is that there has been neuronal loss; glia, if anything, increasing with age. Unfortunately, the range of normal values is very great and a given brain might lose 150 g and still be within normal limits. One solution to this is to assess brain weight in the context of intracranial volume (Davis and Wright, 1977) but this technique can be rather difficult and time-consuming. A useful internal standard is to measure the ratio of the weight of brain stem and cerbellum to total brain weight. In the adult this is normally 1 : 8 and a reduction in the contribution of total brain weight reflects relative hemispheric loss such as might be seen in Alzheimer's disease (AD).

Complementary strategies employ the measurement of volumes. Increased ventricular volume, which may be estimated by filling the ventricles with fluid, measuring brain weight before and after slicing or filling the ventricles with a radio-opaque medium and taking X-rays, in the absence of any obstruction, is a reasonable measure of cerebral tissue loss and may be used to give regional information. A more direct approach, however, and one that can be used with great effect to estimate total neuronal number within a part of the brain, is to measure the volume of that particular region. This is most efficiently done by randomly placing a grid of points on successive brain slices, each a known distance apart. The number of dots landing on the region of interest, for instance, the neocortex, multiplied by the product of the area associated with each dot and the mean slice thickness, gives an estimate of the volume of that structure (Aherne and Dunnill, 1982). This method is substantially quicker than attempting to trace around the pial and white matter boundaries of the cortex.

Alternative methods, such as measurement of displacement (Aherne and Dunnill, 1982), are not generally applicable to the nervous system as regions of interest such as the neorcortex or part of the thalamus are not readily dissected away from the rest of the brain. Measurement of sulcal subarachnoid space is not commonly used on *post-mortem* specimens, although subjective assessment is often made and it can be very useful in the context of neuroimaging.

Histological methods
Some of the most fundamental questions to be addressed in defining a neurodegenerative disease include: (1) Is there neuronal loss? (2) What is the distribution of the loss? and (3) How severe is the loss? (Coleman and Flood, 1987). Subjective estimation of neuronal loss is still the most commonly used approach but this can not be considered reliable. For instance, it was only the advent of a recent quantitative study that revealed that there is neuronal loss in the hippocampus in Huntington's disease (Spargo et al., 1993). The most frequently employed quantitative measure is that of neuronal density; that is, the number of neurons per unit area of section or, preferably, unit volume of tissue. Two issues arise here: (1) How useful a measure is neuronal density in its own right? and (2) Is neuronal density being measured in a reliable, unbiased way?

Neuronal density is a function of many variables other than total nerve cell number. Increase or decrease in volume of the region under study will lead to a decrease or increase in neuronal density, respectively, with no neuronal loss whatsoever. Changes in tissue volume unfortunately occur readily: as part of the disease itself, during fixation, during tissue processing (especially in paraffin wax) and during sectioning and mounting. To complicate matters further, the degree of volume change may, itself, be a function of the process under investigation. For instance, elderly brain shrinks during processing less than young brain does, perhaps because it is stiffer due to the increase in gliosis which takes place in ageing. These effects can be partially accounted for by measuring shrinkage during fixation, processing and during the preparation of sections, but even that cannot take into account shrinkage that has taken place as part of the disease process itself. (Relating neuronal density to intracranial volume may help – see above.)

A solution to these problems that works in many instances is to measure the volume of the area under study, as well as the mean neuronal density throughout it. The product of these two parameters gives the total neuronal number which is evidently independent of any shrinkage at any stage of disease or processing. To be able to implement this system any neuron must be equally likely to be sampled when assessing neuronal density and the whole of the so-called 'reference volume' must be available. This is often not the case in archival or referred material. In addition, the boundaries of the reference volume must be definable and meaningful. This criterion is readily fulfilled for structures such as the inferior olive or certain thalamic nuclei but is very much harder to ascertain with regard to, for instance, neocortical areas where to plot the cytoarchitectonic boundaries would be a formidable task. To be able to look at small, but less well-defined, areas is important as the nervous system is so heterogeneous. For instance, total neuronal counts for the entire neocortex is an entirely valid parameter to measure but small, critical regional losses, affecting either a limited number of cytoarchitectonic regions or only a single lamina, could be missed.

It seems reasonable, therefore, to measure neuronal density when reference volume can not be estimated, but to interpret the findings with caution.

1. An increase in neuronal density can only result from tissue shrinkage. If processing changes are excluded this must arise from dehydration or neuropil loss *in vivo*. The only components of the neuropil likely to disappear are axonal and dendritic processes (neurites). Importantly, coincidental neuronal loss can not be excluded.
2. No significant change in neuronal density is almost impossible to interpret as loss of neurites may balance neuronal loss and, therefore, be indistinguishable from no change.
3. Reduction in neuronal density, unless minor, is difficult to interpret in any way other than as indicative of neuronal loss as long as oedema-inducing processes have been excluded: this being the only process likely to cause an increase in tissue volume and hence reduction in neuronal density without neuronal loss. Importantly, however, a measured reduction in neuronal density may underestimate the severity of neuronal loss as associated neuronal shrinkage may act in the opposite direction (as in 1 above).

Additional problems facing the would be assessor of neuronal death include:

1. Individual cell types may be difficult to distinguish and, in pathological states, standard criteria, such as size, may become unusable.
2. There is large 'normal' variation requiring large numbers to achieve small variances.
3. Most parts of the brain are organized in an anisotropic way. For instance, most cortical structures are layered and even along the length of cortical ribbon there are usually changes from the top to the bottom of a sulcus.
4. In human neuropathology control material is becoming increasingly difficult to acquire.

In conclusion, the counting of neurons is not a trivial task but if properly executed does provide the investigator with invaluable data. Interested readers are referred to other more comprehensive reviews (Gundersen *et al.*, 1988a, b; Warren, 1992).

Cell size may also be of interest and here shrinkage problems are even more of an issue and embedding tissue in resin, as opposed to paraffin wax, will almost certainly become increasingly used as shrinkage in resin is relatively minor. The geometry of some cells can also make measuring of cell bodies difficult as, for instance, in pyramidal cells, it is hard to decide where perikarya ends and apical dendrite begins. Neuron width at the level of the nucleolus is a reasonable parameter to measure but, more recent stereological techniques, when appropriately applied, can provide estimates of cell volume (Gundersen et al., 1988a).

The relationship between one cell type and another may be of interest and this aspect of spatial statistics is only just beginning to be applied to the central nervous system (CNS) but is proving valuable in the study of various aspects of pathogenesis. Methods available include a variety of distance methods and, where features of interest occupy sufficient area, actual and predicted degrees of overlapping can be assessed. Such an approach has recently been used to show that βA4 protein deposits in AD are not associated with blood vessels any more than would be expected by chance. In fact the opposite appears to be the case (Luthert and Williams, 1991).

Pattern is another crucial aspect of the organization of the CNS. It clearly demonstrates a wide variety of patterns and the enormous complexity of the CNS arises from only a relatively modest number of genes and it therefore forms by a relatively small number of 'rules' which manifest themselves in the developing and adult structure of the CNS. Interestingly, in pathology, there are more and more instances where subtle neuronal misarrangements may be of significance and the application of spatial statistics to these problems should be a fruitful area of research in the next few years.

Pattern analysis and spatial frequency analysis can be used to look for periodicities and several distance methods can be employed to assess whether a given feature is arranged randomly, regularly or clumped. Growth phenomena (of cellular and noncellular elements) can be investigated by fractal analysis. Currently most of these types of analysis are being carried out in two dimensions but the prospects for three-dimensional studies are even more exciting. For reviews of some of the above approaches see Aherne and Dunnill (1982) and Upton and Fingleton (1985).

Structural changes within neurons
In addition to shrinking or dying neurons display a range of pathological structural responses that, whilst finite, far exceeds that of any other cell type. A collosal body of knowledge now exists concerning the severity and distribution of disease specificity of these changes. Below will be considered, in broad terms, the techniques available for studying these abnormalities.

Conventional light microscopy stains
Routine light microscopy provides the mainstay of neuropathological examination. With a simple haematoxylin and eosin or cresyl violet stained section abnormalities of nerve cell body size, shape and organization can rapidly be detected as long as the changes are not too subtle. Accumulated abnormal substances may show up through basophilia (Pick bodies or tangles), eosinophilia (Lewy bodies) or by virtue of their pigmentation, for example, lipofuscin (Braak, 1984). Vacuolation, dispersal of Nissl substance, and nuclear and nucleolar abnormalities may also be found.

Classically, a variety of stains have been used on an empirical basis to visualize certain cellular components (Bancroft and Stevens, 1982). The most

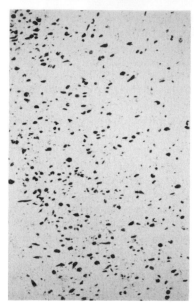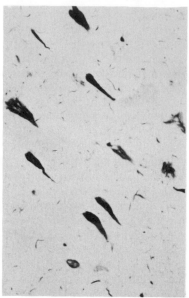

Fig. 9.1 Gallyas stain. Photomicrographs of Alzheimer's disease brain stained with the Gallyas silver method. The left-hand panel shows a low-power view of the full thickness (pia to white matter) of the entorhinal cortex and demonstrates many black neurofibrillary tangles. These are shown at a higher magnification on the right and in the background fine neuropil threads are apparent.

important in the current context are the silver stains (Gallyas, 1971; Wilcock *et al.*, 1990), many of which were developed in the first half of this century (Palmgren, 1948). Neurofilaments possess a site with high affinity for silver salts and this provides the basis for many stains that demonstrate axons and dendrites, both in their normal state and in various stages of degeneration. As cytoskeletal abnormalities of numerous types are common in different dementing illnesses silver stains have been fundamental in the characterization of separate disease states. (The neuronal cytoskeleton is composed largely of neurofilaments and microtubules.) Abnormal neurites (nerve cell processes) and tangles in Alzheimer's disease and Pick bodies in Pick's disease are readily identified with such silver stains. Interest in these methods has recently been rekindled by the growing appreciation of the Gallyas silver method (Gallyas, 1971) (Fig. 9.1). In optimum preparations no normal tissue components stain at all, demonstrating abnormal accumulations of tangles or abnormal neurites in dramatic contrast to the pale background (Fig. 9.1). A modified Bielschowsky stain has the virtue of demonstrating both paired helical filament (PHF) and amyloid abnormalities in Alzheimer's disease.

The staining technique developed by Golgi (DeFelipe and Jones, 1992) and subsequently modified by many others also relies on silver or other metallic salts but differs from the above silver stains in that only a small percentage of neurons are impregnated and, in optimal preparations, most of the dendritic tree and much of the axon will be demonstrated. Unfortunately, satisfactory impregnation is often not achieved in *post-mortem* tissue although many useful data have been acquired with this technique (Probst *et al.*, 1983; Scheibel, 1987).

Many crucial structural changes have been demonstrated not through classical, so-called empirical staining techniques but with immunohistochemistry, which is discussed at length below.

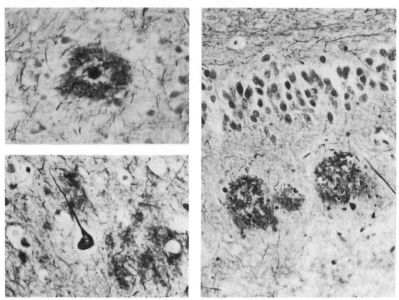

Fig. 9.2 Modified Bielchowsy stain. The top left panel shows a plaque with a central core. The bottom left panel shows a darkly staining neurofibrillary tangle and fuzzy, diffuse amyloid deposits. The right-hand panel shows plaques in the molecular layer of the dentate gyrus. (Dentate granule cells run across the top.)

Electron microscopy

Transmission electron microscopy allows examination of the fine structural detail of the nervous system and with conventional heavy metal stains (lead citrate and uranyl acetate) membranes and many structural proteins can be readily identified. A major draw back is the requirement for rapid fixation, and protracted agonal state together with *post-mortem* delay conspire to render much autopsy material more-or-less uninterpretable. Fortunately, however, some structures of particular interest, notably paired helical filaments in AD, by their very nature, are resistant to degradation and are well-preserved even after long delays. When available, biopsy material provides a solution (Neary *et al.*, 1986) but, even with such surgical material, particularly when the specimen is small, the quality of preservation may be far from ideal. Refinements to electron microscopy include adaptations of immuno-, enzyme and lectin histochemistry (see below).

Scanning electron microscopy reveals the surface structure of tissue and has limited application in *post-mortem* studies of ageing and dementia although interesting results concerning the degeneration of the perivascular innervation in Alzheimer's disease have been generated using this approach. Plaque core structure has also been studied and in a valuable X-ray microanalytical extension of this technique the elemental composition of plaques, tangles and other inclusions can be investigated (Candy *et al.*, 1989).

Confocal microscopy

Confocal microscopy allows thin portions of a section to be examined without interference from the out of focus image above and below (Fine *et al.*, 1988). Typically used with immunofluorescence (see below) fine three-dimensional images can be reconstructed. The main application for this has been in the examination of cells grown *in vitro* but plaque structure and Golgi-impregnated neurons have been studied in this way.

Immunohistochemistry of neuronal proteins
A weakness in conventional, empirical stains is that the chemical nature of the identified structure is frequently unknown or not specific. Immunohistochemistry has gone a long way to solve this problem and a good practically based review of the technique in the context of neurobiology can be found elsewhere (Priestley, 1987).

In brief, an antigen-specific antibody is raised and applied to a section. Following washing away of unbound antibody, that still stuck to the antigen under investigation is demonstrated in a variety of different ways which all rely upon a final step that generates a visualizable product. In light microscopy this is commonly the reaction product generated when diaminobenzidine is converted to a brown deposit by a peroxidase enzyme localized to the primary antibody. In electron microscopy electron dense gold or silver particles are used (Fig. 9.3).

The antigen used to raise the antibody may be a crude extract of the antigen under investigation or, increasingly, a synthetic polypeptide a dozen or so residues in length. With the growing number of proteins for which full sequence data is available it is even possible to look for several different parts of a single molecule (Spargo *et al.*, 1990).

Antibodies may be raised by injection of antigen into, generally, rabbits to generate a polyclonal anti-serum which can be taken by venesection. The anti-serum is likely to recognize many parts of the antigen but may require purification if other antibodies in the circulation of the injected rabbit also bind to sections. Alternatively, injection of antigen into, generally, mice is followed by the fusion of spleen cells with a myeloma cell line to generate single clones

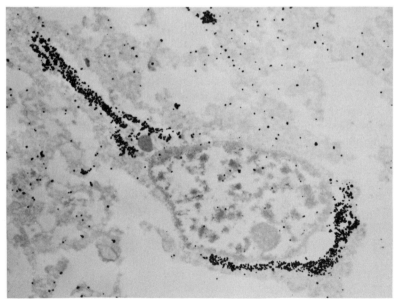

Fig. 9.3 Immunohistochemistry for tau protein. Electron micrograph showing dark dots localizing antibody that has bound to tau protein and which are labelling neurofibrillary tangle material in the cytoplasm of a single pyramidal cell.

of cells in culture which produce monoclonal antibodies directed at single epitopes. Whilst the latter approach is often preferable it is important to recognize that it is epitopes, not specific proteins, that are being recognized and that the same epitope may be present on several proteins. Nonspecific binding for this and other reasons remains a major problem in immunohistochemistry and a full range of appropriate controls and biochemical confirmation of the presence of the protein of interest is always most desirable.

Firstly, and particularly with polyclonal anti-sera, it is important to adsorb the antibody onto the specific antigen of interest prior to staining and check that staining is then greatly reduced or preferably abolished. Secondly, it is important to make certain that nonspecific binding is not taking place and, thirdly, some check must be made that the antibody is specifically recognizing an epitope on the protein of interest and not a similar, or identical, epitope on another protein. The latter problem is best checked by running a protein gel from, in this instance, brain and transferring (blotting) the protein on to nitrocellulose. The resulting blot is incubated with the antibody to check that it binds to a band (or bands) of the appropriate molecular weight(s) and not to anything else. If necessary, the labelled band can be removed and sequenced to make absolutely certain but this is rarely necessary. Unfortunately, the configuration of a protein in a section and on a gel may differ and affect antibody binding, thereby complicating matters.

An exhaustive list of antibodies in use in ageing and dementia would run to several volumes but some of the major structural and 'house-keeping' proteins studied are discussed below.

Neuronal cytoskeletal proteins
Most intraneuronal inclusions are largely composed of abnormal cytoskeletal proteins. Phosphorylated neurofilament epitopes were identified several years ago in plaque neurites and neurofibrillary tangles in Alzheimer's disease (Miller *et al.*, 1986). More recently, attention has focussed more closely upon tau protein. This is a microtubule-associated protein (MAP) and an abnormally phosphorylated form is found in tangles. A monoclonal antibody 'Alz 50' specifically recognizes this form of tau (Love *et al.*, 1988). Whether the neurofilament antibodies are recognizing the same, different or overlapping set of epitopes remains unclear.

Neuronal response proteins
Ubiquitin is a protein with a variety of functions including the degradation of short-lived and abnormal proteins. Possibly because neurons recognize the cytoskeletal proteins discussed above as abnormal, many inclusions contain ubiquitin conjugates and can be visualized with antibodies raised to ubiquitin (Lowe and Mayer, 1990). Not only has ubiquitin immunohistochemistry been of great value in increasing the sensitivity of detection of structural abnormalities, it has also permitted the detection of previously unrecognized structural inclusions (Lowe and Mayer, 1990; Wightman *et al.*, 1992) that remain undetectable by conventional stains and whose primary protein abnormality is unknown.

Synaptic markers
A number of proteins are associated with synaptic vesicles and immunohistochemistry for these proteins gives a general impression of the density of synapses. In Alzheimer's disease, for instance, the deafferentiation of the outer

portion of the molecular layer of the dentate gyrus and other areas has been demonstrated this way (Masliah *et al.*, 1989).

Adhesion molecules
Many membrane-spanning molecules play a crucial rôle in linking cells with one another and with the extracellular matrix. They are critical in development of the nervous system and are being increasingly studied in disease states.

Markers of neurotransmitters and neuromodulators
The volume of published work describing the distribution of neuromodulators, neurotransmitters and their associated enzyme systems in adults, ageing and dementia is truly formidable and the reader is referred to comprehensive texts for specific details (Nieuwenhuys, 1985). Classical neurotransmitters have not been easy to demonstrate immunohistochemically or with enzyme histochemistry and localization of synthetic and/or degradative enzymes (e.g. choline acetyl transferase and acetyl choline esterase respectively for the cholinergic system) has been widely employed. Whilst this approach is of value for demonstrating distribution, classical neurochemical techniques may be better for quantification of transmitter levels (Dodd *et al.*, 1988). Another difficulty is that transmitter-associated enzymes may have a different distribution from the transmitter itself.

Neuropeptides (such as substance P, neuropeptide Y, somatostatin, enkephalin etc.) are localized individually or multiply within different, specific populations of neurons, often in association with a classical transmitter. For instance, the GABAergic inhibitory neurons can be further subdivided according to their complement of peptides. Peptide immunoreactivity also persists for reasonable periods *post-mortem* and is generally tolerant of brief fixation so this technique has found widespread application in neurodegenerative disease as a method for defining the groups of neurons that are either preferentially destroyed or spared in a given condition. This pattern of selective vulnerability is used both to characterize separate diseases and to generate hypotheses as to the pathogenesis of given disorders (see above).

Demonstration of growth factors and associated agents
Another group of intercellular messengers are the growth factors and inhibitors and in this group one might also usefully include proteases and protease inhibitors. A satisfactory balance of these is likely to be essential for the formation, maintenance and turnover of synapses and nerve cell processes and it has been suggested that imbalance of these systems may lead to loss of connectivity and/or trophic support. Immunohistochemistry has prevailed in the demonstration of these agents although, as elsewhere, parallel immunoblotting and corroboration by the demonstration of the appropriate mRNA by *in situ* hybridization and/or Northern blots is of great importance. The proteases provide an interesting group of enzymes as their activity may be demonstrated directly by, for instance, their ability to digest a layer or overlaid photographic emulsion.

Calcium binding proteins
The notion that increased cytoplasmic free calcium concentration is a final common pathway in nerve cell death is gaining widespread support and this has focussed attention upon a set of cytoplasmic proteins with a consensus calcium binding sequence (EF hand) that are differentially expressed in specific populations of neurons (Celio, 1990). Antibodies are now available to

detect these proteins, members of the group including calmodulin, calbindin, parvalbumin and S100 protein, for example, Hof and Morrison (1991).

Transcription factors
Most second messenger systems, such as cyclic adenosine monophosphate (AMP), G-proteins or the inositol phosphate pathway are most readily studied biochemically (Dolphin and Scott, 1991). There is growing interest, however, in so-called third messenger systems or transcription factors. These proteins, or sometimes combinations of proteins, regulate transcription of a set of genes possessing the appropriate promoter or enhancer elements. One particular system, involving the proteins *Fos* and *Jun* has attracted great attention in the nervous system (Sheng and Greenberg, 1990; Morgan and Curran, 1991). These proteins, and related antigens, can be detected immunohistochemically and their mRNA by *in situ* hybridization (see below). Although it is early days as far as ageing and dementia are concerned it seems probable that many studies concerned with the notion that disorders of transcription are pivotal in these states will be appearing over the next five or so years.

Demonstration of receptors
Neurotransmitters, growth factors and other intercellular chemical messengers act at receptors positioned within the plasma membrane of cells. These receptors are usually transmembrane proteins with an extracellular domain that binds the effector molecule and an intracellular domain that upon occupation of the receptor site triggers one or more of a number of second messenger events. Antibodies are available that identify epitopes on several important receptors but many receptors maintain their binding characteristics *post-mortem* and there are two main approaches to their functional (as opposed to antigenic) investigation (Lunt, 1987; Dashwood, 1992; Stewart and Bourne, 1992).

In one approach the tissue is homogenized and binding of the messenger molecule under investigation (the ligand) is carried out in solution. The other is to cut frozen sections and to study binding whilst retaining morphology. This clearly has the advantage of demonstrating regional differences but is rather harder to quantify accurately. The principle of both methods is as follows: various concentrations of radiolabelled ligand are incubated with the homogenate or section for a fixed period of time and then any excess that fails to bind is washed off. The amount of 'total binding', as assessed by quantitative autoradiography (for sections) or scintillation counting, is then measured. 'Nonspecific' binding is measured by incubating the same radiolabelled ligand in the presence of a large excess of unlabelled ligand or some other compound which blocks specific binding to the receptor under investigation. The required specific binding is then simply given by:

$$\text{Specific binding} = \text{Total binding} - \text{Nonspecific binding} \qquad (1)$$

Where sections are used, radiolabelled standards, containing a range of known amounts of radioactivity bracketting the range of specific activities anticipated in the sections, are exposed against autoradiography film, along with the sections. The resulting autoradiograph is then placed upon a light box and the optical density of the standards used to generate a standard curve relating optical density on the film to specific activity of the sample. Optical density (or equivalent) can be measured by a microdensitometer or by viewing the image with a video camera attached to a frame grabber and image analyser. Each point (pixel) on the autoradiograph is represented by a number, typically between 0 and 255. In this way images of binding, including specific binding, can be generated by mathematical manipulation of the pixel values comprising the image. In addition, regions of interest, possibly defined on an image of adjacent histology section, can be outlined and mean and standard deviations of binding calculated.

Quantitative autoradiography is undoubtedly a powerful and elegant technique but there exists a large number of methodological problems, a full discussion of which are beyond the scope of this article (however, see Dashwood, 1992). Some of these include: problems associated with quenching of radioactivity by the tissue versus the standards, limited dynamic range of autoradiography film, variable background fogging of the film, *post-mortem* delay effects and accurate identification of anatomical areas.

DEMONSTRATION OF EXTRACELLULAR LESIONS

It is not only the neurons themselves that can undergo pathological changes. Alterations in the composition of the extracellular space are likely to have profound effects upon neuronal function and accumulation of abnormal protein seems to be a key event in several disorders.

Amyloid
The most important extracellular proteins in dementia are βA4 protein (deposited in large amounts in relation to blood vessels and plaques in Alzheimer's disease) and prion protein (deposited in small amounts in spongiform encephalopathies and related conditions). Both of these proteins form amyloid, that is, they adopt a β-pleated sheet configuration, and they are important markers of disease (Roberts *et al.*, 1988). The βA4 protein requires pretreatment with formic acid to expose the epitopes on the protein to the antibody.

Other extracellular proteins
Other extracellular proteins of interest are type IV collagen and other basement membrane proteins which can be used to demonstrate blood vessels (Luthert and Williams, 1991) and albumin and other plasma proteins which may be used as markers of blood–brain barrier disruption (Luthert, 1992).

CHARACTERIZATION OF REACTIVE CHANGES

Neuronal changes, as discussed above, may be subtle and, more often, pathology can be detected more readily by the brain's cellular reaction to it. The two most important cell types are the astrocyte and the resident macrophage-like cell of the CNS, the microglial cell.

Astroglia
The most widely used antibodies in routine diagnostic neuropathology must be those directed against epitopes on glial fibrillary acidic protein (GFAP). This intermediate filament protein is found almost exclusively in astrocytes (ependymal cells also contain it) and as normal grey matter astrocytes express very little of this protein but do so in abundance when reacting to many different pathological stimuli, immunohistochemistry for GFAP is a valuable tool for showing that something is amiss (Fig. 9.4). Almost without exception, neuronal loss is associated with astrocytosis, so even when it can be difficult to be

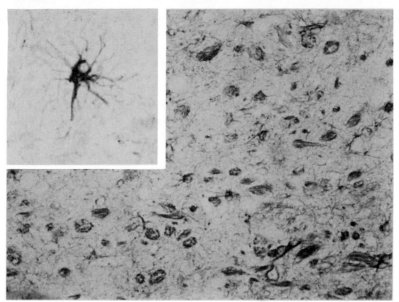

Fig. 9.4 Immunohistochemistry for glial fibrillary acidic protein. Extracellular tangles are labelled with this antibody as astrocyte processes engulf the abnormal extracellular material. The insert shows a high-power photomicrograph of a single astrocyte with no associated tangle.

confident that neurons have died (see below), diffuse astrocytosis may confirm the presence of a pathological process. Normal white matter astrocytes express GFAP so the method is not quite as valuable there, although any major increase is readily appreciated. A Holzer stain remains the best option where white matter gliosis is of crucial interest (Fig. 9.5).

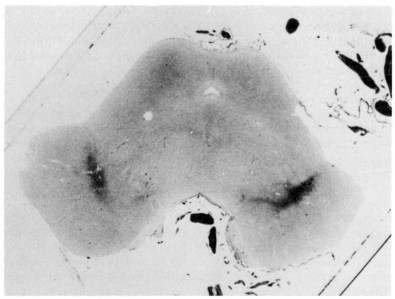

Fig. 9.5 Holzer stain. Macroscopic photograph of an entire section of the mid-brain. Note the dark staining of the substantia nigra which is showing intense reactive gliosis secondary to neuronal loss in a case of corticobasal degeneration.

Microglia

Microglial cells are the other main reactive cell population in the brain and although they are less frequently visualized in routine practise their rôle in the pathogenesis of neurodegenerative disease is currently the subject of intense study. Antibodies are available to various known and unknown epitopes on, mainly activated, microglia and macrophages. The demonstration of microglia is the main application for a technique related to immunohistochemistry, namely, lectin histochemistry. Lectins are naturally occurring plant compounds that bind with varying specificity to sugar residues. One of these, namely Ricinus communis agglutinin has proved to be of particular value in the demonstration of microglia (Mannoji *et al.*, 1986).

Other elements of the immune system

Microglia are the dominant resident immune cell but lymphocytes traffic through the nervous system and in pathological states they may be found in increased number. Precise typing of lymphocyte subsets requires frozen sections as the epitopes are readily destroyed by fixation. At a less refined level, however, T and B cells, for instance, can be discriminated in paraffin wax sections.

DEMONSTRATION OF NUCLEIC ACID

Studies of the nature and distribution of specific nucleic acid sequences fall into several categories. Firstly, there are those directed at genetic issues in familial dementias and these will not be discussed here. The others are concerned either with the potential rôle of viruses in the pathogenesis of ageing and dementing phenomena and/or with the demonstration of abnormalities in the expression of mRNA. The latter predominate as, with the exception of acquired immune deficiency syndrome (AIDS), a viral aetiology of dementing illness is supported by very little evidence. The reader is referred to more specific texts for a full description (Polak and McGee, 1990) but a brief resumé of *in situ* hybridization is given below. Specialist molecular biology text should be consulted for the breadth of other molecular biological techniques that are finding a day-to-day application in the investigation of the pathogenesis of ageing and dementia.

In situ hybridization

The principle of *in situ* hybridization is relatively straightforward. A DNA or RNA probe, which may be labelled in a variety of ways, is constructed such that its sequence is complementary to that being looked for. It is then incubated on the section under conditions which favour hybridization of the probe with the complementary sequence of, for instance, mRNA. Removal of excess, unbound probe, followed by visualization of bound nucleic acid, allows localization of the message.

Two main types of probes are used. One is derived from large (500–5000 base pairs long) cloned segments of DNA. The other is a synthetic oligodeoxyribonucleotide which can now be readily prepared and purchased at a relatively modest cost. These are typically 10–50 nucleotides in length and penetrate tissue better. There are, however, important issues of hybridization efficiency and specificity.

Labelling of a probe can be either isotopic or nonisotopic. The former have the edge in terms of sensitivity but are more hazardous and less convenient. Hybridized sections can be exposed to film, which is useful for general localization to quite small anatomical regions such as the CA fields of the hippocampus, or to a layer of emulsion coating the slide, which is more time-consuming but does, under optimal conditions, allow for cellular localization of the message.

Progress has been made in quantifying the amount of mRNA with radiolabelled probes but these are not trivial studies to carry out. RNA is inherently unstable and *post-mortem* delay, and probably more importantly agonal state, are major determinants to the levels of mRNA remaining. Internal controls can be used but different species of mRNA degrade at different rates. Other important controls are required for nonspecific binding and for binding to closely related but different sequences. Using several oligo probes directed to different portions of the molecule is a useful check on the latter. It is probably these sorts of methodological difficulties that have contributed to the various descriptions of the levels of the message for the differently spliced forms of the amyloid precursor protein in ageing and Alzheimer's disease.

TISSUE ACQUISITION

A chapter on neuropathology and neurochemistry of human CNS disorders would not be complete without a consideration of the difficulties faced in acquiring tissue. Many of the techniques described above are exquisitively sensitive to *post-mortem* delay and to agonal state. The latter term refers to the mode of death. Most elderly and dementing individuals die with bronchopneumonia and may be unconscious, presumably through hypoxia, for many hours or even days. The brain is therefore kept hypoxic and at 37 °C for a considerable period of time during which 'active' degradative processes take place. This is almost certainly considerably more damaging to *post-mortem* studies than is *post-mortem* delay which may be less critical, particularly if the body is rapidly refridgerated after death. Reducing *post-mortem* delay is also difficult. If consent for *post-mortem* is not discussed with relatives before hand hasty requests after death may lead to offence and/or refusal. Similarly, the growing practice of community care means that extra efforts have to be made to facilitate the rapid transfer of bodies to an appropriately equipped mortuary.

None of these problems are insuperable; but they require not only additional funding but also total committment by clinicians, pathologists and technical staff alike. Because of the growing pressure on routine diagnostic and clinical services and the growing range of specialist approaches to handling tissue it is no longer acceptable to immerse everything in 10% formalin, not to mention the declining 'routine' *post-mortem* rate. Specifically funded Brain Banks are providing at least a partial solution. Many of these are disease-related and, in contrast to the general lack of enthusiasm for *post-mortem* examination elsewhere, relatives may see *post-mortems*, in this context, as a very positive end to what is often a heart-breaking terminal phase to these virtually untreatable conditions.

Following *post-mortem* examination for cause of death and any other disease states that may have had a bearing on the patient's clinical state full neuropathological characterization of the extent and nature of any age-related or pathological process is required. Comprehensive clinical data are also essential. To diagnose Alzheimer's disease without clear documentary evidence that the patient was demented is most undesirable. Finally, a word on controls. For reasons outlined above, control material may be even harder to come by than diseased cases. Yet for any study to be of value the control group must be matched for age, sex, agonal state and *post-mortem* delay. In addition they, ideally, should be as well characterized clinically. The fact that an elderly lady first comes to medical attention in the course of her terminal pneumonic illness is no guarantee that she was cognitively normal for her age. It might simply reflect a very caring family.

Despite these difficulties it is clear that study of *post-mortem* tissues is absolutely essential for the further understanding of these important conditions. There is no accurate spontaneous animal model for human dementing illnesses (with the exception of scrapie and spongiform encepathopathies) and although transgenic and *in vitro* studies are of great value, the final testing ground for the resulting models of pathogenesis and potential treatments has to be in humans.

REFERENCES

Aherne, W.A. and Dunnill, M.S. (1982). *Morphometry*. Edward Arnold, London.

Bancroft, J.D. and Stevens, A. (1982). *Theory and Practice of Histological Techniques*. Churchill Livingstone, Edinburgh, London, Melbourne, New York.

Braak, H. (1984). Architectonics as seen by lipofuscin stains. In *Cerebral Cortex*. Edited by Peters, A. and Jones, E.G. (Eds). Vol. 1, pp. 59–104. Plenum Press, New York.

Burns, A., Luthert, P.J., Levy, R. *et al.* (1990). Accuracy of clinical diagnosis of Alzheimer's disease. *British Medical Journal*, **301**, 1026.

Candy, J., Oakley, A., Pullen, R. *et al.* (1989). Trace elements and the pathogenesis of Alzheimer's disease. In *Alzheimer's Disease: Towards an Understanding of the Aetiology and Pathogenesis*, Davies, D.C. (Ed.), pp. 77–88. Karger, London.

Celio, M.R. (1990). Calbindin D-28k and parvalbumin in the rat nervous system. *Neuroscience*, **35**, 375–475.

Coleman, P.D. and Flood, D.G. (1987). Neuron number and dendritic extent in normal aging and Alzheimer's disease. *Neurobiology of Aging*, **8**, 521–45.

Dashwood, M.R. (1992). Pitfalls and problems associated with quantitative *in vitro* receptor autoradiography. In *Quantitative Methods in Neuroanatomy*, Stewart, M.G. (Ed.), pp. 45–66. John Wiley & Sons, Chichester, New York, Brisbane, Toronto, Singapore.

Davis, P.J.M. and Wright, E.A. (1977). A new method for measuring cranial cavity volume and its application to the assessment of cerebral atrophy at autopsy. *Neuropathology and Applied Neurobiology*, **3**, 341.

DeFelipe, J. and Jones, E.G. (1992). Santiago Ramon y Cajal and methods in neurohistology. *Trends in Neurosciences*, **15**, 237–46.

Dekaban, A.S. and Sadowsky, D. (1978). Changes in brains weights during the span of human life: relation of brain weights to body heights and body weights. *Annals of Neurology*, **4**, 345–56.

Dodd, P.R., Hambley, J.W., Cowburn, R.F. and Hardy, J.A. (1988). A comparison of methodologies for the study of functional transmitter neurochemistry in human brain. *Journal of Neurochemistry*, **50**, 1333–45.

Dolphin, A.C. and Scott, R.H. (1991). Identification of G-protein-mediated processes. In *Molecular Neurobiology. A Practical Approach*, Chad, J. and Wheal, H. (Eds), pp. 95–113. IRL Press, Oxford, New York, Tokyo.

Fine, A., Amos, W.B., Durbin, R.M. and McNaughton, P.A. (1988). Confocal microscopy: Applications in neurobiology. *Trends in Neurosciences*, **11**, 346–51.

Gallyas, F. (1971). Silver staining of Alzheimer's neurofibrillary changes by means of physical development. *Acta Neuropathologica Hungarica*, **19**, 1–8.

Gundersen, H.J.G., Bagger, P., Bendtsen, T.F. *et al.* (1988a). The new stereological tools: Disector, fractionator, nucleator and point sampled intercepts and their use in pathological research and diagnosis. *Acta Pathologica, Microbiologica et Immunologica Scandinavica*, **96**, 857–81.

Gundersen, H.J.G., Bendtsen, T.F., Korbo, L. *et al.* (1988b). Some new, simple and efficient stereological methods and their use in pathological research and diagnosis. *Acta Pathologica, Microbiologica et Immunologica Scandinavica*, **96**, 379–94.

Hof, P.R. and Morrison, J.H. (1991). Neocortical neuronal subpopulations labeled by a monoclonal antibody to calbindin exhibit differential vulnerability in Alzheimer's disease. *Experimental Neurology*, **111**, 293–301.

Love, S., Saitoh, T., Quijada, S. *et al.* (1988). Alz-50, ubiquitin and τ immunoreactivity of neurofibrillary tangles, Pick bodies and Lewy bodies. *Journal of Neuropathology and Experimental Neurology*, **47**, 393.

Lowe, J. and Mayer, R.J. (1990). Annotation – Ubiquitin, cell stress and diseases of the nervous system. *Neuropathology and Applied Neurobiology*, **16**, 281–91.

Lunt, G.G. (1987). Neuroreceptors. In *Neurochemistry. A Practical Approach*, Turner, A.J. and Bachelard, H.S. (Eds), pp. 137–60. IRL Press, Oxford, New York, Tokyo.

Luthert, P.J. (1992). Opening of the barrier in cerebral pathology. In *Handbook of Experimental Pharmacology*, Vol. 103, *Physiology and Pharmacology of the Blood–Brain Barrier*, Bradbury, M.W.B. (Ed.), pp. 44–57. Springer-Verlag, Berlin, Heidelberg, New York.

Luthert, P.J. and Williams, J.A. (1991). A quantitative study of the coincidence of blood vessels an A4 protein deposit in Alzheimer's disease. *Neuroscience Letters*, **126**, 110–12.

Mannoji, H., Yeger, H. and Becker, L.E. (1986). A specific histochemical marker (lectin Ricinus communis agglutinin-1) for normal human microglia, and application to routine histopathology. *Acta Neuropathologica (Berl.)*, **71**, 341–3.

Masliah, E., Terry, R.D., DeTeresa, R.M. and Hansen, L.A. (1989). Immunohistochemical quantification of the synapse-related protein synaptophysin in Alzheimer disease. *Neuroscience Letters*, **103**, 234–9.

Miller, C.J., Brion, J.-P., Calvert, R. *et al.* (1986). Alzheimer's paired helical filaments share epitopes with neurofilament side arms. *European Molecular Biology Organization Journal*, **5**, 269–76.

Morgan, J.I. and Curran, T. (1991). Stimulus-transcription coupling in the nervous system: Involvement of the inducible proto-oncogenes *fos* and *jun*. *Annual Reviews of Neuroscience*, **14**, 421–51.

Neary, D., Snowden, J.S., Bowen, D.M. *et al.* (1986). Cerebral biopsy in the investigation of presenile dementia due to cerebral atrophy. *Journal of Neurology, Neurosurgery and Psychiatry*, **49**, 157–62.

Nieuwenhuys, R. (1985). *Chemoarchitecture of the Brain*. Springer-Verlag, Berlin, Heidelberg, New York, Tokyo.

Palmgren, J.J. (1948). A rapid method for selective silver staining of nerve fibres and nerve endings in mounted paraffin sections. *Acta Zoologica (Stockholm)*, **29**, 377–92.

Polak, J.M. and McGee, J.O'D. (1990). *In Situ Hybridization*. Oxford University Press, Oxford, New York, Tokyo.

Priestley, J.V. (1987). Immunocytochemical techniques for the localization of neurochemically characterized nerve pathways. In *Neurochemistry. A Practical Approach*, Turner, A.J. and Bachelard, H.S. (Eds), pp. 65–112. IRL Press, Oxford, New York, Tokyo.

Probst, A., Basler, V., Bron, B. and Ulrich, J. (1983). Neuritic plaques in senile dementia of Alzheimer type: A Golgi analysis in the hippocampal region. *Brain Research*, **268**, 249–54.

Roberts, G.W., Lofthouse, R., Allsop, D. *et al.* (1988). CNS amyloid proteins in neurodegenerative diseases. *Neurology*, **38**, 1534–40.

Scheibel, A.B., Tomiyasu, U. (1978). Dendritic sprouting in Alzheimer's presenile dementia. *Experimental Neurology*, **60**, 1.

Scheibel, A.B. (1987). Structural aspects of the aging brain: Spine system and the dendritic arbor. In *Alzheimer's Disease: Senile Dementia and Related Disorders*, Vol. 7, *Ageing*, Katzman, T.R. and Bick, (Eds), pp. 353–75. Raven Press, New York.

Sheng, M. and Greenberg, M.E. (1990). The regulation and function of *c-fos* and other immediate early genes in the nervous system. *Neuron*, **4**, 477–85.

Spargo, E.S., Everall, I. and Lantos, P.L. (1993). Neuronal loss in the hippocampus in Huntington's disease: A comparison with HIV infection. *Journal of Neurology, Neurosurgery and Psychiatry*, **56**, 487–91.

Spargo, E., Luthert, P.J., Anderton, B.H. *et al.* (1990). Antibodies against different portions of A4 protein identify a subset of plaques in Down's syndrome. *Neuroscience Letters*, **115**, 345–50.

Stewart, M.G. and Bourne, R.C. (1992). Quantitative receptor autoradiography in neurobiology: measurement of binding sites with an image analysis system. In *Quantitative Methods in Neuroanatomy*, Stewart, M.G. (Ed.), pp. 27–43. John Wiley & Sons, Chichester, New York, Brisbane, Toronto, Singapore.

Upton, G. and Fingleton, B. (1985). *Spatial Data Analysis by Example*, Vol. 1, *Point Pattern and Quantitative Data*. John Wiley & Sons, Chichester, New York, Brisbane, Toronto, Singapore.

Warren, M.A. (1992). Simple morphometry of the nervous system. In *Quantitative Methods in Neuroanatomy*, Stewart, M.G. (Ed.), pp. 211–47. John Wiley & Sons, Chichester, New York, Brisbane, Toronto, Singapore.

Wightman, G., Anderson, V.E.R., Martin, J. *et al.* (1992). Hippocampal and neocortical ubiquitin-immunoreactive inclusions in amyotrophic lateral sclerosis with dementia. *Neuroscience Letters,***139**, 269–74.

Wilcock, G.K., Matthews, S.M. and Moss, T. (1990). Comparison of three silver stains for demonstrating neurofibrillary tangles and neuritic plaques in brain tissue stored for long periods. *Acta Neuropathologica (Berl.)*, **79**, 566–8.

Michael D. Kopelman

Neuropsychiatry and Memory Disorders Clinic
Academic Unit of Psychiatry
United Medical and Dental Schools of
Guy's and St Thomas's Hospitals

10 THE EFFECT OF DRUGS ON MEMORY

INTRODUCTION

There is a long history of attempting to ameliorate or reverse the cognitive deficits of dementia, using a variety of different agents. These have employed the use of vasodilator substances (e.g. hydrogenated ergot alkaloids, such as hydergine), central nervous system stimulants, hyperbaric oxygen, high potency vitamin preparations or ribonucleic acid (Kopelman and Lishman, 1986; Whalley, 1989). Results have generally been disappointing, although the occasional success has been sufficient to motivate researchers to undertake further trials (Wittenhorn, 1981; Kopelman and Lishman, 1986; Whalley, 1989). In addition, more specific treatments have been employed or advocated, such as the use of dopamine agonists in the dementias of Parkinson's disease, steroids in subacute sclerosing panencephalitis, amantadine in Creutzfeld–Jakob disease, and AZT in acquired immune deficiency syndrome (AIDS). Nevertheless, recent research, focussing attention on the depletion of various neurotransmitters in Alzheimer and related dementias, has resulted in a shift of emphasis to the possibility of 'replacement' therapy in these disorders. To date, cholinergic depletion in Alzheimer-type dementia is the best documented neurochemical loss, and cholinergic 'replacement' therapy the most fully investigated potential treatment.

There are three issues involved in the development of a purported 'replacement' therapy: (1) establishing that a particular neurotransmitter is depleted in Alzheimer or some other dementia; (2) demonstrating the functional significance of that neurotransmitter depletion; and (3) demonstrating the efficacy of a replacement therapy. These will each be considered in turn with respect to Alzheimer dementia.

NEUROTRANSMITTER DEPLETION IN ALZHEIMER DEMENTIA

Acetylcholine

Several studies have reported a substantial loss of cholinergic neurons in the nucleus basalis, septal nucleus and dorsal band of Broca of the basal forebrain which project to the neocortex, hippocampus and amygdala (Whitehouse, 1982; Arendt *et al.*, 1983; Mann *et al.*, 1984, 1986). There is widespread, cortical and subcortical reduction in choline acetyl transferase levels (Bowen *et al.*, 1976; Perry *et al.*, 1987; Wilcock *et al.*, 1982; Rossor *et al.*, 1984) and this abnormality is associated with a reduction in cholinergic synthesis in biopsy samples (Sims *et al.*, 1980; Francis *et al.*, 1985). Postsynaptic muscarinic receptors appear to be intact, but nicotinic and presynaptic muscarinic receptors appear to be somewhat depleted (Perry *et al.*, 1978; 1987; Mash *et al.*, 1985; Flynn and Mash, 1986). Whether these cholinergic changes proceed from basal forebrain to cortex, or vice-versa, or occur simultaneously remains essentially unresolved (Arendt *et al.*, 1985; Perry, 1986; Mann *et al.*, 1986). However, Esiri *et al.* (1990) have demonstrated that the topographical distribution of cholinergic depletion appears to correlate well with the density of neurofibrillary tangles, and they argued that the disease spreads along cortico-cortical connections and between the neocortex and medial temporal structures.

Noradrenaline
There is a loss of neurons in the locus coeruleus from which ascending adrenergic pathways arise, and this cell loss is greatest in patients under the age of 80 years at the time of their death (Bondareff *et al.*, 1982; Mann *et al.*, 1984). Moreover, there is a reduction in cortical noradrenaline, which also occurs mainly in younger subjects (Mann *et al.*, 1980; Rossor *et al.*, 1984). There is a reduction in the activity of phenylethanolamine-*N*-methyl transferase, which converts adrenaline to noradrenaline, the reduction in the hippocampus being correlated with a measure of *ante-mortem* cognitive impairment (Burke *et al.*, 1987).

Dopamine
Dopamine reduction occurs in the caudate nucleus (Palmer *et al.*, 1986) and in other subcortical sites including the amygdala (Rossor and Iversen, 1986). Concentrations in the cerebral cortex are generally preserved (Rossor and Iversen, 1986), although there may be some depletion of frontal dopamine (Mann *et al.*, 1987). The dopaminergic cells of the ventral tegmental area, projecting to the limbic and frontal areas of the cortex, are markedly depleted in Alzheimer's disease, and neurofibrillary tangles are commonly found in this region (Mann *et al.*, 1987). On the other hand, the cells of the substantia nigra, projecting to the basal ganglia, are relatively unaffected.

Vasopressin
Rossor *et al.* (1980) found only a nonsignificant trend for vasopressin levels to be reduced in Alzheimer's disease, but a more recent study found reduced levels in the hippocampus, nucleus accumbens and globus pallidus (Mazurek *et al.*, 1986).

Serotonin
A variable degree of loss of large neurons in the (serotinergic) raphe nucleus has been reported in association with the presence of neurofibrillary tangles (Mann *et al.*, 1984; Yamamoto and Hirano, 1985). There is a reduction of serotonin levels in the temporal and frontal cortex (Benton *et al.*, 1982; D'Amato *et al.*, 1987), and there is also a reduction in serotoninergic binding sites in these regions (Cross *et al.*, 1986; D'Amato *et al.*, 1987). According to D'Amato *et al.* (1987), the reduction of serotoninergic markers in Alzheimer's disease is comparable in severity with the reduction in cholinergic markers. However, Bowen *et al.* (1992a) report that in half of the cortical areas they assayed, there was no evidence of reduced presynaptic activity.

Glutamate and glycine
Reductions in cerebrospinal fluid (CSF) concentrations of glutamate and glycine have been reported in Alzheimer patients, and glutamate content appeared to show some significant correlations with cognitive measures (Smith

et al., 1985). In that study, other amino acids did not show any significant correlations with cognitive scores. A substantial reduction in free glutamate in the terminal zone of the 'perforant pathway' in the entorhinal cortex has also been reported (Hyman *et al.*, 1987), which was attributed to a degeneration of a specific population of neurons in that region. Ellison *et al.* (1986) found a significant reduction of glutamate in the inferior temporal gyrus, but not in other cortical regions, and Perry *et al.* (1987) failed to find any significant cortical reduction.

Glutamate appears to be the main excitatory neurotransmitter to the pyramidal neurons of the hippocampus (Shepherd, 1988) and Bowen (1990) has reported that degeneration of columns of corticocortical glutamatergic pyramidal cells in circumscribed (parietotemporal) areas of the cerebral cortex occurs early in Alzheimer's disease. Moreover, Bowen *et al.* (1992a) suggest that glutamatergic transmission may normally be the chief factor that sustains the activity of corticocortical neurons in the cortex. Thus the degeneration in the parietotemporal cortex probably reduces excitory input into neurons, and, if the glycine B site of the *N*-methyl-D-aspartate (NMDA) receptor complex is not saturated by endogenous ligand, a partial agonist such as D-cycloserine should promote the effect of the remaining pool of glutamate transmitter on the receptor (Bowen *et al.*, 1992b), widely thought to play a critical role in memory processes (Lynch and Baudry, 1988). On the other hand, Penney *et al.* (1990) have found a substantial loss of NMDA binding sites, and a moderate loss of glutamate binding, in autoradiographic studies of Alzheimer brains, suggesting that the potential for facilitating activity at these receptors may be limited.

Gamma-aminobutyric acid
Gamma-aminobutyric acid (GABA) is the inhibitory neurotransmitter within the interneurons of the hippocampus, producing postsynaptic inhibition within the pyramidal neurons by feedback and feed-forward mechanisms (Shepherd, 1988). GABA shows a reduction of approximately 20 to 30% in the temporal cortex of younger Alzheimer patients (Rossor *et al.*, 1982, 1984). However, GABA may not be significantly diminished in other cortical or subcortical regions, nor in older Alzheimer patients (Rossor *et al.*, 1982, 1984; Ellison *et al.*, 1986). One study found decreased GABA content in the frontal and occipital lobes (Perry *et al.*, 1987), and another obtained a reduction at *post-mortem* in the frontal and temporal lobes (Lowe *et al.*, 1988); and there is evidence that GABA-A and GABA-B receptors are both reduced in the frontal cortex of Alzheimer patients (Chui *et al.*, 1987). However, Lowe *et al.* (1988) failed to find reduced GABA levels *ante-mortem* in biopsy samples from Alzheimer patients, suggesting that this may be a late manifestation of the disorder.

Somatostatin
Many neuritic plaques and many neurons containing tangles are immunoreactive to somatostatin (Morrison *et al.*, 1985; Roberts *et al.*, 1985); and there is evidence of a widespread neocortical reduction in somatostatin levels, which is most profound in the temporal or parietal cortex, but is not found in the basal forebrain or other subcortical structures (Beal *et al.*, 1986; Tamminga *et al.*, 1987). There is also evidence that a reduction in CSF markers of somatostatin correlates with cognitive abnormalities (Soininen *et al.*, 1984; Tamminga *et al.*, 1987). On the other hand, Palmer *et al.* (1988) reported reduced somatostatin levels *post-mortem*, but not in *ante-mortem* biopsy samples. Tissue samples were taken from the temporal lobe in both cases, and the biopsy group had had

Alzheimer symptoms for a mean duration of 3 years against 8 years in the post-mortem group. This suggests that somatostatin depletion, like GABA depletion (Lowe *et al.*, 1988; Palmer *et al.*, 1988), may be a relatively late manifestation of the disorder.

Neuropeptides and amino acids
There is a report that substance P is significantly reduced in the cerebral cortex and hippocampus, especially in the inferior temporal gyrus (Beal and Mazurek, 1987). Neuropeptide Y was found to be reduced in one study in association with changes in somatostatin (Kowall and Beal, 1988) but other studies have found normal neuropeptide Y (Rossor and Iversen, 1986). A further study reported a reduction in corticotrophin-releasing factor in the frontal, temporal and occipital lobes, which was correlated with the reduction of choline acetyl transferase (Whitehouse *et al.*, 1987). In general, levels of cholecystokinin, vasoactive intestinal polypeptide, neurotensin, thyrotropin-releasing hormone, asparate, alanine, taurine and glutathione have all been reported as normal (Rossor and Iversen, 1986; Ellison *et al.*, 1986; Perry *et al.*, 1987).

Summary
There is considerable evidence that cholinergic neurons, enzymes and synthesis are all depleted in Alzheimer patients. There is also evidence of substantial reductions in cortical levels of noradrenaline, serotonin, somatostatin and glutamate, particularly in younger patients. Findings with respect to dopamine, vasopressin, GABA and the neuropeptides are more equivocal. These various findings are summarized in Table 10.1, particularly with respect to findings

Table 10.1   Neurotransmitters in Alzheimer's disease.

1. *Acetylcholine*	
Precursor enzymes, ACh synthesis, and cholinergic neurons	↓ ↓
Muscarinic receptors	Little or no change
Nicotinic receptors	↓
2. *Catecholamines and related substances*	
Noradrenaline and locus coeruleus neurons	↓
Dopamine: Frontal cortex	↓
Other cortex	Little or no change
Caudate, amygdala, tegmentum	↓ ↓
Substantia nigra	Relatively unaffected
Vasopressin (modulates adrenergic activity)	↓ in hippocampus
3. *Serotonin*	
Raphe neurons	↓
Frontal and temporal cortex serotonin	↓ ↓
Frontal and temporal binding sites	↓
4. *Glutamate/GABA*	
Glutamate (excitatory): Entorhinal cortex	↓ ↓
Temporal-parietal cortex	↓
Other cortical regions	Little or no change
GABA (inhibitory): Frontal and temporal cortex	↓ late in disorder
5. *Other neurotransmitters*	
↓ Somatostatin, ? ↓ Substance P, ↓ Corticotrophin-releasing factor	

pertinent to the psychopharmacological studies discussed below. Of the possible role of these substances in human memory, only acetylcholine has been explored in detail, but there is some research on the catecholamines and the glutamate/GABA system. The various findings will be considered in the next section.

THE FUNCTIONAL ROLE OF NEUROTRANSMITTERS IN MEMORY

Acetylcholine and memory

One way of examining the effects of a putative neurotransmitter agent upon human memory is to administer a substance known to antagonize or 'block' the actions of that agent. This has been done most commonly in the cholinergic system by administering hyoscine/scopolamine to healthy subjects, and examining its effects upon aspects of attention and memory (Kopelman, 1986). It should be noted that scopolamine exerts its predominant effects upon the so-called muscarinic receptors in the brain but that, at higher doses, it also antagonizes nicotinic receptors (Weiner, 1980) and, indeed, nicotine has been shown to reverse some of its effects (Wesnes and Revell, 1984).

Variable results have been obtained on tests of attention and information-processing, but many studies reveal impairment. It appears that dual-channel tasks (e.g. dichotic listening) and vigilance tasks conducted over an extended period are particularly sensitive to the effect of cholinergic blockade (Drachman *et al.*, 1980; Wesnes and Warburton, 1983; 1984; Dunne and Hartley, 1985). There appears to be quite a striking dose–response effect, and this is particularly well illustrated in studies by Safer and Allen (1971), Nuotto (1983), Wesnes and Warburton (1984) and Parrott (1986). Dunne and Hartley (1985) and Broks *et al.*, (1988) argued that scopolamine can disrupt attentional processes without affecting overall memory performance. However, various other studies have reported that scopolamine can produce amnesic deficits at doses which do not impair performance in tests of attention or vigilance (Crow and Grove-White, 1973; Crow *et al.*, 1975; Caine *et al.*, 1981; Sunderland *et al.*, 1987; Kopelman and Corn, 1988). A third group of studies have found fairly uniform impairments across different types of test (Parrott, 1986; Wesnes *et al.*, 1988). The most recent studies suggest that the amnesic properties of scopolamine cannot be accounted for by covarying for any effects on attention; and there may be *independent* effects of the drug on memory and attention processes (see below).

There are many studies which have found that cholinergic blockade produces an impairment on learning tests ('explicit memory'), whilst immediate recall of small quantities of information ('primary' or 'working' memory) remains relatively unaffected (e.g. Crow and Grove-White, 1973; Drachman and Leavitt, 1974; Frith *et al.*, 1984; Kopelman and Corn, 1988). Moreover, this learning deficit can be reversed by concurrent administration of a cholinergic agonist or anticholinesterase (Drachman, 1977; Mohs and Davies, 1985). Two studies have included Alzheimer and Parkinson patients, respectively, demonstrating that these groups show lower dose thresholds for the manifestation of scopolamine-induced learning impairments (Dubois *et al.*, 1987; Sunderland *et al.*, 1987). Only the more recent studies have examined the pattern of memory deficits in a detailed fashion, similar to that employed in neuropsychological studies of amnesic or dementing patients (Caine *et al.*, 1981; Beatty *et al.*, 1986; Nissen *et al.*, 1987; Kopelman and Corn, 1988; Rusted, 1988; Rusted and Warburton, 1988; Tröster *et al.*, 1989; Curran *et al.*, 1991; Knopman, 1991).

Caine *et al.* (1981) found impairment on verbal and nonverbal learning tests as well as impairment on a test of immediate forgetting in a small group of subjects. They also showed that the verbal recall impairment could be mitigated by providing semantic or acoustic retrieval cues. Beatty *et al.* (1986) demonstrated a deficit in verbal memory, and impairment on a test of 'short-term' forgetting in which the subject has to perform a (variable) distractor task for a few seconds before recalling a group of three words (the Brown–Peterson test). On the other hand, performance was intact for a task in which subjects were required to retrieve as many words as possible beginning with a particular letter (a verbal fluency task involving retrieval from semantic memory). Beatty *et al.* (1986) suggested that performance in cholinergic blockade differed from that seen in Alzheimer's dementia, but the argument depended upon small differences in error patterns in which ceiling and floor effects were evident. Nissen *et al.* (1987) showed impairment on verbal recall and recognition tests with intact ability at a perceptuomotor learning task (serial reaction time) and at two semantic retrieval tasks.

In a larger study, Kopelman and Corn (1988) compared findings for cholinergic blockade with the results obtained in closely similar studies of Alzheimer and Korsakoff patients. They reported that cholinergic blockade did not have a significant effect upon the more passive aspects of immediate ('primary' or 'working') memory, namely, span tests and a measure of verbal, short-term forgetting in which the 'distractor task' was kept constant throughout. In this, it resembled the Korsakoff syndrome and contrasted with the marked deficits seen in Alzheimer-type dementia. On the other hand, cholinergic blockade did produce impairment at a visuospatial, short-term forgetting test, and at a verbal test in which the distractor task was varied and made more difficult, thereby increasing the 'information-processing load' of the task. 'Secondary memory' refers to the learning of larger quantities of information over intervals longer than a few seconds, and on such tests, cholinergic blockade produced a pattern similar to that seen in the anterograde amnesia of Korsakoff and many Alzheimer patients. There was a pronounced impairment in learning verbal and visuospatial material on both recall and recognition memory tests, a normal forgetting rate once learning had been accomplished (Fig. 10.1), and preservation of the rate at which a perceptuomotor skill was learned. In particular, cholinergic blockade did not affect the response to priming but produced an impairment of cued recall (Fig. 10.2), a pattern commonly found in studies of amnesic patients (Graf *et al.*, 1984) and in some studies of Alzheimer patients (Partridge *et al.*, 1990; Christensen *et al.*, 1992). 'Priming' refers to the general facilitation of a response from having seen a word (or other stimulus) before, whereas 'cued recall' refers to recall of the words (or other stimuli) from a specific list in response to particular cues. However, cholinergic blockade differed from the pattern seen in amnesic or demented patients in that it did not produce any retrograde amnesia, nor did it affect performance at a verbal fluency (semantic memory) task, or the recall of the temporal context of information. Kopelman and Corn (1988) concluded that cholinergic blockade produced a pattern of anterograde amnesia broadly consistent with that seen in the Korsakoff syndrome and many Alzheimer patients, but that it did not mimic the extensive retrograde loss seen in both disorders, nor the full range of 'primary' or 'working' memory deficits which occur in Alzheimer-type dementia.

This latter aspect of memory has been studied in detail in a series of elegant experiments by Rusted (1988) and Rusted and Warburton (1988). Rusted (1988) found that a digit span task and a visuospatial 'mental rotation' task were

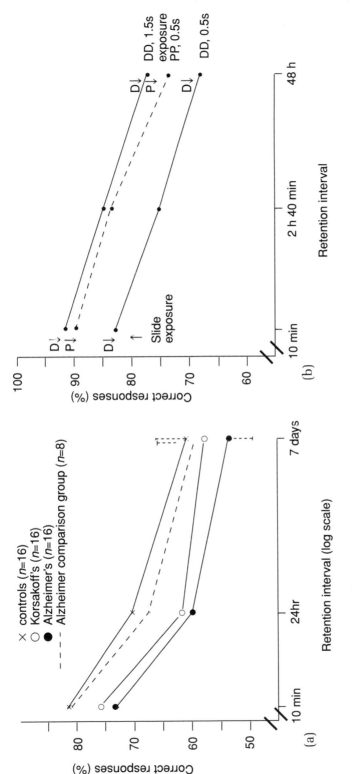

Fig. 10.1 Forgetting rates in Alzheimer dementia, Korsakoff's syndrome and cholinergic blockade. (a) Forgetting rates over the course of a week on a picture recognition test, after Alzheimer and Korsakoff patients' performance had been 'matched' as closely as possible to control subjects by prolonging exposure times for initial presentation of slides (pictures from magazines). Reproduced with permission from *Neuropsychologia*, 1985. (b) Forgetting rates for placebo and cholinergic blockade in healthy subjects: at 0.5 seconds' exposure of slides the drug (DD) group (scopolamine) performed significantly poorer at 10 minutes than the placebo (PP) group, whereas at 1.5 seconds exposure the drug group performed as well as the 0.5 second placebo group. In both drug groups, the rate of forgetting over 48 hours was the same as the placebo group, i.e. a pattern which mimics that seen in organic amnesia and dementia. D = drug. P = placebo. Reproduced with permission from *Brain*, 1988.

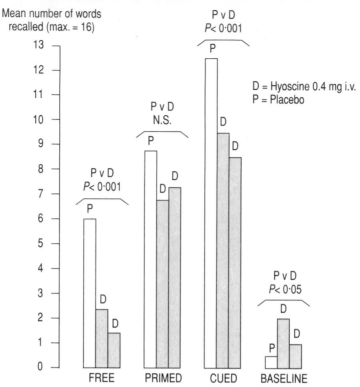

Fig. 10.2 Word list recall in free, primed, cued and baseline conditions. Open bars = placebo (P). Hatched bars = drug: scopolamine (D). Two drug groups were studied. Cholinergic blockade produced significant ($P < 0.001$) impairment on free and cued recall, and no significant impairment on priming, a pattern which mimics that seen in studies of organic amnesia (Graf *et al.*, 1984) and dementia (Partridge *et al.*, 1990). N.S. = not significant. Reproduced with permission from *Brain*, 1988.

unaffected by cholinergic blockade, and also by the performance of either a concurrent verbal articulation task or a concurrent spatial tapping task. Moreover, there were no significant interactions between the effects of cholinergic blockade and the concurrent tasks. On the other hand, performance at a test of immediate free recall was significantly impaired by cholinergic blockade and by both the concurrent tasks. In another experiment, Rusted and Warburton (1988) found a significant effect of cholinergic blockade on an immediate and delayed test of memory for spatial location and at a simple logical reasoning task, but no significant effect on a shape recognition task. Rusted (1988) has interpreted these findings in terms of Baddeley and Hitch's (1974) model of 'working memory', in which a 'central executive' of limited processing resources is subserved by an auditory–verbal 'articulatory loop' and a visuospatial 'scratch-pad'. In Rusted's view, cholinergic blockade produces a selective effect on the 'central executive' component of working memory, consistent with the pattern of impairment in early Alzheimer patients obtained by Morris (1986) and by Baddeley *et al.* (1986), using different tasks. However, she acknowledged that some other factor (perhaps related to the chronicity or severity of cholinergic depletion) needs to be postulated to account for the well-documented impairment of Alzheimer patients on simple span tests. In brief, Rusted (1988) argued that the pattern of deficit in 'working memory' following cholinergic blockade is qualitatively similar to that which occurs in Alzheimer's disease, and that quantitative differences in the extent of impairment account for discrepancies, for example, on span test performance.

With regard to secondary memory, Tröster *et al.* (1989) found that 0.5 to 0.8 mg scopolamine produced dose-related impairments on a variety of measures of verbal and nonverbal memory, consistent with the studies reported above. However, there were no effects upon a test of retrograde memory, although in this study there was also impairment on a verbal fluency test. By contrast, Lines *et al.* (1991) found normal performance on verbal fluency. Knopman (1991) found that scopolamine produced impairment in the free recall of word lists, but did not affect a word-completion priming task, a motor serial reaction task or repetition priming on a tachistoscopic word identification task. These findings would appear to confirm that scopolamine resembles organic amnesia in leaving so-called 'implicit memory' (Schacter, 1987) unaffected, whereas 'explicit memory' is impaired (cf. Kopelman and Corn, 1988). Curran (1991) has also found that priming is spared by scopolamine administration, although Frith *et al.* (1989) have found that scopolamine did affect the rate of learning of a perceptuomotor tracking task.

On the vexed issue of the relationship of memory to attention deficits, Kopelman and Corn (1988) found that cholinergic blockade produced a significant decrement on a subjective measure of arousal and on one of three 'attention' tests administered, but covarying for the latter had negligible effect upon the significant impairments obtained for anterograde memory tests. Likewise, Curran *et al.* (1991) performed an analysis of covariance for subjectively rated sedation and three psychomotor measures against tests of memory, mental rotation, reasoning, vigilance and perceptuomotor skills. They found that subjectively rated sedation was more closely related to performance on the psychomotor tasks than the memory tasks; and that covarying for sedation or psychomotor performance did not affect the significant effects of the drug on immediate recall of paired-associates or immediate and delayed recall of a prose passage. Wesnes *et al.* (1988) found impairments across a battery of memory and attention tests, and subsequent analysis (Wesnes, 1992) using factor analytic techniques suggested the effects of the drug on attention were independent from those on memory. Potter *et al.* (1991) measured event-related potentials (ERPs) during a task requiring continuous recognition memory for visually presented words. They found that, in a placebo condition, correctly recognized words evoked more positive ERPs than did distractor words. Scopolamine caused a substantial impairment in task performance, but it did not reduce the size of these old–new word ERP differences. It was concluded that the old–new ERP effects were unlikely to reflect the level of functioning of cholinergically innovated brain regions contributing to recognition memory (which the authors suggest depends upon familiarity judgements), but may have been more closely associated with retrieval than acquisition processes. Finally, Rusted and Eaton-Williams (1991) examined the separate and combined effects of scopolamine and nicotine on verbal recall, finding that a single dose of nicotine improved recall performance on lengthy but not short word lists, but had no effect on the scopolamine-induced recall deficits observed for both lists of words. These results were interpreted in terms of the independence of attention and memory processes, and the authors suggested that whereas nicotine improves attention, scopolamine has a specific effect upon memory processes.

Table 10.2 summarizes the principal findings in studies of cholinergic blockade.

Table 10.2 Summary of principal cholinergic blockade findings.

Memory process	Finding(s)	Pertinent studies
Working memory (material held over a matter of a few seconds only)	Impairment related to information-processing load of task (with relatively simple tasks spared, e.g. span)	Kopelman and Corn (1988) Rusted (1988) Rusted and Warburton (1988)
'Explicit' memory	Impairment on many tasks involving recall or recognition of verbal or nonverbal material	Many studies including: Crow and Grove-White (1973) Drachman and Leavitt (1974) Frith *et al.* (1984) Kopelman and Corn (1988) Wesnes *et al.* (1988) Tröster *et al.* (1989)
Rate of forgetting from explicit memory	Unaffected	Kopelman and Corn (1988)
Semantic memory (general knowledge, usually tested by verbal fluency in these studies)	Spared if retrieval period is 60 seconds or less for each item,	Nissen *et al.* (1987) Kopelman and Corn (1988) Curran *et al.* (1991) Lines *et al.* (1991)
	but others find impairment	Caine *et al.* (1981) Tröster *et al.* (1989) Dunne (1990)
Priming (usually assessed by 'word-completion' tasks in these studies)	Unimpaired	Kopelman and Corn (1988) Knopman (1991) Curran (1991)
	Equivocal result	Nissen *et al.* (1987)
Procedural memory (skill learning)	Unimpaired	Nissen *et al.* (1987) Kopelman and Corn (1988) Knopman (1991)
	Impaired	Frith *et al.* (1989)
Retrograde memory (predrug or 'remote' memories)	Unimpaired	Kopelman and Corn (1988) Tröster *et al.* (1989)
Relationship of memory impairment to attention deficit	Probably these deficits at least partially independent	Kopelman and Corn (1988) Curran *et al.* (1991) Rusted and Eaton-Williams (1991) Wesnes (1992)

Catecholamines and memory

There have been a number of studies examining the effect of adrenergic agents upon memory and, in particular, investigating vasopressin which may modulate noradrenergic neurotransmission (De Wied and van Ree, 1982). Much of this work derives from animal studies; and there is considerable controversy concerning whether vasopressin exerts a direct action on memory itself or has a secondary effect by a beneficial action on arousal and/or mood (Gash and Thomas, 1983; De Wied, 1984; Sahgal, 1984). Weingartner *et al.* (1981) and Millar *et al.* (1987) both suggested that vasopressin has a direct, beneficial effect on 'explicit' memory in healthy subjects, whereas Snel *et al.* (1987) postulated an action upon 'tonic attentional processes' rather than either the storage or retrieval of memories.

Frith *et al.* (1985) and Clark *et al.* (1986) studied the effect of low doses of clonidine on the grounds that it would inhibit noradrenaline release. Frith *et al.* (1985) found that healthy subjects were impaired by this drug on a paired-associate learning task but that span tests and a measure of semantic memory were unaffected. On the other hand, Clark *et al.* (1986) found that the most striking effects were on subjective arousal, and that there was a significant impairment at both 'focussed' and 'divided' attention tasks. In short, it seems likely that adrenergic agents have a direct effect upon processes mediating 'attention' and 'arousal', but it remains controversial whether they have direct mnemonic effects beyond this.

Gamma-aminobutyric acid benzodiazepines and memory

Benzodiazepines *potentiate* the action of GABA. GABA is an inhibitory neurotransmitter acting at interneurons within the hippocampus, and this potentiation produces an *impairment* of memory. GABA is depleted in late Alzheimer's disease (see above), but the severe depletion of glutamate, the excitatory neurotransmitter (Hyman *et al.*, 1987) within the entorhinal cortex, may be more critical for the memory loss.

There have been many studies of the actions of benzodiazepines on memory, in part prompted by their use in dentistry and anaesthetics (see e.g. O'Boyle *et al.*, 1987, and excellent reviews by Curran, 1986, 1991). As in studies of cholinergic blockers, 'primary' memory is usually unaffected as measured on, for example, span tasks or the 'recency component' of free recall (e.g. Ghoneim and Mewaldt, 1975; Brown *et al.*, 1982; Curran *et al.*, 1987). However, when subjects are given a larger quantity of information to learn or when recall is tested after a delay, benzodiazepines produce an anterograde impairment in 'explicit' memory (e.g. Ghoneim and Mewaldt, 1975, 1977; Curran *et al.*, 1987). This is sensitive to both recall and recognition testing (Brown *et al.*, 1982) and is similar in many ways to that produced by hyoscine/scopolamine (Frith *et al.*, 1984), except that it is reversed by a benzodiazepine antagonist (Dorow *et al.*, 1987) but not by a cholinergic agent (Ghoneim and Mewaldt, 1977; Preston *et al.*, 1989). Tasks involving verbal material are more consistently affected than those involving pictorial material (Curran, 1986). Once learning has been accomplished, the rate of forgetting is normal (Brown *et al.*, 1983), and these drugs do not produce any retrograde deficit (Ghoneim and Mewaldt, 1975, 1977), and may even facilitate the recall of material learned immediately before drug administration (Brown *et al.*, 1982; Ghoneim *et al.*, 1984). Retrieval of semantic knowledge is slowed by these drugs (Brown *et al.*, 1983; Ghoneim *et al.*, 1984), but the overall level of performance is not significantly affected (Brown *et al.*, 1983). Curran (1991) reported that flumazenil has differential effects in reversing the sedating and amnesic properties of diazepam, lorazepam and midazolam; and Curran *et al.* (1991) and File *et al.* (1992) concluded that sedation contributes to, but does not completely account for, the amnesic effects of benzodiazepines.

Brown *et al.* (1982) and Lister and Weingartner (1987) both pointed to the similarity between many aspects of the anterograde amnesia produced by benzodiazepines and that of the organic amnesic syndrome. However, several recent studies point to possible differences between benzodiazepine-induced amnesia and the pattern seen in cholinergic blockade and in organic disease. Taylor *et al.* (1987) found that diazepam produced impairment on a task requiring judgements about visual rotation; and Brown *et al.* (1989) found that lorazepam suppressed the normal facilitation ('priming') provided by presenting the first three letters of words to be recalled on a list learning task ('word completion priming'). Taylor *et al.*'s result contrasted with the normal visual rotation performance obtained by Rusted (1988) in her cholinergic blockade study, and Brown *et al.*'s result contrasted with normal 'priming' obtained by Kopelman and Corn (1988) in cholinergic blockade, by Graf *et al.* (1984) in organic amnesia and by Partridge *et al.* (1990) in Alzheimer dementia. Subsequently, Knopman (1991) and Curran and various colleagues (Curran, 1991) have also found impaired word completion priming by lorazepam, whilst scopolamine and oxazepam left priming intact. These findings were taken to imply that lorazepam, and possibly some (but not all) other benzodiazepines, has a qualitatively different effect from the classical amnesic syndrome, as it affects both 'explicit' memory and priming (also known as 'implicit' memory).

Summary

We now have substantial understanding of the pattern of memory impairment produced by two groups of drugs: the cholinergic antagonists, such as scopolamine, and the benzodiazepines. In general, they produce anterograde amnesic deficits similar to those produced by organic amnesia or dementia, but they do not produce retrograde amnesia. As in organic amnesia and some studies of dementia, word-completion priming and the rate of 'long-term' forgetting are preserved in scopolamine studies. In addition, the degree of impairment produced by scopolamine on 'working memory' appears to depend on the 'information-processing load' of the particular task. A surprising finding is that lorazepam, unlike scopolamine and some other benzodiazepines, appears to impair measures of priming. It seems unlikely that the amnesic properties of either the anticholinergic agents or the benzodiazepines can be wholly explained by an effect upon attention processes. By contrast, it seems likely that any effect of the catecholamines on memory is attributable to actions upon attention, arousal or mood. Little is known about the cognitive properties of other neurotransmitter systems.

'REPLACEMENT' THERAPY IN ALZHEIMER PATIENTS

Cholinergic agents

Trials of cholinergic 'replacement' therapy have involved the administration of oral choline or lecithin (precursors of acetylcholine), of the infusion of the anticholinesterase, physostigmine (which inhibits the breakdown of acetylcholine) or, occasionally, of dimethylaminoethanol or arecoline (a cholinomimetic which acts directly on cholinergic receptors). More recently, there have been trials of RS-86, oral physostigmine, tetrahydroaminoacridine (THA), various drug combinations and nicotine.

The earliest trials of cholinergic agents in amnesic or dementing patients occurred in the late 1970s, and there were initially a few promising findings (e.g. by Peters and Levin (1977) in a postherpes encephalitis patient). However, reports soon began to appear of negative or negligible results when these substances were administered to Alzheimer patients (e.g. Boyd *et al.*, 1977; Etienne *et al.*, 1978; Signoret *et al.*, 1978; Smith *et al.*, 1978). By the time Bartus *et al.* (1982) published their review of the trials in Alzheimer-type dementia, they were able to report that of 17 trials using cholinergic precursors (choline or lecithin), 10 reported no effect, six reported nonsignificant trends towards improved cognitive performance, and only one study claimed statistically significant gains. Subsequent trials have, in general, produced equally disappointing results. For example, a careful study of prolonged (6 months') lecithin administration failed to find any overall benefit of the drug (Little *et al.*, 1985), a result which has been replicated (Heyman *et al.*, 1987). Two trials of the muscarinic agonist, RS-86, also failed to show any significant benefit relative to placebo in Alzheimer patients (Bruno *et al.*, 1986; Hollander *et al.*, 1987), although one of the studies claimed that there was a 'clinically meaningful' improvement in 6 out of 12 patients (Hollander *et al.*, 1987). A study finding a small but statistically significant benefit of intravenous arecoline on a picture recognition task (Christie *et al.*, 1981) was replicated by Tariot *et al.* (1988), but the latter authors noted more striking effects upon aspects of psychomotor activity and mood.

Trials employing intravenous physostigmine or oral THA have appeared to be somewhat more successful. Johns *et al.* (1983) suggested that improvement was likeliest when the dose was titrated in order to identify the optimum dose for each individual subject, and when recognition rather than recall memory tests were employed. Both these substances are anticholinesterases, preventing the breakdown of acetylcholine, and Johns *et al.* (1983) pointed out that these substances differ from choline and lecithin in not requiring intact presynaptic neurons (in which acetylcholine synthesis occurs) in order to achieve their effect. Johns *et al.* (1983) suggested that this might account for the apparently greater promise of anticholinesterases in the trials they reported up to the date of their review. For example, Christie *et al.* (1981) reported significant improvement in 11 Alzheimer patients on a picture recognition test 15 minutes after the start of an intravenous infusion of physostigmine. Davis and Mohs (1982) obtained significant benefits in 10 patients from oral physostigmine on a picture and a word recognition test. Thal *et al.* (1983) reported significant improvement from combined physostigmine and lecithin on a word learning test in six patients. Muramato *et al.* (1984) obtained significant improvement from varying doses of physostigmine on a copying task in three patients. On the other hand, several more recent studies have failed to show any significant benefit from physostigmine, although a trend towards improvement is often obtained (Mohs *et al.*, 1985; Gustaffson *et al.*, 1987; Stern *et al.*, 1987). It is particularly interesting that Gustaffson *et al.* (1987) obtained an increase in cerebral blood flow following intravenous physostigmine, although there were no significant cognitive benefits.

More recent studies have focussed upon the use of THA, a longer acting anticholinesterase, usually in combination with lecithin. Kaye *et al.* (1982) used combined THA and lecithin and found only a nonsignificant trend towards improvement in 10 patients on two verbal learning tasks. However, 'dramatic' benefits with statistically significant improvements on test scores were claimed by Summers *et al.* (1986) in a widely cited study from administration of oral THA at doses of 150 to 200 mg daily, in combination with 10.9 g lecithin daily, to 15 Alzheimer patients. However, there were a number of technical faults in that trial. In particular, it appears that the authors did not actually report the results of the 'blind' phase of their trial, but 'pooled' the findings from a 'blind' and a 'nonblind' phase (Kopelman, 1987). Moreover, there was a curious finding, pointed out by Small et al. (1987), whereby performance on placebo was always exactly the same as in the 'baseline' condition.

Chatellier and Lacomblez (1990) administered a mean dose of 114 mg THA or placebo daily plus 1200 mg lecithin daily over a 4-week treatment period and a 4-week control period, without washout at crossover, in 67 outpatients with probable Alzheimer dementia, of whom 60 completed the study. On the Mini-Mental State Examination (MMSE) and the Stockton Geriatric score, there were no significant differences between THA and placebo. A visual analogue rating scale was completed by a relative and by the physician in charge; on the physician's rating, there was a slight and statistically significant improvement on THA. However, the authors concluded that, at doses lower than 125 mg a day, there was no significant benefit of THA on the symptoms of Alzheimer dementia. Moreover, during a 4-month follow-up period, there were no significant differences between changes obtained on THA or placebo. Hepatitis was induced in 9 out of 67 patients in this series. It should be noted that the mean MMSE score in these patients was 13.75 at baseline, implying that the patients were quite severely demented in this study.

Gauthier and 22 others (1990) studied 52 patients with a clinical diagnosis of probable Alzheimer dementia, and administered the maximum daily dose of THA tolerated by each patient (up to 100 mg per day), determined in a prestudy phase, over a period of 8 weeks. Results were compared with those obtained during 8 weeks on placebo in a crossover design. Lecithin was administered concurrently at a daily dose of 4.7 g. Patients were seen every 2 weeks by an investigator who was blind to the phase of treatment, and who conducted assessments on the MMSE, a disability rating scale, a global impression score and a measure of activities of daily living. Thirty-nine patients completed the double-blind phase of the study (a patient to investigator ratio of 1.7 : 1!). There was a significant improvement on the MMSE of 1.2 points half-way through the THA treatment period, but this was considered 'of doubtful clinical importance in view of the lack of change in scores on other cognitive, functional, and behavioral scales'. No significant differences were obtained between THA and placebo at the end of the 8-week treatment phases. The authors noted that they had administered lower doses of THA and lecithin than Summers et al. (1986), but they had done so because of dose-related hepatotoxicity in preliminary studies.

Eagger et al. (1991) studied 89 patients, of whom 65 completed the trial. Patients were randomly assigned to THA at a dose up to 150 mg daily plus 10.8 g lecithin daily or placebo plus lecithin. After 13 weeks treatment and 4 weeks washout, subjects were assigned to the other treatment. The main outcome measures were the MMSE, an abbreviated mental test score and a rating of the activities of daily living. In addition, some computerized and conventional psychological tests were included. The main finding was a highly significant benefit of THA over placebo in terms of MMSE score. Comparing the data in the treatment phase with the results in the placebo phase, there was a mean gain of 1.54 points during THA treatment, and a mean decline of 1.16 points from baseline during the placebo treatment. Findings on the abbreviated mental test score showed a significant improvement on THA in the same direction, and there were also significant gains on a computerized test of dot localization and a test requiring subjects to follow a simple rule and reverse it. There were no significant gains on the measures of activities of daily living, or on any of the other computerized tests, or on measures of paired-associate learning, visual recognition memory, story recall or the recall of pictures of objects. The authors argued that the improvement on the MMSE constituted a change equivalent to the deterioration in score which might be expected over a period of 6 months, and they argued that THA had exerted its benefits on perceptual and attentional processes rather than on memory itself. In this connection, it should be noted that THA probably has both nicotinic and muscarinic actions (Nordberg et al., 1990). Subsequently, Eagger et al. (1992) reported that, on those tests in which benefit was obtained, improvement occurred during the first 2 weeks, reached a maximum at 1 month, and was maintained during the rest of the 3-month treatment period. Although encouraging, the size of the gains reported were relatively small (cf. the two previous studies), and account needs to be taken of the substantial number of cognitive and other assessments in which no benefits were found.

Following reports that nicotinic cholinergic receptors may be depleted in the temporal lobes of Alzheimer patients (Flynn and Mash, 1986; Perry et al. 1987), whilst postsynaptic 'muscarinic' cholinergic receptors are preserved (Mash et al. 1985; Perry et al., 1987), there have been two studies of the effect of nicotine administered to Alzheimer patients. One of these studies reported 'a modest facilitation of memory' (Newhouse et al., 1986), and the other an improvement in tests of attention and information-processing (Jones, 1990; Sahakian et al., 1989), consistent with earlier work in healthy subjects (Wesnes and Revell, 1984). Jones and her colleagues (Sahakian et al. 1989; Jones, 1990) obtained significant benefits on a modified version of the Wesnes and Warburton (1984) vigilance task and on the ability to detect a flickering light in a critical flicker fusion task. No benefits were obtained at a task requiring recall of spatial sequences over intervals of 0 to 16 seconds. The authors interpreted this result in terms of nicotinic mechanisms being involved in attention and information-processing, rather than memory, processes. Although consistent with other researchers' findings (e.g. Rusted and Eaton-Williams, 1991), their study lacked sufficient measures of memory to conclude this, but included some intriguing behavioural observations suggesting that nicotine may have some direct effects on memory as well (Jones, 1990, pp. 173–4, 176–7).

Finally, there have been several studies in animals indicating that cholinergic brain implants can reverse the memory deficits induced by normal ageing, cholinergic lesions, or prolonged alcohol ingestion with associated cholinergic neuron loss (e.g. Gage et al., 1984; Arendt et al., 1988). Such findings provide further evidence for the role of the cholinergic system in memory processes and some hope that pharmacological intervention may eventually be successful. However, following the disappointing and/or equivocal results from dopaminergic implants in humans for Parkinson's disease, cholinergic implants in humans have not yet been tried. The nearest thing that has been attempted is the direct infusion of a cholinergic agonist, bethamecol, into the cerebrospinal fluid through an intraventricular cannula, but this appears not to have produced any significant benefits (Penn et al., 1988; Whitehouse, 1988).

The positive findings for the administration of cholinergic agents to Alzheimer patients are summarized in Table 10.3.

Table 10.3 Cognitive benefits from administration of cholinergic agents in Alzheimer patients: findings in selected studies.

Study	Drug	Test/assessment showing benefit
Christie *et al.* (1981)	Arecoline	Picture recognition memory
	Physostigmine	Picture recognition memory
Davis and Mohr (1982)	Physostigmine	Picture recognition and word recognition memory
Thal *et al.* (1983)	Physostigmine and lecithin	Word learning and recall
Muramato *et al.* (1984)	Physostigmine	Copying and drawing
Summers *et al.* (1986)	THA and lecithin	Global assessment scale
		Alzheimer's Deficit Scale
		Orientation test
		Names learning test
Jones (1990)	Nicotine	Vigilance/'information-processing' task (detecting sequences of odd or even digits)
		Detection of flicker on critical flicker fusion task
Chatellier and Lacomblez (1990)	THA and lecithin	Visual analogue global rating scale by physician
Gauthier *et al.* (1991)	THA and lecithin	Mini-Mental State Examination (MMSE)
Eagger *et al.* (1991, 1992)	THA and lecithin	MMSE
		Abbreviated mental test score
		Computerized dot localization
		Rule-reversal task.

THA = tetrahydroaminoacridine.

Adrenergic agents, serotonin reuptake inhibitors and thiamine

As discussed above, vasopressin is thought to modulate the action of the noradrenergic neurotransmitter system, and it is controversial whether any cognitive benefits it produces are mediated by an action on attention or memory. There have been several studies of its effects in patients who have dementing or other memory disorders. Several have reported negative results (e.g. Fewtrell *et al.*, 1982), whilst others have obtained an improvement in mood or attention which might account for any benefit in memory (e.g. Oliveros *et al.*, 1978). The most impressive results have been obtained in studies in which either the patients had diabetes insipidus, in which vasopressin is deficient (e.g. Laczi *et al.*, 1982, 1983), or a conditioning procedure was employed, i.e. a closer analogue of De Wied's animal studies (e.g. Anderson *et al.*, 1979).

In Alzheimer patients, Tariot *et al.* (1988) have conducted a trial of L-deprenyl, a monamine oxidase inhibitor which is metabolized to amphetamine and methamphetamine. They obtained a small but statistically significant improvement in performance at a free recall test in their subjects, associated with increased energy and social interaction and diminished anxiety. The authors suggested that the drug may have enhanced 'effort' or attention.

In a series of papers, McEntee, Mair and colleagues have argued that noradrenergic depletion may be a critical factor in producing the memory deficit of the alcoholic Korsakoff syndrome; and they have reported that a low dose of clonidine produces a small but statistically significant benefit in Korsakoff patients at tests of memory and attention (McEntee and Mair, 1980; Mair and McEntee, 1986). A puzzle is that they obtained this benefit in Korsakoff patients at the same dose of clonidine at which Frith *et al.* (1985) obtained impairment in healthy subjects. Following these findings, O'Donnell *et al.* (1986) reported that a week's administration of oral methylphenidate (an adrenergic agonist) produced a statistically significant improvement in six Korsakoff patients on a verbal recall task (the 'selective reminding' test). However, O'Carroll *et al.* (1992) have recently failed to replicate McEntee and Mair, not obtaining any significant improvements on a number of cognitive measures using clonidine and placebo in a crossover trial involving 18 Korsakoff patients.

Somewhat similarly, two studies have examined the effect of 5-hydroxytryptamine (5HT) reuptake inhibitors on alcohol-induced memory impairment. Weingartner *et al.* (1983) found that zimelidine reversed the memory impairment in healthy volunteers after administration of ethanol. Likewise, Martin *et al.* (1989) reported that fluvoxamine improved memory performance in five patients with Korsakoff's syndrome, and that the improvements were correlated significantly with reductions in CSF 5-HIAA. However, at least three studies have failed to find significant gains on cognitive tasks following the administration of 5-HT reuptake inhibitors to Alzheimer patients (Dehlin *et al.*, 1985; Cutler *et al.*, 1985; Lawlor *et al.*, 1988).

In this connection, there is evidence that the mamillary bodies and the dorsomedial nucleus of the thalamus show neuritic plaques and/or neurofibrillary tangles in 95% of patients with Alzheimer's disease (Grossi *et al.*, 1989), and that transketolase activity is substantially reduced in Alzheimer patients (Gibson *et al.*, 1988). Although there are some important differences, there are also some close resemblances between the neuropsychological patterns of amnesia in Korsakoff's syndrome and Alzheimer dementia (Kopelman, 1985, 1989, 1991). A preliminary trial of oral thiamine in moderately severe Alzheimer patients showed small but statistically significant benefits on the MMSE relative to placebo (Blass *et al.*, 1988), comparable in size to those obtained using THA. However, behavioural ratings did not show any change in response to thiamine.

Glutamate/gamma-aminobutyric acid

Piracetam (1-acetamide-2-pyrrolidine) is a cyclical derivative of GABA with a chemical structure very similar to GABA. It is believed to increase cerebral energy metabolism (as measured by the turnover of adenosine triphosphate, glucose and oxygen), and animal studies suggested that it might improve learning (Bartus *et al.*, 1983). However, findings in studies of Alzheimer patients have been disappointing (McDonald, 1982; Branconnier, 1983). On the basis of animal studies, it was also believed that it might potentiate the action of cholinergic agents, when administered together, but a careful study of combined piracetam and lecithin failed to find any significant benefit in Alzheimer patients (Growdon *et al.*, 1986). To the author's knowledge, there have not yet been any trials of piracetam in Huntington patients, in whom GABA is also depleted.

As discussed above, benzodiazepines appear to facilitate the action of GABA and cause amnesia. Benzodiazepine-induced amnesia has been put forward as a 'model' of the anterograde memory deficit in the Korsakoff syndrome (Brown *et al.*, 1982; Lister and Weingartner, 1987), but, as far as the author is aware, there have not yet been any clinical trials of benzodiazepine antagonists in this condition. A study employing a GABA antagonist in Alzheimer dementia failed to demonstrate any benefit (Mohr *et al.*, 1986).

As mentioned above, Bowen and colleagues (Bowen, 1990; Bowen *et al.*, 1992a, b) have suggested that a partial agonist of the glycine B site on the NMDA receptor, such as D-cycloserine, might facilitate the effect of the remaining pool of glutamate, the excitatory neurotransmitter on this receptor. These receptor sites are concentrated within the CA1/CA4 regions of the hippocampus known to be important in memory processes (Zola-Morgan *et al.*, 1986; Squire, 1987; Lynch and Baudry, 1988). Wesnes (1992) has reported beneficial effects of D-cycloserine in reversing scopolamine-induced memory impairments in elderly subjects, and a trial of D-cycloserine is now being undertaken by Proctor, Bowen and others in Alzheimer patients.

Summary
Cholinergic agents, particularly the anticholinesterases (physostigmine and THA), have been reported to produce benefits upon tests of picture and word recognition memory, word list and name learning, copying and drawing, orientation, and various global indexes of cognitive functioning including the MMSE. However, the benefits have been small, and there have been many failures to replicate. Promising results have also been reported from the administration of a monoamine oxidase inhibitor (L-deprenyl), a serotonin reuptake inhibitor (fluvoxamine) and thiamine, but these findings require replication. D-Cycloserine is currently under assessment as it is claimed that it should promote the action of glutamate on the NMDA receptor in the hippocampal CA1/CA4 regions (Bowen *et al.*, 1992a, b).

CONCLUSIONS
Although the focus of attention in Alzheimer research is currently on molecular genetics, one goal of such studies is to identify deficient enzymes and biochemical processes which require replacement or augmentation. Consequently, the investigation of replacement therapies, based on knowledge of depleted neurotransmitters and of the functional roles of those transmitters, remains a valid research approach, especially in view of the disappointing results of administering other substances (Kopelman and Lishman, 1986).

Depletions of acetylcholine, noradrenaline, serotonin and glutamate seem important in the neurochemistry of Alzheimer's disease, and depletion of GABA may be a late development. Cholinergic depletion is the most consistent finding in Alzheimer dementia, and various studies of cholinergic blockade have now elucidated that cholinergic depletion would be expected to produce a substantial anterograde amnesia, although retrograde amnesia has to be explained in different terms (Kopelman, 1992a, b). The depletion of glutamate, an excitatory neurotransmitter within the NMDA hippocampal system, may also be important in producing the anterograde amnesia in Alzheimer dementia; and administration of benzodiazepines produces amnesia, possibly by the potentiation of GABA, the inhibitory neurotransmitter within the hippocampal interneurons. Less is known about the specific cognitive effects of other neurotransmitters, but the catecholamines appear to act primarily upon attention, arousal and mood.

In view of this, the results of clinical trials of 'replacement' substances are disappointing. A possible criticism is that the cognitive actions of the replacement agents upon specific memory processes have not been analysed (Table 10.3) with anything like the care or precision of studies of substances which impair memory (Table 10.2). However, it seems unlikely that major effects of the replacement agents would have failed to show through even on the assessments which were employed. Much more importantly, the replacement agents may be relatively impotent in the presence of substantial neuronal loss or synaptic degeneration; and methods of arresting those processes may need to be developed before neurotransmitter 'replacement' can become effective.

POSTSCRIPT

Since this chapter was written, the results of the American collaborative study of THA in 215 Alzheimer patients have been published (Davies *et al.*, 1992). At the end of a six-week trial, there was a significantly smaller decline in scores on the Alzheimer's Disease Assessment scale on THA relative to placebo, but findings on other measures failed to reach statistical significance, a result broadly in line with the studies reviewed above.

REFERENCES

Anderson, L.T., David, R., Bonnet, K. and Dancis, J. (1979). Passive avoidance learning in Lesch-Nyhan disease: effect of l-desamino-8-arginine-vasopressin. *Life Sciences*, **24**, 905–10.

Arendt, T., Allen, Y., Sindon, J. *et al.* (1988). Cholinergic-rich brain transplants reverse alcohol-induced memory deficits. *Nature*, **332**, 448–50.

Arendt, T., Bigle, V., Arendt, A. and Tennstedt, A. (1983). Loss of neurons in the nucleus basalis of Meynert in Alzheimer's disease, paralysis agitans and Korsakoff's disease. *Acta Neuropathologica (Berlin)*, **61**, 101–8.

Arendt, T., Bigle, V., Tennstedt, A. and Arendt, A. (1985). Neuronal loss in different parts of the nucleus basalis is related to neuritic plaque formation in cortical target areas in Alzheimer's disease. *Neuroscience*, **14**, 1–14.

Baddeley, A. and Hitch, G. (1974). Working memory. In *Recent Advances in Learning and Motivation*, Vol. 8, Bower, G. (Ed.). Academic Press, New York.

Baddeley, A.D., Logie, R., Bressi, S. *et al.* (1986). Dementia and working memory. *Quarterly Journal of Experimental Psychology*, **38A**, 603–18.

Bartus, R.T., Dean, R.L. and Beer, B. (1983). An evaluation of drugs for improving memory in aged monkeys: implications for clinical trials in humans. *Psychopharmacology Bulletin*, **19**, 168–84.

Bartus, R.T., Dean, R.L., Beer, B. and Lippa, A.S. (1982). The cholinergic hypothesis of geriatric memory dysfunction. *Science*, **217**, 408–17.

Beal, M.F. and Mazurek, M.F. (1987). Substance P-like immuno-reactivity is reduced in Alzheimer's disease cerebral cortex. *Neurology*, **37**, 1205–9.

Beal, M.F., Mazurek, M.F., Svendsen, C.N. *et al.* (1986). Widespread reduction of somatostatin-like immunoreactivity in the cerebral cortex in Alzheimer's disease. *Annals of Neurology*, **20**, 489–95.

Beatty, W.W., Butters, N. and Janowsky, D.S. (1986). Patterns of memory failure after scopolamine treatment: implications for cholinergic hypotheses of dementia. *Behavioural and Neurological Biology*, **45**, 196–211.

Benton, J.S., Bowen, D.M., Allen, S.J. *et al.* (1982). Alzheimer's disease as a disorder of the isodendritic core. *Lancet*, **i**, 456.

Blass, J.P., Gleason, P., Brush, D. *et al.* (1988). Thiamine and Alzheimer's disease. *Archives of Neurology*, **45**, 833–5.

Bondareff, W., Mountjoy, C.Q. and Roth, M. (1982). Loss of neurons of origin of the adrenergic projection to the cerebral cortex (nucleus locus ceruleus) in senile dementia. *Neurology*, **32**, 164–8.

Bowen, D.M. (1990). Treatment of Alzheimer's disease: molecular pathology versus neurotransmitter-based therapy. *British Journal of Psychiatry*, **157**, 327–30.

Bowen, D.M., Francis, P.T., Pangalos, M. *et al.* (1992a). Treatment strategies for Alzheimer's disease. *Lancet*, **339**, 132–3.

Bowen, D.M., Francis, P.T., Procter, A.W. and Young, A.B. (1992b). Treatment of Alzheimer's disease. *Journal of Neurology, Neurosurgery and Psychiatry* (in press).

Bowen, D.M., Smith, C.B., White, P. and Davidson, A.N. (1976). Neurotransmitter-related enzymes and indices of hypoxia in senile dementia and other abiotrophies. *Brain*, **99**, 459–96.

Boyd, W., Graham-White, J., Blackwood, G. *et al.* (1977). Clinical effects of choline in Alzheimer senile dementia. *Lancet*, **ii**, 711.

Branconnier, R.J. (1983). The efficacy of the cerebral metabolic enhancers in the treatment of senile dementia. *Psychopharmacology Bulletin*, **19**, 212–19.

Broks, P., Preston, G.C., Traub, M. *et al.* (1988). Modelling dementia: effects of scopolamine on memory and attention. *Neuropsychologia*, **26**, 685–700.

Brown, J., Brown, M.W. and Bowes, J.B. (1983). Effects of Lorazepam on rate of forgetting, on retrieval from semantic memory and on manual dexterity. *Neuropsychologia*, **21**, 501–12

Brown, M.W., Brown, J. and Bowes, J. (1989). Absence of priming coupled with substantially preserved recognition in lorazepam induced amnesia. *Quarterly Journal of Experimental Psychology*, **41A**, 599–617.

Brown, J., Lewis, V., Brown, M. *et al.* (1982). A comparison between transient amnesias induced by two drugs (Diazepam or Lorazepam) and amnesia of organic origin. *Neuropsychologia*, **20**, 55–70.

Bruno, G., Mohr, E., Gillespie, M. *et al.* (1986). Muscarininc agonist therapy of Alzheimer's disease: a clinical trial of RS-86. *Archives of Neurology*, **43**, 659–61.

Burke, W.J., Chung, H.D., Nakra, B.R.S. *et al.* (1987). Phenylethanolamine-*N*-methyltransferase activity is decreased in Alzheimer's disease brains. *Annals of Neurology*, **22**, 278–80.

Caine, E.D., Weingartner, H., Ludlow, C.L. *et al.* (1981). Qualitative analysis of scopolamine-induced amnesia. *Psychopharmacology*, **74**, 74–80.

Chatellier, G. and Lacomblez, L. (1990). Tacrine (tetrahydoaminoacridine; THA) and lecithin in senile dementia of the Alzheimer type: a multicentre trial. *British Medical Journal*, **300**, 495–9.

Christensen, H., Maltby, N., Jorm, A.F. *et al.* (1992). Cholinergic blockade as a model of the cognitive deficits in Alzheimer's disease. *Brain*, **115**, 1681–99.

Christie, J.E., Shering, A., Ferguson, G. and Glen, A.I.M. (1981). Physostigmine and arecholine: effects of intravenous infusions in Alzheimer presenile dementia. *British Journal of Psychiatry*, **138**, 46–50.

Chui, D.C.M., Penney, J.B. and Young, A.B. (1987). Cortical GABA$_B$ and GABA$_A$ receptors in Alzheimer's disease: a quantitative autoradiographic study. *Neurology*, **37**, 1454–9.

Clark, C.R., Geffen, G.M. and Geffen, L.B. (1986). Role of monoamine pathways in attention and effort. *Psychopharmacology*, **90**, 35–9.

Cross, A.J., Crow, T.J., Ferrier, I.N. and Johnson, J.A. (1986). The selectivity of serotonin S2 receptors in Alzheimer-type dementia. *Neurobiology of Aging*, **7**, 3–7.

Crow, T.J. and Grove-White, I.G. (1973). An analysis of the learning deficit following hyoscine administration to man. *British Journal of Pharmacology*, **49**, 322–7.

Crow, T.J., Grove-White, I.G. and Ross, D.G. (1975). The specificity of the action of hyoscine on human learning. *British Journal of Clinical Pharmacology*, **2**, 367–8.

Curran, H.V. (1986). Tranquillising memories: a review of the effects of benzodiazepines on human memory. *Biological Psychology*, **23**, 179–213.

Curran, H.V. (1991). Benzodiazepines, memory and mood: a review, *Psychopharmacology*, **105**, 1–8.

Curran, H.V., Schifano, F. and Lader, M. (1991). Models of memory dysfunction? A comparison of the effects of scopolamine and lorazepam on memory, psychomotor performance and mood. *Psychopharmacology*, **103**, 83–90.

Curran, H.V., Schiwy, W. and Lader, M. (1987). Differential amnesic properties of benzodiazepines: a dose–response comparison of two drugs with similar elimination half-lives. *Psychopharmacology*, **92**, 358–64.

Cutler, N.R., Haxby, J., Kay, A.D. *et al.* (1985). Evaluation of zimelidine in Alzheimer's disease. *Archives of Neurology*, **42**, 744–8.

D'Amato, R.J., Zweig, R.M., Whitehouse, P.J. *et al.* (1987). Aminergic systems in Alzheimer's disease and Parkinson's disease. *Annals of Neurology*, **22**, 229–36.

Davis, K.I., Thal, L.J., Gamzu, E.R. *et al.* (1992). A double-blind placebo-controlled multicenter study of tacrine for Alzheimer's disease. *New England Journal of Medicine*, **397**, 1253–9.

Davis, K.L. and Mohs, R.C. (1982). Enhancement of memory processes in Alzheimer's disease with multiple-dose intravenous physostigmine. *American Journal of Psychiatry*, **139**, 1421–4.

De Wied, D. (1984). The importance of vasopressin in memory. *Trends in Neuroscience*, **7**, 62–4.

De Wied, D. and van Ree, J.M. (1982). Neuropeptides, mental performance and ageing. *Life Sciences*, **31**, 709–19.

Dehlin, O., Hedenrud, B., Jansson, P. *et al.* (1985). A double-blind comparison of alaproclate and placebo in the treatment of patients with senile dementia. *Acta Psychiatrica Scandinavica*, **71**, 190–6.

Dorow, R., Berenberg, D., Duka, T. and Sauerbrey, N. (1987). Amnesic effects of lormetazepam and their reversal by the benzodiazepine antagonist R-15–17 88. *Psychopharmacology*, **93**, 507–14.

Drachman, D.A. (1977). Memory and cognitive function in man: does the cholinergic system have a specific role? *Neurology*, **27**, 783–90.

Drachman, D.A. and Leavitt, J. (1974). Human memory and the cholinergic system. *Archives of Neurology*, **30**, 113–21.

Drachman, D.A., Noffsinger, D., Sahakian, B.J. *et al.* (1980). Ageing, memory, and the cholinergic system. *Neurobiology of Ageing*, **1**, 39–43.

Dubois, B., Danze, F., Pillow, B. *et al.* (1987). Cholinergic-dependent cognitive deficits in Parkinson's disease. *Annals of Neurology*, **32**, 26–30.

Dunne, M.P. (1990). Scopolamine and sustained retrieval from semantic memory. *Journal of Psychopharmacology*, **4**, 13–18.

Dunne, M.P. and Hartley, L.R. (1985). The effects of scopolamine upon verbal memory: evidence for an attentional hypothesis. *Acta Psychologica*, **58**, 205–17.

Eagger, S.A., Levy, R. and Sahakian, B.J. (1991). Tacrine in Alzheimer's disease. *Lancet*, **337**, 989–92.

Eagger, S., Morant, N., Levy, R. and Sahakian, B. (1992). Tacrine in Alzheimer's disease. Time course of changes in cognitive function and practice effects. *British Journal of Psychiatry*, **160**, 36–40.

Ellison, D.W., Beal, M.F., Mazurek, M.F. *et al.* (1986). A *post-mortem* study of aminoacid neurotransmitters in Alzheimer's disease. *Annals of Neurology,* **20**, 616–21.

Esiri, M.M., Pearson, R.C.A., Steele, J.E. *et al.* (1990). A quantitative study of the neurofibrillary tangle and the choline acetyltransferase activity in the cerebral cortex and the amygadala in Alzheimer's disease. *Journal of Neurology, Neurosurgery and Psychiatry,* **53**, 161–5.

Etienne, P., Gauthier, S., Johnson, G. *et al.* (1978). Clinical effects of acetylcholine in Alzheimer's disease. *Lancet,* **i**, 508–9.

Fewtrell, W.D., House, A.O., Jamie, P.F. *et al.* (1982). Effects of vasopressin on memory and new learning in a brain-injured population. *Psychological Medicine,* **12**, 423–5.

File, S.E., Sharma, R. and Shaffer, J. (1992). Is lorazepam-induced amnesia specific to the type of memory or to the task used to assess it? *Journal of Psychopharmacology,* **6**, 76–80.

Flynn, D.D. and Mash, D.C. (1986). Characterisation of L-(3H) nicotine binding in human cortex: comparison between Alzheimer's disease and the normal. *Journal of Neurochemistry,* **47**, 1948–54.

Francis, P.T., Palmer, A.M., Sims, N.R. *et al.* (1985). Neurochemical studies of early-onset Alzheimer's disease. *New England Journal of Medicine,* **313**, 7–11.

Frith, C.D., Richardson, J.T.E., Samuel, M. *et al.* (1984). The effects of intravenous diazepam and hyoscine upon human memory. *Quarterly Journal of Experimental Psychology,* **36A**, 133–44.

Frith, C.D.J., Ferrier, I.N. and Crow, T.J. (1985). Selective impairment of paired associate learning after administration of a centrally-acting adrenergic agonist (clonidine). *Psychopharmacology,* **87**, 490–3.

Frith, C.D., McGinty, M.A., Gergel, I. and Crow, T.J. (1989). The effects of scopolamine and clonidine upon the perfomance and learning of a motor skill. *Psychopharmacology,* **98**, 120–5.

Gage, F.H., Bjorklund, A., Stenevi, U. *et al.* (1984). Intrahippocampal septal grafts ameliorate learning impairments in aged rats. *Science,* **225**, 533–5.

Gash, D.M. And Thomas, G.J. (1983). What is the importance of vasopressin in memory processes? *Trends in Neurosciences,* **6**, 197–8.

Gauthier, S., Bouchard, M., Lamontagne, A. *et al.* (1990). Tetrahydroaminoacridine–lecithin combination treatment in patients with intermediate-stage Alzheimer's disease. Results of a Canadian double-blind, crossover, multicenter study. *New England Journal of Medicine,* **322**, 1272–6.

Ghoneim, M.M. and Mewaldt, S.P. (1975). Effects of diazepam and scopolamine on storage, retrieval, and organisational processes in memory. *Psychopharmacologia (Berlin),* **44**, 257–62.

Ghoneim, M.M. and Mewaldt, S.P. (1977). Studies on human memory: the interactions of diazepam, scopolamine, and physostigmine. *Psychopharmacology,* **52**, 1–6.

Ghoneim, M.M., Mewaldt, S.P. and Henriches, J.R. (1984). Dose–response analysis of the behavioural effects of diazepam: 1 learning and memory. *Psychopharmacology,* **82**, 291–5.

Gibson, G.E., Sheu, K.-F.R., Blass, J.P. *et al.* (1988). Reduced activities of thiamine-dependent enzymes in the brains and peripheral tissues of patients with Alzheimer's disease. *Archives of Neurology,* **45**, 836–40.

Graf, P., Squire, L.R. and Mandler, G. (1984). The information that amnesic patients do not forget. *Journal of Experimental Psychology: Learning, Memory and Cognition,* **11**, 501–18.

Grossi, D., Lopez, O.L. and Martinez, A.J. (1989). Mamillary bodies in Alzheimer's disease. *Acta Neurologica Scandinavica*, **80**, 41–5.

Growdon, J.H., Corkin, S., Huff, F.J. and Rosen, T.J. (1986). Piracetam with lecithin in the treatment of Alzheimer's disease. *Neurobiology of Ageing*, **7** 269–76.

Gustaffson, L., Edvinsson, L., Dahlgren, N. *et al.* (1987). Intravenous physostigmine treatment of Alzheimer's disease evaluated by psychometric testing, regional cerebral blood flow (rCBF) measurement, and EEG. *Psychopharmacology*, **93**, 31–5.

Heyman, A., Schmechel, D., Wilkinson, W. *et al.* (1987). Failure of long-term high-dose lecithin to retard and the progression of early-onset Alzheimer's disease. *Journal of Neutransmission*, **24** (Suppl.), 279–86.

Hollander, E., Davidson, M., Mohs, R.C. *et al.* (1987). RS-86 in the treatment of Alzheimer's disease: cognitive and biological effects. *Biological Psychiatry*, **22**, 1067–78.

Hyman, B.T., Van Hoesen, G.W. and Damasio, A.R. (1987). Alzheimer's disease: glutamate depletion in the hippocampal perforant pathway zone. *Annals of Neurology*, **22**, 37–40.

Johns, C.A., Greenwald, B.S., Mohs, R.C. and Davis, K.L. (1983). The cholinergic treatment strategy in ageing and senile dementia. *Psychopharmacology Bulletin*, **19**, 185–97.

Jones, G. (1990). The Cholinergic Hypothesis of Dementia. PhD thesis, University of London.

Jones, D.M.M., Jones, M.E.L., Lewis, M.J. and Spriggs, T.L.B. (1989). Drugs and human memory: effects of low doses of nitrazepam and hyoscine on retention. *British Journal of Clinical Pharmacology*, **7**, 479–83.

Kaye, W.H., Sitaram, N., Weingartner, H. *et al.* (1982). Modest facilitation of memory in dementia with combined lecithin and anticholinesterase treatment. *Biological Psychiatry*, **51**, 275–9.

Knopman, D. (1991). Unaware learning versus preserved learning in pharmacologic amnesia: similarities and differences. *Journal of Experimental Psychology, Learning, Memory and Cognition*, **17**, 1017–29.

Kopelman, M.D. (1985). Rates of forgetting in Alzheimer-type dementia and Korsakoff's syndrome. *Neuropsychologia*, **23**, 623–38.

Kopelman, M.D. (1986). The cholinergic neurotransmitter system in human memory and dementia: a review. *Quarterly Journal of Experimental Psychology*, **38A**, 535–73.

Kopelman, M.D. (1987). Oral tetrahydraminacridine in the treatment of senile dementia, Alzheimer's type. *New England Journal of Medicine*, **316**, 1604 (letter).

Kopelman, M.D. (1989). Remote and autobiographical memory, temporal context memory, and frontal atrophy in Korsakoff and Alzheimer patients. *Neuropsychologia*, **27**, 437–60.

Kopelman, M.D. (1991). Frontal dysfunction and memory deficits in the alcoholic Korsakoff syndrome and Alzheimer-type dementia. *Brain*, **114**, 117–37.

Kopelman, M.D. (1992a). The 'new' and the 'old': components of the anterograde and retrograde memory loss in Korsakoff and Alzheimer patients. In *The Neuropsychology of Memory*, 2nd edition, Squire, L.R. and Butters, N. (Eds). Guildford Press, New York.

Kopelman, M.D. (1992b). Storage, forgetting, and retrieval in the anterograde and retrogade amnesia of Alzheimer dementia. In *Memory Functioning in*

Dementia, Backman, L. (Ed.), pp. 45–71. Elsevier Science Publishers, Amsterdam.

Kopelman, M.D. and Corn, T.H. (1988). Cholinergic 'blockade' as a model for cholinergic depletion: a comparison of the memory deficits with those of Alzheimer-type dementia and the Alcoholic Korsakoff syndrome. *Brain*, **111**, 1079–110.

Kopelman, M.D. and Lishman, W.A. (1986). Pharmacological treatments of dementia (non-cholinergic). *British Medical Bulletin*, **42**, 101–5.

Kowall, N.W. and Beal, M.F. (1986). Cortical somatostatin, Neuropeptide Y, and NADPH diaphorase neurons: Normal anatomy and alterations in Alzheimer's disease. *Annals of Neurology*, **23**, 105–14.

Laczi, F., Valkusz, Z., Laszlo, F.A. *et al.* (1982). Effects of lysine-vasopressin and 1 deamino 8D arginine vasopressin on men in healthy individuals and diabetes insipidus patients. *Psychoneuroendocrinology*, **7**, 185–93.

Laczi, R., van Ree, J.M., Wagner, A. *et al.* (1983). Effects of desglycinamide–arginine–vasopressin (DG AVP) on memory processes in diabetes insipidus in patients and non-diabetic subjects. *Acta Endocrinologica (Copenhagen)*, **102**, 205–12.

Lawlor, B.A., Mellow, A.M., Sunderland, T. *et al.* (1988). A pilot study of serotonergic system responsivity in Alzheimer's disease. *Psychopharmacology Bulletin*, **24**, 127–9.

Lines, C.R., Preston, G.C., Broks, P. and Dawson, C.E. (1991). The effects of scopolamine on retrieval from semantic memory. *Journal of Psychopharmacology*, **5**, 234–7.

Lister, R.G. and Weingartner, H.J. (1987). Neuropharmacological strategies for understanding psychobiological determinants of cognition. *Human-Neurobiology*, **6**, 119–27.

Little, A., Levy, R., Chuaqui-Kidd, P. and Hand, D. (1985). A double blind placebo controlled trial of high dose lecithin in Alzheimer's disease. *Journal of Neurology, Neurosurgery and Psychiatry*, **48**, 736–42.

Lowe, S.L., Francis, P.T., Procter, A.W. *et al.* (1988). Gamma-aminobutyric acid concentration in brain tissue at two stages of Alzheimer's disease. *Brain*, **111**, 785–99.

Lynch, G. and Baudry, M. (1988). Structure–function relationships in the organization of memory. In *Perspectives in Memory Research*, Gazzaniga, M.S. (Ed.). MIT Press, Cambridge, Massachusetts.

Mair, R.G. and McEntee, W.J. (1986). Cognitive enhancement in Korsakoff's psychosis by clonidine: a comparison with L-dopa and ephedrine. *Psychopharmacology*, **88**, 374–80.

Mann, D.M.A., Lincoln, J., Yates, P.O. *et al.* (1980). Changes on monamine containing neurones of the human CNS in senile dementia. *British Journal of Psychiatry*, **136**, 533–41.

Mann, D.M.A., Yates, P.O. and Marcyniuk, B. (1984). Alzheimer's presenile dementia, senile dementia of Alzheimer type, and Down's syndrome in middle age form: an age related continuum of pathological changes. *Neuropathology and Applied Neurobiology*, **10**, 185–207.

Mann, D.M.A., Yates, P.O. and Marcyniuk, B. (1987). Dopaminergic neurotransmitter changes in Alzheimer's disease and Down's syndrome at middle age. *Journal of Neurology, Neurosurgery and Psychiatry*, **50**, 341–4.

Mann, D.M.A., Yates, P.O. and Marcyniuk, B. (1986). A comparison of nerve cell loss in cortical and subcortical structures in Alzheimer's disease. *Journal of Neurology, Nuerosurgery and Psychiatry*, **49**, 310–12.

Martin, P.R., Adinoff, B., Eckardt, M.J. *et al.* (1989). Effective pharmacotherapy of alcoholic amnestic disorder with fluvoxamine. *Archives of General Psychiatry*, **46**, 617–21.

Mash, D.C., Flynn, D.D. and Potter, L.T. (1985). Loss of M2 muscarinic receptors in the cerebral cortex in Alzheimer's disease and exceptional cholinergic denerveation. *Science*, **228**, 1115–17.

Mazurek, M.F., Beal, M.F., Bird, E.D. and Martin, J.B. (1986). Vasopressin in Alzheimer's disease: a study of *post-mortem* brain concentrations. *Annals of Neurology*, **20**, 665–70.

McDonald, R.J. (1982), Drug treatment of senile dementia. In *Psychopharmacology of Old Age*, Wheatley, D. (Ed.). Oxford University Press, Oxford.

McEntee, W.J. and Mair, R.G. (1980). Memory enhancement in Korsakoff's psychosis by clonidine: further evidence for a noradrenergic deficit. *Annals of Neurology*, **7**, 466–70.

Millar, K., Jeffcoate, W.J. and Walden, C.P. (1987). Vasopressin and memory improvement in normal short-term recall and reduction of alcohol-induced amnesia. *Psychological Medicine*, **17**, 335–41.

Mohr, E.M., Bruno, G., Foster, N. *et al.* (1986). GABA-antagonist therapy for Alzheimer's disease. *Clinical Neuropharmacology*, **9**, 257–63.

Mohs, R.C. and Davis, K.L. (1985). Interaction of choline and scopolamine in human memory. *Life Sciences*, **37**, 193–7.

Mohs, R.C., Davis, B.M., Johns, C.A. *et al.* (1985). Oral physostigmine treatment of patients with Alzheimer's disease. *American Journal of Psychiatry*, **142**, 28–33.

Morris, R.G. (1986). Short-term forgetting in senile dementia of the Alzheimer's type. *Cognitive Neuropsychology*, **3**, 77–97.

Morrison, J.H., Rogers, J., Scherr, S. *et al.* (1985). Somatostatin immunoreactivity in neuritic plaques of Alzheimer patients. *Nature*, **314**, 90–2.

Muramato, O., Sugishita, M. and Ando, K. (1984). Cholinergic system and constructional praxis: a further study of physostigmine in Alzheimer's disease. *Journal of Neurology, Neurosurgery and Psychiatry*, **47**, 485–91.

Newhouse, P.A., Sunderland, T., Thompson, K. *et al.* (1986). Intravenous nicotine in a patient with Alzheimer's disease. *American Journal of Psychiatry*, **143**, 1494–9 (letter).

Nissen, M.J., Knopman, D.S. and Schachter, D.L. (1987). Neurochemical dissociation of memory systems. *Neurology*, **37**, 789–94.

Nordberg, A., Adem, A., Nilsson-Hakansson, L. *et al.* (1990). New approaches to clinical and *postmortem* investigations of cholinergic mechanisms. In *Progress in Brain Research*, Vol. 84, Aquilonius, S.M. and Gillberg, P.G. (Eds). Elsevier Science Publishers, The Netherlands.

Nuotto, E. (1983). Psychomotor, physiological and cognitive effects of scopolamine and ephedrine in healthy man. *European Journal of Clinical Pharmacology*, **24**, 603–9.

O'Boyle, C., Barry, H., Fox, E. *et al.* (1987). Benzodiazepine-induced event amnesia following a stressful surgical procedure. *Psychopharmacology*, **91**, 244–7.

O'Carroll, R.E., Moffoot, A., Ebmeier, K.P. *et al.* (1992). Korsakoff's syndrome, cognition and clonidine. *Psychological Medicine* (in press)

O'Donnell, V.M., Pitts, W.M. and Fann, W.E. (1986). Noradrenergic and cholinergic agents in Korsakoff's syndrome. *Clinical Neuropharmacology*, **9**, 65–70.

Oliveros, J.C., Jandali, M.K., Timsit-Berthier, M. *et al.* (1978). Vasopressin in amnesia. *Lancet*, **i**, 42 (letter).

Palmer, A.M., Proctor, A.W., Stratmann, G.L. and Bowen, D.M. (1986). Excitatory amino acid-releasing and cholinergic neurones in Alzheimer's disease. *Neuroscience Letters*, **66**, 199–204.

Palmer, A.M., Stratmann, G.C., Proctor, A.W. and Bowen, D.M. (1988). Possible neurotransmitter basis of behavioural changes in Alzheimer's disease. *Annals of Neurology*, **23**, 616–20.

Parrott, A.C. (1986). The effects of transdermal scopolamine and 4 dose levels of oral scopolamine (0.15, 0.3, 0.6, and 1.2 mg) upon psychological performance. *Psychopharmacology*, **89**, 347–54.

Partridge, F.M., Knight, R.G. and Feehan, M.J. (1990). Direct and indirect memory performance in patients with senile dementia. *Psychological Medicine*, **20**, 111–18.

Penn, R.D., Martin, E.M., Wilson, R.S. *et al.* (1988). Intraventricular bethanechol infusion for Alzheimer's disease: results of double-blind and escalating-dose trials. *Neurology*, **38**, 219–22.

Penney, J.B., Maragos, W.F., Greenamyre, J.T. *et al.* (1990). Excitatory amino acid binding sites in the hippocampal region of Alzheimer's disease and other dementias. *Journal of Neurology, Neurosurgery and Psychiatry*, **53**, 314–20.

Perry, E.K., Tomlinson, B.E., Blessed, G. *et al.* (1978). Correlation of cholinergic abnormalities with senile plaques and mental test scores in senile dementia. *British Medical Journal*, **ii**, 1457–9.

Perry, E.K. (1986). The cholinergic hypothesis – ten years on. *British Medical Bulletin*, **42**, 63–9.

Perry, T.L., Yong, V.W., Bergeron, C. *et al.* (1987). Amino acids, glutathione, and glututhione transferase activity in the brains of patients with Alzheimer's disease. *Annals of Neurology*, **21**, 331–6.

Peters, B.H. and Levin, H.S. (1977). Memory enhancement after physostigmine treatment in the amnesic syndrome. *Archives of Neurology*, **34**, 215–19.

Potter, D.B., Pickles, C.D., Roberts, R.C. and Rugg, M.D. (1991). The effects of scopolamine on event-related potentials in a continuous recognition memory task. *Journal of Psychophysiology*, **29**, 29–37.

Preston, G.C., Ward, C., Lines, C.R. *et al.* (1989). Scopolamine and benzodiazepine models of dementia: cross-reversals by Ro 15-1788 and physostigmine. *Psychopharmacology*, **98**, 487–94.

Roberts, G.W., Crow, T.J. and Polak, J.M. (1985). Location of neuronal tangles in somatostatin neurones in Alzheimer's disease. *Nature*, **314**, 92–4.

Rosser, M.N., Garrett, N.J., Johnson, A.L. *et al.* (1982). A *post-mortem* study of the cholinergic and GABA systems in senile dementia. *Brain*, **105**, 313–30.

Rossor, M. and Iversen, L.L. (1986). Non-cholinergic neurotransmitter abnormalities in Alzheimer's disease. *British Medical Bulletin*, **42**, 70–4.

Rossor, M.N., Iversen, L.L., Reynolds, G.P. *et al.* (1984). Neurochemical characteristics of early and late onset types of Alzheimer's disease. *British Medical Journal*, **288**, 961–4.

Rossor, M.N., Iversen, L.L., Mountjoy, C.Q. *et al.* (1980). Arginine vasopressin and choline acetyl transferase and choline acetyl transferase in brains of patients with Alzheimer-type dementia. *Lancet*, **ii**, 1369–70.

Rusted, J.M. (1988). Dissociative effects of scopolomine on working memory in healthy young volunteers. *Psychopharmacology*, **96**, 487–92.

Rusted, J. and Eaton-Williams, P. (1991). Distinguishing between attentional and amnesic effects in information processing: the separate and combined effects of scopolamine and nicotine on verbal free recall. *Psychopharmacology*, **104**, 363–6.

Rusted, J.M. and Warburton, D.M. (1988). The effects of scopolamine on working memory in healthy young volunteers. *Psychopharmacology*, **96**, 145–52.

Safer, D.J. and Allen, R.P. (1971). The central effects of scopolamine in man. *Biological Psychiatry*, **3**, 347–55.

Sahakian, B., Jones, G., Levy, R. *et al.* (1989). The effects of nicotine on attention, information processing, and short-term memory in patients with dementia of the Alzheimer type. *British Journal of Psychiatry*, **154**, 797–800.

Sahgal, A. (1984). A critique of the vasopressin–memory hypothesis. *Psychopharmacology*, **83**, 215–28.

Schacter, D.L. (1987). Implicit memory: history and current status. *Journal of Experimental Psychology: Learning, Memory and Cognition*, **13**, 501–18.

Shepherd, G.M. (1988). A basic circuit of cortical organization. In *Perspectives in Memory Research*, Gazzaniga, M.S. (Ed.). MIT Press, Cambridge, Massachusetts.

Signoret, J.L., Whiteley, A. and Lhermitte, F. (1978). Influence of choline on amnesia in early Alzheimer's disease. *Lancet*, **ii**, 837.

Sims, N., Bowen, D., Smith, C. *et al.* (1980). Glucose metabolism and acetylcholine synthesis in relation to neuronal activity in Alzheimer's disease. *Lancet*, **i**, 333–4.

Small, G.W., Spar, J.E.E. and Plotkin, D.A. (1987). Oral tetrahydroaminoacridine in the treatment of senile dementia, Alzheimer's type. *New England Journal of Medicine*, **316**, 1604 (letter).

Smith, C.C.T., Bowen, D.M., Francis, P.T. *et al.* (1985). Putative amino acid transmitters in lumbar CSF and patients with histologically-verified Alzheimer's dementia. *Journal of Neurology, Neurosurgery and Psychiatry*, **48**, 469–71.

Smith, C.M., Swash, M., Exton-Smith, A. *et al.* (1978). Choline therapy in Alzheimer's disease. *Lancet*, **ii**, 318.

Snel, J., Taylor, J. and Wegman, M. (1987). Does DGAVP influence memory, attention and mood in young healthy men? *Psychopharmacology*, **92**, 224–8.

Soininen, H.S., Jolkkonen, J.T., Reinikainen, K.J. *et al.* (1984). Reduced cholinesterase activity and somatostatin-like immunoreactivity in the CSF of patients with dementia of the Alzheimer-type. *Journal of the Neurological Sciences*, **63**, 167–72.

Squire, L.R. (1987). *Memory and Brain*. Oxford University Press, Oxford.

Stern, Y., Sano, M. and Mayeux, R. (1987). Effects of oral physostigmine in Alzheimer's disease. *Annals of Neurology*, **22**, 306–10.

Summers, W.K., Majovski, L.V., Marsh, G.M. *et al.* (1986). Oral tetrahydroaminoacridine in long-term treatment of senile dementia, Alzheimer type. *New England Journal of Medicine*, **315**, 1241–5.

Sunderland, T., Tariot, P.N., Cohen, R.M. *et al.* (1987). Anticholinergic sensitivity in patients with dementia of the Alzheimer-type and age-matched controls: a dose–response curve. *Archives of General Psychiatry*, **44**, 418–25.

Tamminga, C.A., Foster, N.L., Fedio, P. *et al.* (1987). Alzheimer's disease: low cerebral somatostatin levels correlate with impaired cognitive function and cortical metabolism. *Neurology*, **37**, 161–5.

Tariot, P.N., Cohen, R.M., Welkowitz, J.A. *et al.* (1988). Multiple-dose arecoline infusions in Alzheimer's disease. *Archives of General Psychiatry*, **45**, 901–5.

Taylor, J., Hunt, E. and Coggan, P. (1987). Effect of diazepam on the speed of mental rotation. *Psychopharmacology*, **91**, 369–71.

Thal, L.J., Fuld, P.A., Masur, D.M. and Sharpless, N.S. (1983). Oral physostigmine and lecithin improve memory in Alzheimer's disease. *Annals of Neurology*, **13**, 491–6.

Tröster, A.I., Beatty, W.W., Staton, R.D. and Rorabaugh, A.G. (1989). Effects of scopolamine on anterograde and remote memory in humans. *Psychobiology*, **17**, 12–18.

Weiner, N. (1980). Atropine, scopolamine, and related antimuscarinic drugs. In *Goodman and Gilman's The Pharmacological Basis of Therapeutics*, Gilman, A.G., Goodman, L.S. and Gilman, A. (Eds). 6th edition, pp. 120–37. Macmillan, New York, and Balliere Tindall, London.

Weingartner, H., Gold, P., Ballenger, J.C. *et al.* (1981). Effects of vasopressin on human memory functions. *Science*, **211**, 601–3.

Weingartner, H., Rudorfer, M.V., Buchsbaum, M.S. and Linnoila, M. (1983). Effects of serotonin on memory impairments produced by ethanol. *Science*, **221**, 472–3.

Wesnes, K. (1992). The design, validity and applications of scopolamine model of dementia. Paper presented at the *British Psychological Society Annual Conference*, p. 13 (abs).

Wesnes, K. and Revell, A. (1984). The separate and combined effects of scopolamine and nicotine on human information processing. *Psychopharmacology*, **84**, 5–11.

Wesnes, K., Simpson, P. and Kidd, A. (1988). An investigation of the range of cognitive impairments induced by scopolamine 0.6 mg sc. *Human Psychopharmacology*, **82**, 27–41.

Wesnes, K. and Warburton, D.M. (1983). Effects of scopolamine on stimulus sensitivity and response bias in a visual vigilance task. *Neuropsychobiology*, **9**, 154–7.

Wesnes, K. and Warburton, D.M. (1984). Effects of scopolamine and nicotine on human rapid information processing performance. *Psychopharmacology*, **82**, 147–50.

Whalley, L.J. (1989). Drug treatments of dementia. *British Journal of Psychiatry*, **155**, 595–611.

Whitehouse, P.J., Price, D.L., Struble, R.G. *et al.* (1982). Alzheimer's disease and senile dementia: loss of neurons in the basal forebrain. *Science*, **215**, 1237–9.

Whitehouse, P.J., Vale, W.W., Zweig, R.M. (1987). Reductions in corticotrophin releasing factor-like immunoreactivity in cerebral cortex in Alzheimer's disease. *Neurology*, **37**, 905–9.

Whitehouse, P.J. (1988). Intraventricular bethanechol in Alzheimer's disease: a continuing controversy. *Neurology*, **38**, 307–8.

Wilcock, G.K., Esiri, M.M., Bowen, D.J. and Smith, C.C.T. (1982). Alzheimer's disease: correlation of cortical choline acetyltransferase activity with the severity of dementia and histological abnormalities. *Journal of Neurological Sciences*, **57**, 407–17.

Wittenborn, J.R. (1981). Pharmacotherapy for age-related behavioural deficiencies. *Journal of Nervous and Mental Diseases*, **169**, 139–56.

Yamamoto, T. and Hirano, A. (1985). Nucleus raphe dorsalis in Alzheimer's disease: neurofibrillary tangles and loss of large neurons. *Annals of Neurology*, **17**, 573–7.

Zola-Morgan, S., Squire, L.A. and Amaral, D.G. (1986). Human amnesia and the medial temporal region: enduring memory impairment following a bilateral lesion limited to field CA1 of the hippocampus. *Journal of Neuroscience*, **6**, 2950–67.

Tony Hope

University of Oxford Department of Psychiatry
and

Vikram Patel

The Maudsley and Bethlem Royal Hospitals

11 ASSESSMENT OF BEHAVIOURAL PHENOMENA IN DEMENTIA

INTRODUCTION

Dementia is frequently associated with behavioural changes (Burns *et al.*, 1990). Until recently, such changes have largely been seen as secondary to cognitive impairment and unworthy of further study (Fairburn and Hope, 1988). However, it is these behavioural changes rather than the disturbances of memory that often pose the greatest burden on carers and are the most common reason for psychiatric referral, treatment with psychotropic drugs and hospitalization (Teri *et al.*, 1989; Steele *et al.*, 1990). In this chapter, some conceptual issues surrounding the definition and classification of disturbed behaviour in people with dementia and the methods used in assessing behaviour will be discussed.

WHAT IS BEHAVIOUR?

Behaviour is notoriously difficult to define; the *Encyclopaedia of Psychology* (Eysenck *et al.*, 1972) offers eight definitions and asserts that there are many more. Any single definition needs to be supplemented with details of what is excluded from the definition and examples of what is included. We suggest, in the context of dementia, that behaviour refers to observable acts which can be measured. Examples of the phenomena we would include within this definition are aggressive behaviour, sleep, sexual behaviour, eating and activity disturbances ('wandering'). Within the concept of aggressive behaviour we include verbally aggressive behaviour such as verbal abuse. This certainly seems clinically sensible since verbal aggression is an observable act, although unlike physical aggression, its assessment involves taking into account the meaning of what is said. We are excluding a number of aspects which are occasionally included within the term 'behaviour'. Thus, physiological events, such as changes in heart rate, are not included because they are not *acts*. Most psychiatric phenomenology, such as delusions, hallucinations and mood disorders are excluded because they are neither observable, nor acts. These phenomena are primarily inner experiences and are assessed by what a person reports about the experience. But, unlike the case of verbally aggressive behaviour, these verbal reports are not *acts* which constitute the phenomenology. In the case of depressed mood, some behaviour such as motor retardation contribute to the overall concept. However, the core of the concept of depressed mood remains the subjective experience. For this reason, depressed mood is not behaviour whereas motor retardation would be. We also exclude cognitive abilities and impairments from the definition. Although these may be assessed by how people behave (e.g. how they perform certain tasks), such behaviour is the means for assessment rather than the meaning of the concept.

Thus, we suggest four mutually exclusive categories of phenomena: physiological phenomena; psychiatric phenomenology; cognitive abilities/ impairments; and behaviour. Although these are, we believe, different categories, there are some grey areas. It is not clear, for example, whether the disturbances of sleep should be regarded as physiological responses, or as behaviour. We include sleep disturbances in the category of behaviour for the purpose of this review. Incontinence is also difficult to classify. It is usually related to physical illness and disability and not therefore within any of the above categories. We do not include a discussion of incontinence in this review.

Particular types of behaviour can be further defined in two different ways: topographic or functional (Barlow and Hersen, 1984). The former stresses the observable aspects of the behaviour with minimal subjective inference on the part of the observer, whereas the latter emphasizes the purposes and consequences of the behaviour (Slater, 1980). Functional definitions require a judgement of why an act has occurred or what effects it has. These two ways of defining types of behaviour are poles of a spectrum rather than separate categories. For example, many definitions of aggressive behaviour include the concept of 'intent to harm' (e.g. Moyer, 1976). This is at the functional pole. A definition of this kind poses particular difficulties in the cognitively impaired, where the capacity to think, reason and rationalize is impaired and the assessment, or even the meaning of 'intention' is problematic (Patel and Hope, 1992a). We think it is more appropriate to define aggressive behaviour through specifying a range of component types of behaviour such as kicking, hitting and so on. Such concepts are closer to the topographical end of the spectrum than is the definition of aggressive behaviour as intent to harm. However, there is still some judgement necessary about the purpose of the act. Closer still to the topographical pole would be a definition of 'kicking' in terms of specified movements of the leg. This has the theoretical advantage of being freer from interpretation on the part of the observer. However, it is so removed from our normal, more global recognition of 'kicking' that it is unlikely to be either valid or reliable. As a general rule, we would favour the use of definitions towards the topographical end of the spectrum without going so far as to define a type of behaviour simply in terms of its component movements.

BEHAVIOUR OR PERSONALITY CHANGE?

There is one further semantic question which needs to be addressed. What is the relationship between a change in behaviour and a change in personality (Hope, 1992)? For example, if a formerly mild mannered person, on developing dementia, shows frequent aggressive behaviour, should we say that his personality has changed?

The concept of personality is used to refer to an individual's enduring and persistent responses across a variety of situations (Harre and Lamb, 1983). If, in the above example, the aggressive behaviour occurred in a wide variety of situations, the person might be described as having undergone a personality change. On this view, personality change is one end of a spectrum of changes in behaviour, i.e. it is behaviour change which occurs over a wide range of settings. However, there are good reasons for avoiding the term 'personality change' altogether in the setting of dementia. Firstly, 'organic personality change' has become strongly associated with the view that it is the result of damage to the frontal lobes (Lishman, 1987). Little is known at present of the relationship between behaviour change and brain damage in dementia. Secondly, we think of personality as part of the core of the person. Thus it would be unusual to say that we do not like someone's personality although we like the person. To say that the person with dementia who is sometimes aggressive has an aggressive personality is inextricably linked with making a judgement about him as a person. Since the behaviour is likely to be the result of brain damage, such a judgement seems unfair. Thirdly, to talk of the 'aggressive personality' of someone who is cognitively impaired and who may have very little understanding of his or her behaviour is misleading. It is preferable, therefore, to talk of specific changes in behaviour as this opens the way to posing important empirical questions such as: how can we assess the change? what is the aetiology? and, what methods of treatment should we try? without making too many assumptions.

TYPES OF BEHAVIOURAL PHENOMENA IN DEMENTIA

We will classify behavioural disturbances under six main categories, including one miscellaneous group. Each category will be briefly discussed before turning to the question of the assessment of behavioural disturbance.

Aggressive behaviour
Aggressive behaviour is common in dementia and of major clinical importance. In order to avoid making assumptions about intention, we defined aggressive behaviour as overt acts which involve the delivery of noxious stimuli to (but are not necessarily aimed at) another organism, object or self, and which are clearly not accidental (Patel and Hope, 1992a). Factor analytic studies support a distinction between verbal and physical aggression (Cohen-Mansfield and Billig, 1986; Patel and Hope, 1992b). An additional factor of 'antisocial behaviour' has also been identified (Patel and Hope, 1992b). Being uncooperative or resisting help, irritability and other forms of verbal aggression are the most common types of aggressive behaviour (Patel and Hope, 1992c; Hammel et al., 1990). Amongst physical behaviour, biting, scratching, kicking and hitting are frequent, whereas destroying property and sexual aggression are uncommon. Serious injuries are rarely inflicted on victims (Patel and Hope, 1992c). Although aggressive behaviour is normally assessed and classified in terms of the nature of the aggressive act, it has been suggested that the setting in which it occurs may relate more usefully to aetiology and management (Ware et al., 1990). Thus, whether a person is verbally or physically aggressive may be of less aetiological significance than that the behaviour occurs during intimate care.

Activity disturbances
This term, coined by Reisberg et al. (1987), is preferable to 'wandering' and 'agitation'. The term 'wandering' means different things to different people (Hope and Fairburn, 1990). Agitation is a broad behavioural term connoting excess motor activity which is often nonpurposeful (Barnes and Raskind, 1980). This term has been used to describe a range of distinct types of behaviour from excessive walking to aggression; or indeed 'any other behaviour which does not conform to norms of social conduct' (Cohen-Mansfield et al., 1989). A further problem is that it implies that the person feels 'agitated', which

requires a judgement about the person's inner experience. Factor analytic studies have clearly demonstrated that aggressive behaviour and activity disturbances are two distinct constructs (Cohen-Mansfield, 1989). Activity disturbances can be classified according to their severity and characteristic and include behaviour such as pottering, checking and walking inappropriately at night (Hope and Fairburn, 1990). It is noteworthy that reduced activity and apathy are common behavioural changes in dementia (Devenand et al., 1988), although they have received little attention, probably because they do not pose as great a burden on carers.

Eating behaviour
Disturbances of eating and changes in weight are common in dementia and are often of clinical significance. Up to 50% of the hospitalized elderly have been found to be malnourished (Sandman et al., 1987). Decreased food intake is the most common disturbance of eating behaviour and is usually associated with a loss in weight. It has been suggested that this drop in weight is unique to Alzheimer's disease (compared with multi-infarct dementia) and is not accounted for by malabsorption (Singh et al., 1988). Increased intake, changes in food preference (especially for sweet foods) and disturbances of chewing and swallowing (Morris et al., 1989) and eating of inedible foods, such as faeces (Ghaziuddin and McDonald, 1985), have also been described amongst people with dementia.

Disturbances of diurnal rhythm
This category deals with alterations in the sleep-wake cycle. Normal ageing is associated with reduction in total sleep time, reduced slow wave sleep and daytime fatigue (Moran et al., 1988). These changes are heightened in dementia and are often associated with an increased frequency and duration of nighttime awakenings (Vitiello et al., 1990). Changes in dominant occipital electroencephalographic (EEG) rhythm and sleep disturbances are seen even in early, mild dementia and these variables along with random eye movement (REM) sleep time and density discriminate well between patients with dementia and depression (Reynolds et al., 1983). As dementia progresses, there is reduction in REM sleep with an increase in daytime sleep, and finally a complete disorganization of the sleep-wake cycle (Vitiello and Prinz, 1989). The worsening of activity disturbances in the latter part of the day ('sundowning'), nocturnal activity disturbances (such as excessive walking at night) and inappropriate robing and disrobing might be related to disturbances of diurnal rhythm.

Sexual behaviour
Reduced sexual drive with impotence has been reported as being frequent in male patients (Zeiss et al., 1990), but this needs further investigation. Of more concern to carers is inappropriate sexual behaviour (such as masturbation in public) and sexual aggression, although studies so far have indicated that these are rare (Cooper, 1987; Patel and Hope, 1992c). Behaviour which has been placed in this category includes inappropriate sexual speech, hugging, kissing, self-exposure and attempted fondling (Jensen, 1989).

Other miscellaneous behavioural disturbances
There is a range of behaviour which does not clearly fit into any of the above categories. Screaming, defined as 'shouting or howling that is loud, shrill or piercing' (Cohen-Mansfield et al., 1990) has been studied as a unique type of

behavioural disturbance although others have included it within aggressive behaviour (e.g. Patel and Hope, 1992b). Many people pick at their clothes or the surrounding furniture. Whilst walking aimlessly about the house, it is quite common for people with dementia to pick up small objects as they pass by and place them carefully in another position. There are several other types of odd behaviour which are quite commonly observed although their significance is unclear (Hope and Fairburn, 1992).

ASSESSMENT OF BEHAVIOURAL DISTURBANCES

Much of the current literature on behaviour disturbances in dementia is handicapped by the lack of reliable and valid methods of assessing the behaviour. The majority of studies have involved unstructured descriptions of behaviour in small series of cases. This is especially true in treatment studies (e.g. Greenwald et al., 1986). The emphasis has been on descriptive analysis rather than precise measurement. It has been estimated that unstructured reporting records five times fewer episodes of aggressive behaviour than do structured daily ward reports (Lion et al., 1981). The last few years, however, have seen the development of a variety of methods for the assessment of disturbed behaviour in dementia (Table 11.1). In clinical practice, anyone with dementia who shows disturbed behaviour needs a thorough assessment of their physical health. Evaluation of family relationships is also vital because disturbed relationships can create a hostile and stressful environment for the demented patient who, because of impaired cognition, is unable to cope and responds with disruptive behaviour (Silliman et al., 1988).

We are concerned, in this chapter, with methods of rating and describing the behaviour itself rather than with establishing its cause. We will consider these methods under four headings: collecting information from the patient; collecting information from carers; direct observation; and indirect objective measures.

Collecting information from the patient
Self-report inventories were designed in an attempt to relate personality constructs to behaviour. These are of little value in dementia, mainly because of the cognitive impairment, but partly, also, because these measures do not correlate well with behaviour (Edmunds and Kendrick, 1980). A recent study showed that there was significant underreporting of information when patients were compared with carers even in patients with mild dementia (Ballard et al., 1991).

An alternative approach is the interview-based rating scale. Semistructured interviews such as the Geriatric Mental State (Copeland et al., 1976) and the Sandoz Clinical Assessment-Geriatric (SCAG) (Shader et al., 1974) are instruments that have been frequently used in the assessment of behavioural phenomena and treatment outcome. The SCAG has 19 items (including behaviour, mood and cognitive abilities) and is rated on the basis of a single interview with the patient. Such instruments lay emphasis on the current mental state of the patient and have the disadvantage of either relying on the patients' own reports of disturbed behaviour or the observed behaviour during the relatively short period of the interview (Palmstierna and Wistedt, 1987). In addition, these instruments have only a few items dealing with disturbed behaviour and are therefore of limited value in behavioural assessment.

The Behavioural Pathology in Alzheimer's Disease (BEHAVE-AD) (Reisberg et al., 1987) is rated on the basis of an interview with the patient. It is designed

Table 11.1 Behavioural assessment instruments for use in persons with dementia.

Instrument	Behavioural item content	Type of instrument	Setting
Present behavioural examination (Hope and Fairburn, 1992)	Seven separate behavioural domains, section on mental and physical health	Interview-based rating scale	Community
Behave-Alzheimer's disease (Reisberg et al. 1987)	Global psychiatric phenomenology 7/25 items behavioural	Semistructured interview with carer	Any
Behaviour and mood disturbance scale (Greene et al., 1982)	Global behaviour and mood	Rating scale	Community
Behaviour severity rating scale (Swearer et al. 1988)	Global behaviour and mood	Rating scale	Any
Confusion inventory (Evans, 1987)	Wide range of psychopathology <50% items behavioural	Rating scale	Any
Nurses observation scale for geriatric patients (nos–ger) (Spiegel et al., 1991)	10/30 items behavioural; rest, mood and activities of daily living	Rating scale	Institutional
Cohen-Mansfield agitation inventory (Cohen-Mansfield, 1989)	Aggressive behaviour, activity disturbances, eating behaviour (1 item)	Rating scale	Institutional
Memory and behaviour problems checklist (and revised MBPC) (Zarit et al., 1985)	Aggressive behaviour, activity disturbances, apraxias and activities of daily living	Rating scale	Institutional/community
Disruptive behaviour rating scale (Mungas et al., 1989)	Aggressive behaviour, activity disturbances	Rating scale	Institutional
Rating of aggressive behaviour in the elderly (RAGE) (Patel and Hope, 1992b)	Aggressive behaviour	Rating scale	Institutional
Ryden aggression scale (Ryden, 1988)	Aggressive behaviour	Rating scale	Community
Overt aggression scale (OAS) (Yudofsky et al., 1986) Modified OAS (Kay et al., 1988)	Aggressive behaviour	Rating scale	Institutional
Staff observation aggression scale (Palmstierna and Wistedt, 1987)	Aggressive behaviour	Rating scale	Institutional
Short observation method (MacDonald et al., 1985)	General behaviour (not specifically for behavioural disturbances)	Direct observation	Institutional
Agitation behaviour mapping instrument (Cohen-Mansfield et al., 1989)	Activity disturbances, aggressive behaviour	Direct observation	Institutional

principally to evaluate treatment outcome. It has 25 items, of which only seven are behavioural; the remaining items measure mood and other psychopathology such as delusions and hallucinations. There are some data on inter-rater reliability (Patterson *et al.*, 1990), but no data on test–retest reliability or validity.

Collecting information from carers
In most studies carers are the principal source of information on behaviour. Information can be collected using semistructured or structured interviews or rating scales. There are few data on the nature of biases that may operate in carer reports. Some carers may be more (or less) prone to report difficulties than others. The severity of the behavioural disorder reported may reflect individual carer tolerance as much as the actual severity of the behaviour itself (Teri *et al.*, 1989). Patterson *et al.* (1990) found a remarkably high prevalence of psychotic symptoms reported by carers of demented patients, and question whether carers may exaggerate less pathological experiences such as illusions due to lack of clinical sophistication. Investigator rated semistructured interviews are likely to be more valid than rating scales completed by the carer, but they are time-consuming for the research worker. Some instruments have been developed principally for patients living at home with a principal carer, usually a relative, whereas others are designed to be completed by nursing staff looking after patients in institutional care. We will first discuss those instruments which cover a wide range of behaviour and then those which focus on a limited range.

The only semistructured interview developed principally for studying behaviour in dementia is the Present Behavioural Examination (PBE) (Hope and Fairburn, 1992). This interview is designed to be administered to the principal carer and covers behaviour over the preceding 28 days. There are seven behavioural domains (similar to the classification presented above). There is also a section on mental and physical health. This interview can be used in its entirety or its subsections can be used on their own, for example, the eating (Morris *et al.*, 1989) and aggressive behaviour subsections (Ware *et al.*, 1990). The PBE consists of 121 main behavioural items. Each is defined, as is the rating system to be used. Many items are rated on a seven-point frequency rating scale. The PBE has been designed for obtaining data on behaviour in dementia, to investigate the course and nature of abnormal behaviour and to study the relationships between abnormal behaviour and other features of dementia (such as degree of cognitive impairment).

The Behaviour and Mood Disturbance Scale (Greene *et al.*, 1982) is an ordinal rating scale for use by the primary carer in home-based patients. Its purpose is to measure behaviour likely to cause stress to carers. It has 31 items, of which less than half are behavioural. The items are rated on a five-point loosely defined scale (e.g. 'never', 'always'). Factor analysis of the items revealed three factors: apathetic–withdrawn, active–disturbed and mood disturbance. Data on its test–retest reliability and construct validity are presented. The Behaviour Severity Rating Scale (Swearer *et al.*, 1988) was designed to examine the relationships between behavioural disturbance and disease severity. It has nine behavioural and two mood items, but no psychometric data are available at present. In the study by Swearer and colleagues, the scale was rated on the basis of a telephone interview with the carer.

Most rating scales have been designed to be used by nursing staff with patients in hospital. The vast majority of such scales have been designed principally to give guidance on the type and amount of care which the patient is likely to require. These scales cover 'activities of daily living' such as the ability to carry out tasks of self-care. Behavioural items in the sense used in this chapter are usually few. Nevertheless, such 'global' scales have been frequently used to rate behaviour, presumably because more specific scales have only recently been developed. (For a comprehensive review of such global scales see Israel et al., 1984.) With the increasing availability of new and more specific rating scales, the use of global scales for studies of behaviour is to be discouraged. The Confusion Inventory (Evans, 1987) is a checklist developed to study the 'sundowning' phenomenon (i.e. worsening of some behavioural disturbances in the evening). It has 48 'psychomotor' and 'psychosocial' indicators of mental confusion. Less than half the items represent behavioural disturbance and there are few psychometric data. The Nurses Observation Scale for Geriatric Patients (NOSGER) (Spiegel et al., 1991) has been developed recently. It consists of 30 items, of which only 10 measure behaviour (five 'social behaviour' and five 'disturbing behaviour'). The other items are concerned with memory, mood and activities of daily living.

A number of rating scales have been designed specifically to measure 'agitated' behaviour in dementia. This term usually incorporates elements of aggressive behaviour together with activity disturbances. We will briefly review three examples.

1. *The Cohen-Mansfield Agitation Inventory* (Cohen-Mansfield, 1989): This is designed to be rated by nurses at the end of each 8-hour shift over a 24-hour period (i.e. three sets of ratings). There are 29 behavioural items organized around four factors: verbal agitation; aggression; physical nonaggressive behaviour; and hiding/hoarding. The scale includes items on abnormal eating behaviour. A seven-point frequency rating is used ranging from never to several times each hour over a 1 week period. There are some data available on inter-rater reliability.

2. *The Memory and Behaviour Problems Checklist* (Zarit et al., 1985): This scale includes items on aggressive behaviour, activities of daily living, apraxias and four items on 'spatial disorientation' (wandering, getting lost indoors, getting lost in familiar streets, inability to recognize familiar surroundings). The items on spatial disorientation have been used in a study of the relationship of visuospatial dysfunction to wandering (Henderson et al., 1989). The Revised Memory and Behaviour Problems Checklist has 64 items in three categories: depressive, disruptive and behaviour related to memory impairment. In addition, carer reactions to each behaviour are rated in order to identify stressful behaviour (Teri and Logsdon, 1990).

3. *The Disruptive Behaviour Rating Scale* (Mungas et al., 1989): This consists of four items ('dimensions of disruptive behaviour'), each rated on a five-point scale, two of which concern aggressive behaviour and two activity disturbances. The severity of the behaviour is measured on the basis of the nature of the intervention in response to the behaviour. Ratings are made on behaviour over a 7-day period. A checklist which includes 13 items on aggressive behaviour and seven items on activity disturbances is used as an aid to the ratings. A 'Total Disruptive Score' is obtained by adding the four ratings. Data are available on inter-rater reliability, concurrent and discriminant validity.

There are four rating scales which focus specifically on aggressive behaviour.

1. *The Rating of Aggressive Behaviour in the Elderly (RAGE)* (Patel and Hope, 1992b): This has been designed to be rated by nursing staff at the end of a 3-day period of observation of in-patients. It consists of 23 items, most of which are rated on a four-point scale of frequency. A 'Global Aggression Score' can be obtained by adding all the ratings. The psychometric properties of the scale

have been extensively investigated (inter-rater and test–retest reliability, content and clinical validity) and it is sensitive to change. Inter-rater reliability is significantly improved with the use of a ward checklist. The RAGE is recommended for longitudinal assessment of the natural history of aggressive behaviour, for treatment trials, and in the study of the relationships between aggressive behaviour and other variables. The RAGE has been used to study the rates of aggressive behaviour found in a hospitalized psychogeriatric population (Patel and Hope, 1992c). Forty-five per cent of the sample of 90 patients were considered to have been at least mildly aggressive over the 3-day observation period; this included 15% of the sample who were rated to be moderately or severely aggressive.

2. *The Ryden Aggression Scale* (Ryden, 1988): This has been designed specifically for use in the community. It consists of 25 items divided into three subscales: physical aggression (16 items); verbal aggression (four items); and sexual aggression (five items). It is rated by the carer over a period ranging from a week to a year. Test–retest reliability and discriminant data are available. The RAS has been used to study the predictors and consequences of aggressive behaviour in community-based patients (Hamel *et al.*, 1990).

3. *The Overt Aggression Scale (OAS)* (Yudofsky *et al.*, 1986): This consists of four items on aggressive behaviour, with emphasis on physical aggression. It has been designed for use in a general psychiatric setting, and has maximum reliability for patients who have been admitted as an emergency and for patients transferred from maximum security units. This scale gives a rating for individual aggressive episodes rather than providing an overall rating of aggressive behaviour over a period of time. It is particularly suited to differentiating assaultative patients in general psychiatric settings, but its value in the elderly requires further clarification. The Modified Overt Aggression Scale (Kay *et al.*, 1988) overcomes some of the psychometric weaknesses of the OAS in four ways: by upgrading the nominal rating scale to an ordinal five-point scale representing increasing levels of aggression; by providing operational definitions for each category of behaviour; by adding items on suicidal behaviour; and by introducing a total weighted score. Data on inter-rater reliability and discriminant validity indicate that it has superior psychometric properties than the OAS.

4. *The Staff Observation Aggression Scale* (Palmstierna and Wistedt, 1987; Nilsson *et al.*, 1988): This has been designed to assess the degree and frequency of violent and aggressive acts in psychogeriatric patients, but like the Overt Aggression Scale, it provides an analysis of individual aggressive episodes. As with the OAS and the Disruptive Behaviour Rating Scale the nature of staff intervention is used as an indicator of the severity of the behaviour itself. This is problematic since such interventions are often determined by ward policies. The rating for exactly the same behaviour is therefore likely to vary from unit to unit (Soloff, 1987).

Two personality inventories have been used to study behaviour in people with dementia. One is the inventory of Brooks and McKinlay (1983) which is designed as analogue scales with bipolar adjectives (such as 'even tempered' and 'quick tempered' or 'irritable' and 'easy going'). This inventory is designed to be completed by the relative and has been used by Petry *et al.* (1988, 1989) to compare patients with dementia with nondemented controls. The other is the scale of Blessed *et al.* (1968) which includes 11 items (out of a total of 35 items) which are concerned with changes in personality.

There are no rating scales which focus on disturbances of eating behaviour, diurnal rhythm or sexual behaviour.

Direct observation

Direct observation provides potentially the gold standard for behavioural assessment (Barlow and Hersen, 1984). It requires, however, considerable preparation, allowing for control of factors such as observer reactivity and bias and careful identification and definition of target behaviour. Research workers need to be aware of the issue of reliability of the procedure. Observers need adequate training and practice, and pilot observations are recommended. In an elderly population, special attention needs to be directed to ensure that the level of arousal during the periods of observation is adequate and representative of the general level (Hussain, 1981).

Observational procedures require a number of steps to be taken. The first step is the identification of the target behaviour, i.e. the behaviour of interest to the clinician or research worker. Occasionally, this may not be immediately apparent, and furthermore a general category may mask specific behavioural disturbances. Interviews with carers and unstructured ward observations can be used to identify which specific types of behaviour cause concern or pose a threat to the carer of the patient. Once identified, the target behaviour needs to be defined, using either the topographical or functional approaches (see above). The definition should capture the behaviour of interest. The definition must be objective (i.e. referring to the observable characteristics of the behaviour, avoiding references to internal states), clear (i.e. unambiguous and easily understood) and complete (i.e. specifying the critical parts of the behaviour and providing typical examples) (Barlow and Hersen, 1984). The coding system, too, must be objective and unambiguous. The next step is to select the observation setting. This will be particularly important if the behaviour is situation specific. The setting needs to be relevant to the behaviour of interest and feasible as a place to undertake the observations. Then, one needs to select the observer. The observer or observers will need to be trained and interobserver reliability assessed. The duration of observation will need to be chosen and this choice will depend on a number of factors. High frequency behaviour and behaviour requiring the use of complex coding systems are best observed in short sessions in order to limit observer fatigue. Infrequent behaviour may require longer periods of observation with more than one observer in sequence. Behaviour can be measured in terms of frequency, duration and quality. Selecting the appropriate response dimension depends on the purpose of the study and the nature of the behaviour. Freely occurring discrete behaviour, such as kicking, can be measured in terms of frequency whereas more continuous behaviour such as walking, may be best measured in terms of duration. For more complex ratings, the use of multiple observers and audiovisual recordings of behaviour is recommended. Five types of observation procedures can be distinguished: real-time observations in which both event frequency and duration are recorded as they occur in noninterrupted, natural time flow; event or frequency recording to measure the frequency of discrete behaviour; duration recording to measure the time a behaviour lasts; momentary time sampling where an observer observes how the subject is behaving at predetermined points in time (e.g. on the minute every minute); and interval recording where an observation session is divided into brief observe–record intervals and each interval is scored if the target behaviour occurs during any part of the interval (for further discussion see Barlow and Hersen, 1984).

There have been few studies of people with dementia which have used direct observation although we believe that the potential of this method for studying behaviour has not yet been fully realized. We have used direct observation in two single case studies. One involved the assessment of a patient with activity disturbance (Hope *et al.*, 1991). Four behavioural codes were used: walking, trailing (i.e. following someone), sitting and standing. Continuous real-time observation was employed over 30-minute observation periods. The patient was observed before, during and after pharmacological intervention (in this case, dexamphetamine). In addition to providing data concerning the efficacy of dexamphetamine, the preliminary observations also helped in clarifying the nature of the behavioural disturbance. In the second study, stuctured observations of a patient with Pick's disease who showed a marked increase in eating were carried out in a standardized setting (Hope and Allman, 1991) in which almost unlimited food was available. Behaviour was observed before, during and after treatment with fluvoxamine. A different use of direct observation is exemplified by the development of the RAGE (see above), where observational data were used as the validating criterion for the rating scale (Patel and Hope, 1992b). Burton (1980) used direct observation to study the impact of occupational therapy sessions on disturbed behaviour on a psychogeriatric ward. Patients were observed for 5 seconds at quarter minute intervals over a 1-hour period and interobserver reliabilities were estimated. The study was able to demonstrate that certain types of intervention produced an improvement in some behaviour. Observational data have been used to assess the efficacy of operant procedures in a group of institutionalized elderly aggressive patients (Vaccaro, 1988). MacDonald *et al.* (1985) developed the Short Observation Method for studying activities and contacts of the elderly in residential settings. Observations were recorded using an event sampling technique for nine 'activity' codes (e.g. sitting, moving etc) and four 'contacts' (e.g. with a nurse, resident etc.) over a 1-hour period in the late morning which was found to be representative of behaviour over a 24-hour period. This method has been used to compare the effects of different philosophies of care for the institutionalized patients with dementia (Lindesay *et al.*, 1991). Snyder *et al.* (1978) used 'behaviour mapping' (Cohen-Mansfield, 1989) to study wandering. They observed and followed patients recording the location and duration of specific types of behaviour over 18 10-minute sessions. They found that even those who were thought to be 'continuous wanderers' spent much of the time sedentary and that these 'wanderers' were more likely to scream and socialize with other residents than nonwanderers. Cohen-Mansfield *et al.* (1989) have used the Agitation Behaviour Mapping Instrument which records specific observed behaviour as well as social and physical aspects of the environment. Systematic observations of the type and frequency of 'agitated behaviours' including activity disturbance and aggressive behaviour were carried out. Stratified random time sampling was used, with each patient observed for three consecutive minutes of each hour over a 24-hour period. With training, high interobserver agreement was reported. More detailed observation studies are being undertaken by Keene (personal communication) who is using video recordings to observe aggressive behaviour during washing and dressing. Detailed analysis of the recordings is being used to try and identify the behavioural components which precede the aggressive behaviour.

Indirect objective measures
Some types of behaviour can be measured using objective methods which are not dependent on direct observation. For example, pedometers and electronic monitoring have been used to assess hyperactivity (excessive walking) (Rindlisbacher and Hopkins, 1992). Electroencephalographic recordings, particularly using portable apparatus which can be used in people's own homes, can give more information about the pattern and nature of sleep than could be provided

by direct observation. Electroencephalographic recordings in the laboratory have been used to study sleep in Alzheimer's disease (Vitiello and Prinz, 1989). Physiological markers of diurnal rhythms such as plasma melatonin and human growth hormone release (Moran *et al.*, 1988) and body temperature (Touitou *et al.*, 1986) have also been used, but it is unclear how these markers are themselves affected in dementia. Weight change and biochemical indices of nutrition might be used in studying eating behaviour although changes in the absorption of food could make such measures unreliable indicators of the eating behaviour itself. Relationships have been reported between serum testosterone levels and sexually aggressive behaviour although this needs validation (Cooper, 1987).

FUTURE DIRECTIONS

A major transition is occurring in the way in which behavioural disturbances in dementia are being approached. Until recently, such disturbances were seen either as uninteresting consequences of cognitive impairment, or as general aspects of the 'personality change' accompanying dementia. These perspectives are being replaced by identifying behavioural changes as being of interest in their own right. Crucial to the further study of behavioural disturbances is the development over recent years of standardized assessment methods which focus on the behaviour; this opens up the possibility of studies looking at aetiological factors and therapeutic interventions.

A discussion of the wide variety of different causes of disturbed behaviour in dementia is beyond the scope of this chapter. We wish to emphasize what has been a relatively neglected aspect: the possibility that much disturbed behaviour is the direct result of brain damage and not simply secondary to cognitive impairment. The two most promising approaches are post-mortem studies and drug studies. In an important preliminary study, Palmer *et al.* (1988) found an association between aggressive behaviour and 5-hydroxytryptamine (5-HT) reduction in a small series of people with Alzheimer's disease. The aggressive behaviour was determined retrospectively from the case notes. This work needs to be extended using subjects prospectively assessed by means of reliable and valid methods. *In vivo* brain scanning techniques such as single photon emission tomography (SPECT), positron emission tomography (PET) and magnetic resonance imaging (MRI) may considerably enhance the study of the correlations between behaviour, cerebral function and brain damage. The development of new drugs with well-defined neurotransmitter effects, coupled with improved methods of assessment for specific types of behaviour, should lead to further developments in the biological basis of behavioural disturbance. Thus, it may be possible using these drugs to dissect out the contributions of different neurotransmitter systems to different types of behaviour.

Another area for research using the new methods of assessment is the evaluation of various therapeutic interventions for disturbed behaviour. So far, most treatment studies have used unstructured reporting of behaviour. With the availability of standardized methods of assessment, such research will yield more reliable data on treatment efficacy. The detailed study of behaviour is relevant not only to the study of organic theories of aetiology and pharmacological treatments but also to looking at interpersonal determinants of behaviour. The time is ripe for the development of new approaches to treatment for behaviour problems. On the one hand, we might hope for different drug treatments targetted to specific behavioural disturbances; on the other, new training programmes might be developed from the detailed observation of interpersonal interactions.

Future directions in the area of assessment itself is likely to focus on the development of objective methods of rating behaviour without relying on information collected from carers. These methods could include the use of techniques of direct observation and indirect objective measures of behaviour. Video recording is likely to be used increasingly to study behaviour in detail. The development of new methods of assessment and its consequent fuelling of our understanding of the nature of behavioural phenomena in dementia presents a challenging goal for future research.

REFERENCES

Ballard, C.G., Chitiramohan, R.N., Handy S. *et al.* (1991). Information reliability in dementia sufferers. *International Journal of Geriatric Psychiatry*, **6**, 313–16.

Barlow, D.H. and Hersen, M. (1984). *Single Case Experimental Designs: Strategies for Studying Behaviour Change*. Pergamon Press, Oxford.

Barnes, R. and Raskind, M. (1980). Strategies for diagnosing and treating agitation in the aged, *Geriatrics*, **3**, 111–19.

Blessed, G., Tomlinson, B.E. and Roth, M. (1968). The association between quantitative measures of dementia and of senile change in the cerebral grey matter of elderly subjects. *British Journal of Psychiatry*, **114**, 797–811.

Brooks, D.N. and McKinlay, W. (1983). Personality and behaviour change after severe blunt head injury: a relatives view. *Journal of Neurology, Neurosurgery and Psychiatry*, **46**, 336–44.

Burns, A., Jacoby, R. and Levy, R. (1990). Psychiatric phenomena in Alzheimer's disease. IV. Disorders of behaviour. *British Journal of psychiatry*, **157**, 86–94.

Burton, M. (1980). Evaluation and change in a psychogeriatric ward through direct observation and feedback. *British Journal of Psychiatry*, **137**, 566–71.

Cohen-Mansfield, J. (1989). Agitation in the elderly. *Advances in Psychosomatic Medicine*, **19**, 101–13.

Cohen-Mansfield, J. and Billig, N. (1986). Agitated behaviours in the elderly. I. A conceptual review. *Journal of the American Geriatrics Society*, **34**, 711–21.

Cohen-Mansfield, J., Marx, M.S. and Werner, P. (1989). Full moon: does it influence agitated nursing home residents? *Journal of Clinical Psychology*, **45**, 611–14.

Cohen-Mansfield, J., Werner, P. and Marx, M.S.(1990). Screaming in nursing home residents. *Journal of American Geriatrics Society*, **38**, 785–92.

Cooper, A.J. (1987). Medroxyprogesterone acetate treatment of sexual acting out in men suffering from dementia. *Journal of Clinical Psychiatry*, **43**, 368.

Copeland, J.R.M., Kelleher, M.J., Kellett, J.H. *et al.* (1976). A semi-structured clinical interview for the assessment of diagnosis and mental state in the elderly: The Geriatric Mental State Schedule I: Development and Reliability. *Psychological Medicine*, **6**, 439–49.

Devenand, D.P., Sackeim, H.A. and Mayeux, R. (1988). Psychosis, behavioural disturbance, and the use of neuroleptics in dementia. *Comprehensive Psychiatry*, **29**, 387–401.

Edmunds, G. and Kendrick, D.C. (1980). *The Measurement of Aggression*. Ellis Horwood Limited, Chichester.

Evans, L.K. (1987). Sundown syndrome in the institutionalized elderly. *Journal of the American Geriatrics Society*, **35**, 101–8.

Eysenck, H., Arnold, W. and Meili, R. (1972). *Encyclopaedia of Psychology*, Vol. 1. Search Press, London.

Fairburn, C.G. and Hope, R.A. (1988). Changes in behaviour in dementia: A neglected research area. *British Journal of Psychiatry*, **152**, 406–7.

Ghaziuddin, N. and McDonald, C. (1985). A study of adult coprophagics. *British Journal of Psychiatry*, **147**, 312–13.

Greene, J.G., Smith, R., Gardiner, M. and Timbury, G.C. (1982). Measuring behavioural disturbance of elderly demented patients in the community and its effects on relatives: a factor analytic study. *Age and Ageing*, **11**, 121–16.

Greenwald, B.S., Marin, D.B. and Silverman, S.M. (1986). Serotoninergic treatment of screaming and banging in dementia. *Lancet*, **ii**, 1464–5.

Hamel, M., Gold, D.P., Andres, D. *et al.* (1990). Prediction and consequences of aggressive behaviour by community-based dementia patients. *Gerontologist*, **30**, 206–11.

Harre, R. and Lamb R. (1983). *The Encyclopedic Dictionary of Psychology*. Blackwell Scientific Publications, Oxford.

Henderson, V.W., Mack, W. and Williams, B.W. (1989). Spatial disorientation in Alzheimer's disease. *Archives of Neurology*, **46**, 391–4.

Hope, R.A. (1992). Behaviour and personality change in dementia. In *Dementia and Normal Aging*, Huppert, F. *et al.* Cambridge University Press (in press).

Hope, R.A. and Allman, P. (1991). Hyperphagia in dementia: fluvoxamine takes the biscuit. *Journal of Neurology, Neurosurgery and Psychiatry*, **54**, 88.

Hope, R.A. and Fairburn, C.G. (1990). The nature of wandering in dementia: a community-based study. *International Journal of Geriatric Psychiatry*, **5**, 239–45.

Hope, R.A. and Fairburn, C.G. (1992). The Present Behavioural Examination (PBE): The development of an interview to measure current behavioural abnormalities. *Psychological Medicine*, **22**, 223–30.

Hope, R.A., Patel, V. and Series, H. (1991). Dexamphetamine may reduce hyperactivity in dementia: a case study using direct observation. *International Journal of Geriatric Psychiatry*, **6**, 165–9.

Hussain, R.A. (1981). *Geriatric Psychology: A Behavioural Perspective*. Van Nostrand Reinhold Company, New York.

Israel, L., Kozarevic, D. and Sartorius, N. (1984). *Source Book of Geriatric Assessment*, Vols 1 and 2. Karger, Basle.

Jensen, C.F. (1989). Hypersexual agitation in Alzheimer's disease. *Journal of the American Geriatrics Society*, **37**, 917.

Kay, S.R., Wokenfeld, F. and Murrill, L.M. (1988). Profiles of aggression among psychiatric patients. I. Nature & Prevalence. *Journal of Nervous and Mental Disease*, **176**, 539–46.

Lindesay, J., Briggs, K., Lawes, M. *et al.* (1991). The Domus philosophy: A comparative evaluation of a new approach to residential care for the demented elderly. *International Journal of Geriatric Psychiatry*, **6**, 727–36.

Lishman, W.A. (1987). *Organic Psychiatry*, 2nd edition. Blackwell Scientific Publications, Oxford.

Lion, J.R., Snyder, W. and Merrill, G.L. (1981). Under-reporting of assaults on staff in a state hospital. *Hospital and Community Psychiatry*, **32**, 497–8.

MacDonald, A.J., Craig, T.K.J. and Warner, L.A.R. (1985). The development of a short observation method for the study of activity and contacts of old people in residential settings. *Psychological Medicine*, **15**, 167–72.

Moran, M.G., Thompson II, T.L. and Nies, A.S. (1988). Sleep disorders in the elderly. *American Journal of Psychiatry*, **145**, 1369–78.

Morris, C.H., Hope, R.A. and Fairburn, C.G. (1989). Eating habits in dementia. A descriptive study. *British Journal of Psychiatry*, **154**, 801–6.

Moyer, K.E. (1976). *The Psychobiology of Aggression*. Harper and Row, New York.

Mungas, D. Weiler, P., Franzi, C. and Henry, R. (1989). Assessment of disruptive behaviour associated with dementia: The Disruptive Behaviour Rating scales. *Journal of Geriatric Psychiatry and Neurology*, **2**, 196–202.

Nilsson, K., Palmstierna, T. and Wistedt, B. (1988). Aggressive behaviour in hospitalized psychogeriatric patients. *Acta Psychiatrica Scandinavica*, **78**, 172–5.

Palmer, A.M., Stratmann, G.C., Proctor, A.W. and Bowen, D.M. (1988). Possible neurotransmitter basis of behavioural changes in Alzheimer's disease. *Annals of Neurology*, **23**, 616–20.

Palmstierna, T. and Wistedt, B. (1987). The Staff Observation Aggression Scale: Presentation and evaluation. *Acta Psychiatrica Scandinavica*, **76**, 657–63.

Patel, V. and Hope, R.A. (1992a). Aggressive behaviour in dementia: A review. *International Journal of Geriatric Psychiatry* (in press).

Patel, V. and Hope, R.A. (1992b). A rating scale for aggressive behaviour in the elderly (the RAGE). *Psychological Medicine*, **22**, 211–21.

Patel, V. and Hope, R.A. (1992c). Aggressive behaviour in a hospitalized psychogeriatric population. *Acta Psychiatrica Scandinavica*, **85**, 131–5.

Patterson, M.B., Schnell, A.H., Martin, R.J. *et al.* (1990). Assessment of behavioural and affective symptoms in Alzheimer's disease. *Journal of Geriatric Psychiatry and Neurology*, **3**, 21–30.

Petry, S., Cummings, J.L., Hill, M.A. and Shapira, J. (1988). Personality alterations in dementia of the Alzheimer type. *Archives of Neurology*, **45**, 1187–90.

Petry, S., Cummings, J.L., Hill, M.A. and Shapira, J. (1989). Personality alterations in dementia of the Alzheimer type: A three year follow-up study. *Journal of Geriatric Psychiatry and Neurology*, **2**, 203–7.

Reisberg, B., Borenstein, J., Salob, S.P. *et al.* (1987). Behavioural symptoms in Alzheimer's disease: phenomenology and treatment. *Journal of Clinical Psychiatry*, **48** (5 Suppl.), 9–15.

Reynolds, C.F., Spiker, D.G., Hanin, I. and Kupfer, D.J. (1983). Electroencephalographic sleep, aging and psychopathology: new data and the state of the art. *Biological Psychiatry*, **18**, 139–55.

Rindlisbacher, P. and Hopkins, R.W. (1992). An investigation of the sundowning syndrome. *International Journal of Geriatric Psychiatry*, **7**, 15–24.

Ryden, M.B. (1988). Aggressive behaviour in persons with dementia who live in the community. *Alzheimer Disease and associated disorders*, **2**, 342–5.

Sandman, P.-O., Adolfsson, R., Nygren, C. *et al.* (1987). Nutritional status and dietary intake in institutionalized patients with Alzheimer's disease and multiinfarct dementia. *Journal of the American Geriatrics Society*, **35**, 31–8.

Shader, R.I., Salzman, C. and Harmatz, J.S. (1974). A new scale for clinical assessment in geriatric patients (SCA-G). *Journal of the American Geriatrics Society*, **22**, 107–13.

Silliman, R.A., Sternberg, J. and Fretwell, M.D. (1988). Disruptive behaviour in demented patients living within disturbed families. *Journal of the American Geriatrics Society*, **39**, 617–18.

Singh, S., Mulley, G.P. and Losowsky, M.S. (1988). Why are Alzheimer patients thin? *Age and Ageing*, **17**, 21–8.

Slater, P.J.B. (1980). The ethological approach to aggression. *Psychological Medicine*, **10**, 607–9.

Snyder, L.H., Rupprecht, P., Pyrrek, J. *et al.* (1978). Wandering. *The Geront-ologist*, **18**, 272–80.

Soloff, P.H. (1987). Emergency management of the violent patient. In *The American Psychiatric Association Annual Review No. 6*, Hales, R.E. and Frances, A.J. (Eds). American Psychiatric Press, Washington.

Spiegel, R., Brunner, C., Ermini-Funfschilling, D. *et al.* (1991). A new behavioural assessment scale for geriatric out- and in-patients: the NOSGER (Nurses Observation Scale for Geriatric patients). *Journal of the American Geriatrics Society*, **39**, 339–47.

Steele, C., Rovner, B., Chase, G.A. and Folstein M. (1990). Psychiatric symptoms and nursing home placement of patients with Alzheimer's disease. *American Journal of Psychiatry*, **147**, 1049–51.

Swearer, J.M., Drachman, D.A., O'Donnell, B.F. and Mitchell, A.L. (1988). Troublesome and disruptive behaviours in dementia. Relationships to diagnosis and disease severity. *Journal of the American Geriatrics Society*, **36** 784–90.

Teri, L., Borson, S., Kiyak, H.A. and Yamagishi, M. (1989). Behavioural disturbance, cognitive dysfunction and functional skill. Prevalence and relationships in Alzheimer's disease. *Journal of the American Geriatrics Society*, **37**, 109–16.

Teri, L. and Logsdon, R. (1990). Assessment and management of behavioural disturbances in Alzheimer's disease. *Comprehensive Therapy*, **16**, 36–42.

Touitou, Y., Reinberg. A., Bodnan, A. *et al.* (1986). Age-related changes in both circadian and seasonal rhythms of rectal temperature with special reference to senile dementia of Alzheimer type. *Gerontology*, **32**, 110–18.

Vaccaro, F.J. (1988). Application of operant procedures in a group of institutionalized aggressive geriatric patients. *Psychology and Aging*, **3**, 22–8.

Vitiello, M. V. and Prinz, P.N. (1989). Alzheimer's disease: sleep and sleep/wake patterns. *Clinics in Geriatric Medicine*, **5**, 289–99.

Vitiello, M.V., Prinz, P.N., Williams, D.E. *et al.* (1990). Sleep disturbances in patients with mild-stage Alzheimer's disease. *Journal of Gerontology*, **45**, M131–8.

Ware, C.J.G., Fairburn, C.G. and Hope, R.A. (1990). A community-based study of aggressive behaviour in dementia. *International Journal of Geriatric Psychiatry*, **5**, 337–42.

Yudofsky, S.C., Silver, J.M., Jackson, W. *et al.* (1986). The Overt Aggression Scale for the objective rating of verbal and physical aggression. *American Journal of Psychiatry*, **143**, 35–9.

Zarit, S.H., Orr, N.K. and Zarit, J.M. (1985). *The Hidden Victims of Alzheimer's Disease; Families Under Stress.* New York University Press, New York.

Zeiss, A.M., Davies, H.D., Wood, M. and Tinklenberg, J.R. (1990). The incidence and correlates of erectile problems in patients with Alzheimer's disease. *Archives of Sexual Behaviour*, **19**, 325–31.

Joanna Moriarty

and

Enid Levin

National Institute for Social Work Research Unit

12 SERVICES TO PEOPLE WITH DEMENTIA AND THEIR CARERS

INTRODUCTION

Earlier chapters have focussed upon the diagnosis and clinical description of dementia. In this chapter we turn to the way in which services deal with its impact upon everyday lives. Some are targetted exclusively upon people with dementia, others provide help to the elderly population as a whole. In order to give an impression of their range and style, we have adopted a broad brush approach. In deciding whether to lay the emphasis upon residential or community services, we were guided by the fact that from the time of onset, even if a person with dementia ultimately enters residential care, he or she will have spent time in the community. The central premise of this chapter is that the nature of dementia requires services to be wide-ranging, comprehensive and complementary.

THE RELATIONSHIP BETWEEN FAMILY CARE AND SERVICES

Within the literature, a key distinction is often made between *formal* services and those provided *informally** by family, friends and neighbours. In the USA, families have been estimated to provide 80–90% of medically related and personal care, household tasks, transport and shopping for the frail elderly (Brody, 1985). Studies elsewhere (Midre and Synak, 1989; Henrard, 1991) have suggested that even in Northern European countries where government programmes of housing, domiciliary and residential care are comparatively well developed, the role of family and friends has remained crucial.

Help from family and friends is often used as a portmanteau term covering anything from doing the shopping each week to the 24-hour care of a profoundly disabled person. The majority of studies have shown that, where the second sort of help is required, it is nearly always provided by spouses and children, and by one person in particular (Sinclair *et al.*, 1990).

One study supporting this picture is that of Penning and Chappell (1990) who examined the relationships between self-care, informal and formal care in a sample of 743 noninstitutionalized elderly Canadians. They argued that functional disability (such as difficulty in dressing, bathing and shopping) and

---

*While rejecting the term 'informal' carer as inappropriate and inaccurate, the distinction between formal and informal care is used here merely to clarify the distinction between care provided by statutory, voluntary, not for profit and privately arranged services and sources of help from within the network of family and friends.

the availability of support through the marital relationship were the strongest correlates of informal care.

The juxtaposition of care by family and friends with services is less clear because few studies have examined their joint use. Chappell and Blandford (1991) suggested that, although two basic models have been proposed, neither has been shown to be entirely satisfactory.

The first centres around *complementarity*. Litwak (1985) argued that there was a division of tasks between those best performed by primary groups (the household, wider family, friends and neighbourhood) and those most suited to formal organizations. George (1987) argued that tasks were not so much divided as shared: the formal system entered when the person cared for was so deteriorated that the informal system required assistance or where elements of the informal system were missing.

The second suggest that formal services *substitute* for informal services and are used only as a last resort (Cantor, 1985).

Chappell and Blandford themselves studied a stratified random sample of 1826 Canadians over the age of 60 years living in the community. Some received formal or informal assistance, either jointly or separately, others did not. They concluded that the formal care system stepped in both when health deteriorated sufficiently and when elements of the informal network were not available. The formal system almost never provided care by itself to elderly people in the community.

THE EXTENT OF SERVICE USE BY PEOPLE WITH DEMENTIA

There are a growing number of studies suggesting that the global impairment characteristic of the dementia syndrome and the likelihood of progressive deterioration mean help from both informal and formal sources is likely to be required. One example is that of Coyne *et al.* (1990). Among 242 referrals living in New Jersey with a diagnosis of Alzheimer's disease or a related disorder, they found that increased age and decreased self-care abilities were minimally, but significantly, related to the greater use of community services. However, even among a group likely to be using formal services, uptake was still limited.

Livingston *et al.* (1990a) also noted that people with dementia were likely to have higher levels of contact with services. Every household in an area of inner city London was visited in order to establish prevalence rates for dementia and depression (Livingston *et al.*, 1990b). The sample consisted of 705 people, 35 of whom were identified as having dementia by using the well-validated Short Comprehensive Assessment and Referral Evaluation (Short-CARE) interview schedule (Gurland *et al.*, 1984).

The authors categorized community services into six types: contact with a general practitioner, hospital visits, district nurses and health visitors, home helps, day centres, meals on wheels and other home-based services (included together). Only 5% of the total sample received four or more services. In the month preceding the interview, people with dementia were more likely to have greater contact with services provided by the local authority than the rest of the sample for whom general practitioners were the most usual source of contact. However, the study noted that home help and meals on wheels services were provided at a rate twice that of the national average.

PRINCIPLES UNDERLYING SERVICE DELIVERY

The shift in emphasis by successive governments in the UK in favour of transferring care from institutional to community settings is well known and has been described with clarity and concision by Bebbington and Charnley (1990). Before the 1980s, the dominant paradigm of social welfare for elderly people was the *continuum of care*, by which increasing disability was matched by a progression from domiciliary care to residential and then geriatric care. Now, services were to be directed at people requiring intensive support if they were not to be taken into long-term care. These ideas culminated in the government's White Paper *Caring for People* (1989) and the *National Health Service and Community Care Act* 1990.

Community care has been seen as a valid recognition of the right of people with dementia to live as independently as possible in familiar surroundings. It has also been seen as a mechanism for taking into account the projected rise in the numbers of the very elderly within the population. Some authors have argued that these developments have been influenced by the ideology of the 'New Right' (Jack, 1991) which opposes a dependency culture which it was felt resulted from universalist policies.

Such changes are not confined to the UK. One study in Australia of people with dementia (Brodaty and Gresham, 1989) aimed to reduce distress and the rate of placements in institutions by improving the quality of life for patients and carers. Similarly a Californian study (Lieberman and Kramer, 1991) sought to enhance the coping skills of families of people with dementia, pointing out that developing in-home care was an 'affordable alternative to institutionalization'.

APPROACHES TO COMMUNITY CARE

One of the best known approaches in the UK has been the Kent Community Care Scheme (Challis and Davies, 1986) which has now been replicated in other areas and with different client groups (Challis *et al.*, 1988, 1989). Under these schemes, case managers were allocated budgets, equivalent to two-thirds of the cost of residential care, with which to provide services for frail elderly people at home or about to be discharged home from long-term hospital care. Services were arranged through a variety of sources, hence the terms *welfare pluralism*, or *the mixed economy of welfare*. *Caring for People* (1989) acknowledged the value of this approach as an effective method of targetting resources and planning services.

The theoretical impetus behind this model originated in the USA, where case management was seen as an effective way of coordinating complex mixes of services. Official documents now use the term *care* management, as *case* was felt to imply that it was an individual who was being managed, not his or her care (SSI/SWSG, 1991).

The essential principles revolve around:

>   Case finding
>   Assessment
>   Care planning
>   Service arrangement
>   Monitoring

This is a cyclical process in which needs are assessed, services are delivered in response, and needs are reassessed. The care manager is not only an arranger of services but is in a position to evaluate their effectiveness.

Any professional will be faced with a quandary if the options he or she suggests are not accepted by the person with dementia. It has been argued (Fisher, 1990/1991) that care managers will have particular problems in securing agreement for their actions and, within a consumerist philosophy, intervening for the client's protection. Doubtless these issues will be addressed following completion of the evaluation of the Lewisham Case Management Scheme by the Personal Social Services Research Unit at the University of Kent. This study seeks to compare two matched groups of people with dementia, the first in receipt of standard services, the second with a care manager.

More conventional models of service delivery have been the focus of other studies. Among these is earlier work carried out within the National Institute for Social Work Research Unit (Levin et al., 1989). One hundred and fifty elderly people from three study areas were identified as 'confused' by professionals such as general practitioners, nurses, social workers and home helps. Full assessments carried out by two psychiatrists suggested that of the 150 almost 80% showed evidence of dementia. As well as assessing the elderly people, their carers were also interviewed. Both elderly people and carers were followed up 1 year later. One of the central findings was to question the ability of any single service to meet the complex health and social needs of a person with dementia. It was suggested that there were 10 key requirements for services which centred around early identification, comprehensive assessments, treatment and review, information and counselling, help with practical household and personal care tasks, services which gave carers the opportunity for a break, such as day care, financial support and, if desired, access to permanent residential care.

Based in Cambridge, the Hughes Hall Project for Later Life chose not only to establish prevalence rates and examine the course of dementia, but also to take an experimental approach to see whether it was possible to enable people to remain at home for longer through the provision of help from a newly established multidisciplinary resource team. They argued that the group who would benefit most from intensive community services were those wishing to continue to care for severely demented people (O'Connor et al., 1990).

Coming somewhere between innovatory and standard models of service provision has been the development of a programme of Quadruple Support to people with dementia (Lodge and McReynolds, 1984). Central to this process was the setting up of a multidisciplinary community dementia team, consisting of representatives from health and social services and voluntary organizations. Other components were monitoring through volunteer visits, a support group for carers and day care. Generic services, such as community nurses, home helps and meals on wheels were required. 'Alternative' residential care involving housing associations, health and social services and voluntary organizations were also needed (Lodge and McReynolds, 1990).

Our recent study of respite services for carers living with confused elderly people (Levin et al., 1992) compared services in three areas. In Area One, the psychogeriatric service was the lead agency for services with people with dementia. The psychogeriatricians favoured domiciliary visits and had a high level of coverage. The community psychiatric nurses played the main role in monitoring, arranging and coordinating services. The service in Area Two was, at the time of the study, headed by a social worker and included people employed by the health authority, social services department and workers from voluntary organizations. Each team member took a broadly common perspective but varying approaches and skills could be incorporated into each referral's plan of care. The psychogeriatric service in Area Three was based in a district general hospital. Strong emphasis was placed on thorough, multi-professional assessment and diagnosis. Close cooperation meant that the longer term care of elderly people with dementia tended to pass to the local social services department.

Thus, while each team was committed to multiprofessional assessment, to a community-based approach and support for carers, as well as for the elderly people themselves, there were differences. One factor remained constant: the central role of the elderly person's general practitioner. This was the key source of referral to specialists and a means of regular monitoring.

OVERLAPPING OR COMMON APPROACHES?

Psychogeriatricians and social workers both have responsibilities for assessing the person with dementia and arranging for services. In recent years they have been joined by increasing numbers of community psychiatric nurses. *Caring for People* (1989) made it clear that social workers, community nurses and home help organizers are all suitable as care managers. Each of these professionals may work from divergent standpoints. At the same time, when more than one is involved in the care of a person with dementia, there are bound to be issues of overlap (Marshall, 1990). An interesting solution to this issue has been that of Jones *et al.* (1992) who advocated the establishment of a core curriculum for all professionals working with people with dementia.

COMMUNITY NURSING AND HOME CARE

The tasks of assessment and arranging access to services are clearly integral to providing a successful service to elderly people with dementia, but they must be provided in conjunction with practical services on a day-to-day basis.

In the UK, the contribution in numerical terms alone of domiciliary services, such as home helps, meals on wheels and community nurses, to people with dementia cannot be overestimated. However, it has been argued that a concentration on those living alone has been at the expense of those with carers.

Community nursing services include within their wider remit help with daily living activities relating to personal care. Traditionally, home help services have concentrated on domestic tasks. In recent years, there has been criticism that demarcations of this sort may encourage artificially created divisions. In recognition of the need to acknowledge the wider needs of clients and to provide an alternative to long-term residential care, some local authorities have redesignated home help services home *care* services (Sinclair *et al.*, 1990). Where a distinction has been made between home care and home help services (Barton *et al.*, 1990), home care clients were more incapacitated.

Although some sheltered housing schemes provide help for people with dementia, this is too broad-based a service to be given the attention it merits in the space available here.

OTHER HOME-BASED CARE

The need for other home-based services has also been felt to be important. These can range from providing companionship to taking on a considerable physical workload. The focus may be minimizing risk for people with dementia living on their own (Pearson, 1992), or assisting, or taking over from, the carer (Thornton, 1989). In the UK, Crossroads Care Attendant Schemes are used widely across the country, but not all schemes cover people with dementia. Our own study (Levin et al., 1992) suggested that this type of service had yet to be part of mainstream provision and was patchily available. Only a third of the elderly people overall had a sitter/carers' support worker and the amount of time allocated was limited. More positively, people with varying severity of dementia were using the service. It was seen as a way of introducing services to people who were newly diagnosed and of enabling people who were severely cognitively impaired to be left safely at home while their carer was out.

DAY CARE

In Northern European countries and the USA, day care has been seen as one of the major services for people with dementia. In her review, Tester (1989) suggested that its rapid growth in the UK had outpaced a proper evaluation of its effectiveness. Theoretically, day *hospitals* assign more importance to assessment and therapeutic interventions than day *centres* where the social aspect of the service is emphasized. She supported a distinction being made between *day care*, a service offering:

> communal care, with paid or voluntary care givers present, in a setting outside the user's own home . . . available for at least four hours during the day . . .

and *day facilities*, which should provide company, educational and leisure services.

In the UK and the Netherlands, it has been estimated that 86% of people attending psychogeriatric day hospitals have a diagnosis of dementia. Comparable figures are unavailable for day centres, but the numbers of those with dementia are increasing (Nies et al., 1991).

In our sample, 70% of the elderly people attended some form of day care. It was, after consultations with general practitioners and psychogeriatricians, the single most frequently used service (Levin et al., 1992). However, this figure must partly be attributed to the type of sample, consisting of people already in contact with services.

One model projecting day care as the major service for people with dementia is that of Gilleard (1992). He proposed that psychogeriatric day units should assume the central role within community psychogeriatric services, offering specialized therapeutic services as well as respite (in the narrower sense of overnight, institutional) care, education and support for carers.

In contrast to this model, some models for day care provision have favoured smaller scale operations whereby three or four people with dementia attend day care in the day carers' own homes and the focus is on social interaction and a home-like atmosphere, rather than a structured programme (Burningham, 1991). Such schemes are recent developments and, as yet, no comparisons between this and more conventional service styles have been evaluated.

RELIEF CARE

Neither home-based nor day care generally offer carers of people with dementia a break of at least 24 hours – an idea increasingly seen as a *raison d'être* for providing short-term admissions (Allen, 1983). The variety of different terms describing such a service – rotating, intermittent, relief and respite care – bear witness to the differing purposes and attitudes underlying provision of the service. Compared with day and home-based breaks, a certain amount of ambivalence exists about the purpose but it is essentially an intermediate service, half-way between care entirely within community settings and long-term residential care.

In our study (Levin et al., 1992), whatever the theoretical aim behind the service, so far as the carers were concerned, they were heavily reliant upon it if they were to be able to go on holiday, redecorate, convalesce following illness, or just relax at home for a while. Two-thirds of the 287 carers had used relief care at least once; half of these used it regularly with a minimum of one break every 3 months. By contrast, just 10% of those without relief care could remember an occasion in the previous year when another family member or friend had taken over their caring responsibilities for longer than 24 consecutive hours.

Relief care in institutions has been the subject of varying degrees of criticism. (See Twigg et al., 1990, for some examples.) First developed in Scandinavia, in recent years efforts have been made in the UK to set up schemes providing short-term care for elderly or disabled people in a normal family environment (Robinson, 1991). These are, at the time of writing, not widely available to people with dementia and our own study (Levin et al., 1992) certainly suggested that its users were less dependent. People with severe dementia were given relief care in hospitals or local authority homes.

Some services have tried to provide home-based care for longer periods (Thornton, 1989). Even more rare are agencies arranging holiday breaks for people with dementia, either with or without their carer (Micklewood, 1991).

RESIDENTIAL CARE

The seminal work in Newcastle (Kay et al., 1964) showed that more people with dementia lived in the community than in institutions. At the same time, the concentration of people with dementia in long-term residential care is high. Sixty per cent of residents in US nursing homes have Alzheimer's disease (Brody et al., 1989). Gilleard (1992) cited studies from Australia, Sweden and England all suggesting that high proportions of people with moderate or severe dementia were in some form of residential care. Even in Japan, where the majority of people with dementia are looked after at home, the projected rapid rise in the numbers of the elderly, a decrease in three generational households and change in the ratio of women in paid employment to the elderly with dementia, has seen calls for a rise in the currently limited availability of continuing residential care (Ogawa, 1989).

Gilleard (1992) made it clear that we must answer the question of whether the thrust of services for people with dementia is to be on community or residential settings by first taking into account the fact that, aside from issues of prevalence, the number of people with dementia in the community is, to a large extent, dependent upon the rate of institutionalization of the elderly. This can be inferred by comparing the Netherlands, where until recently much of the expenditure on services for the elderly went into nursing homes and as many as 10% of the elderly as a whole were in residential care, with the UK where the comparable figure is 4% (Nies et al., 1991).

Discussion on the provision of long-term residential care would be incomplete without raising the issue of its quality. Using observational techniques, higher rates of activity and staff contact were found in a unit run according to the domus philosophy, which aims to maintain residents' independence and residual capacities (Lindesay et al., 1991), and in NHS nursing homes (Clark and Bowling, 1989), than in traditional continuing care hospital wards.

The question of the levels of provision of residential care and its quality have been closely interlinked with the pressure on containing the costs of residential care. In the UK, where through income support the social security budget had funded almost 60% of elderly people living in private or voluntary residential and nursing homes, expenditure has risen from £10 in 1979 to £1.2 billion in 1990 (Oldman, 1991). One of the principles of the *NHS and Community Care Act* was to try and reduce what has been described as this 'perverse incentive' to enter residential care. Although alternative funding arrangements, such as insurance for long-term care, are beginning to be offered, Oldman noted that experience in the USA, Germany, France and Japan showed that such schemes have limited success. Where people meet the costs of their care directly, the sums required can absorb all their financial resources. This is termed 'spend down'. In the USA Liu and Manton (1989) are among those who have shown that people in nursing homes are more likely to spend down to the point where they reach Medicaid eligibility.

Even where community services can provide alternatives and the reluctance on the part of some elderly people and their carers to enter residential care is strong, it will always remain a necessary alternative for some. As part of this debate, Foster (1991) has argued that we must accept good residential provision as an integral part of care in the community. She proposed a model of shared care where family-based and residential care need not be mutually exclusive and family members can continue to play a part in caring after the elderly person's entry to residential care.

EFFECTIVENESS OF SERVICES

Any study of services will have been influenced, even constrained, by issues such as time available, purpose and intended audience. The topic is made more complex by the fact that there is no single, ideal method of studying services' effectiveness; each has its advantages and disadvantages. Indeed, a study's usefulness is enhanced if it is able to incorporate more than one approach.

Studies of effectiveness will also be influenced to some extent by sampling. Those reliant upon samples recruited through advertising or local contacts may not necessarily be representative of all those using services. Random community samples may be more representative but are also likely to contain higher numbers of people neither wishing for, not in receipt of, any other services.

Before considering how services may be assessed, it should be noted that there are an increasing number of studies which seek to measure the effectiveness of services by examining their impact upon the mental health of carers. This is, however, more properly the concern of the following chapter.

Consumer views

In a heterogeneous group, such as carers, opinions may differ. For instance, nonresident children may have different needs and expectations from spouses. This should be acknowledged when using carers' opinions to define the need for services.

Carers' views have often been sought by groups supporting or advocating the needs of carers. In these cases, as in Wyn Thomas (1990), disadvantages, such as the small size of the sample or monitoring views at one point only, must be set against the quality of responses and the accessible way in which they are reported.

A tendency of these studies is that, in the absence of any other means of evaluating a service, they result in very high levels of global satisfaction and an inability to show clear distinctions between the 'good' and the 'less good'. One interesting way of incorporating satisfaction measures was described by Ehrlich and White (1991) where carers' views incorporated into the quality assurance programme of a scheme offering day and home-based care to people with Alzheimer's disease.

Insofar as people with dementia are concerned, it has been argued that an increasing number of studies chart the views of *carers*, but few have sought the views of those *receiving* care (Barer and Johnson, 1990). Naturally, people with dementia will have especial problems in giving views on services but we found (Levin *et al.*, 1992) that where specific details were lacking, the response to atmosphere sometimes remained.

Uptake of services

A perplexing picture for those involved in examining services is that, while on the one hand there are many studies suggesting that services are appreciated and may be underprovided, on the other, take up may be low.

Pollitt *et al.* (1989) reported on interviews with 34 mildly demented Cambridge residents and their carers. They attributed low take up of services to carers' ability to manage without assistance, desire for independence and reluctance to admit to needing help. More importantly, some carers saw their relatives' condition as consistent with normal ageing. Pollitt *et al.* argued that until carers made the 'conceptual leap' leap from seeing the condition of the person with dementia as normal to abnormal, it was difficult to offer services designed to prevent the build up of crises.

Montgomery and Borgatta (1989) assigned 541 elderly people to one of five treatment groups or one control group. Almost 60% were so impaired as to be unable to be interviewed. Within 1 year, a quarter were dead – a measure, the authors suggested, of just how late in their 'caring career' families had come forward. Given families' independence and disinclination to use services, the authors concluded that, unless people with dementia are located early enough, it will be hard to demonstrate the effectiveness of any preventative services.

These studies both suggest that take up levels cannot be used in isolation as a measure to demonstrate effectiveness. The characteristics of those to whom services are offered must be taken into account, as should factors such as household composition, carer's age, health and socioeconomic status. In addition Coyne (1991) has suggested that the dissemination of information *about* services to carers is an important aspect of take up, because it plays a part in subsequent service use.

Services as part of a package

An evaluation of the worth of specific services must take into account the wider context of other forms of provision. In our study, the most frequent package of respite was day and relief care (Levin *et al.*, 1992). Only in one area was day, home-based and relief care more readily available. Those without relief care were generally less dependent. Other nonrespite services such as community nurses, carers' groups and so on were also used. While services were offered in standard packages, with little help at the weekends, the carers in our sample were heavily reliant upon services and reported that help from other family members was essentially supportive, rather than directly taking over care of the elderly person.

Costs of services

One way in which comparisons between services can be made is by the incorporation of costings. Wimo *et al.* (1990) used cost–utility analyses to compare patients attending a psychogeriatric day centre with those in residential care. They concluded that, while the costs of institutional care were reduced, this was offset by increased costs for day and home care. However, when the patients' well being was taken into account, day care was a cost-effective service.

The effects of services on outcome

As was suggested earlier, the question which seems to have assumed key importance is whether services can be shown to prevent or reduce rates of institutionalization.

The work of Challis and Davies (1986) and Challis *et al.* (1988) suggested that the needs of frail elderly people were met more effectively through case managers (the term still used by the scheme) able to provide a range and style of service which differed from existing provision. This was indicated by the number of people remaining at home, their carers' greater well being and the scheme's cost effectiveness.

Taking this work as its model but dealing specifically with dementia, the Home Support Scheme (Askham and Thompson, 1990) compared two groups, one in receipt of standard services, the other receiving enhanced home support. With a degree of circumspection due to the small size of the sample, the authors suggested that, although across the sample as a whole a home support scheme was no more effective than existing provision in enabling people to remain at home, this type of service *did* seem to be helpful for people without carers who were not yet at a level requiring 24-hour supervision.

A number of studies have provided a tentatively optimistic picture in relation to the provision of respite services for carers as a means of delaying institutionalization. Carers recruited to the Philadelphia Geriatric Center Respite Demonstration Program (Lawton *et al.*, 1989) were offered institutional or in-home respite, day care, or a combination of services. Over a year, families with respite care had maintained their relative at home for a significantly longer period (22 days). Similarly, Montgomery and Borgatta (1989) reported that families receiving respite and carer education separately or together delayed the use of nursing home placements. People whose families used a package of respite care and education and support provided by the Family Support Unit in Middlesborough survived significantly longer in the community (Donaldson *et al.*, 1988).

Whatever the services which are offered, entry to continuing residential care will also be influenced by the characteristics of the person with dementia and his or her carer. As the issue of carer stress is to be covered in the following chapter, it will suffice here to comment that this has been shown to play a role in predicting admission to permanent residential care (Levin *et al.*, 1989; Leiberman and Kramer, 1991). Some studies have suggested that the cognitive or behavioural characteristics of the person with dementia influence outcome. Knopman *et al.* (1988) suggested severity of dementia, impaired communication skills, incontinence, poor hygiene and irritability were frequent precursors to admission.

The study by Levin *et al.* (1992) dealt with a group of elderly people already on the margins of residential care, as illustrated by their scores on the Behavioural Rating Scale of the Clifton Assessment Procedures for the Elderly (Pattie and Gilleard, 1979). The mean score on follow-up came into the category taken to indicate severe impairment, at a dependency level commonly found in continuing care hospital wards or nursing homes. The three study areas had different styles and levels of service provision but this did not affect outcome 1 year later. Thirty-three per cent had died, 19% were in permanent residential care but almost 50% were still at home. As in previous work (Levin *et al.*, 1989), while relief care was predictive of institutionalization, given that this service was used by the more dependent elderly people, it is notable that two-thirds of those using relief care at first interview were still at home.

The number of elderly people whose care had died or had entered residential care themselves was small ($n = 21$) but it is worth noting that, of these, only one elderly person remained in the community. To return to an earlier theme in the chapter, if people with severe dementia are to be cared for successfully in community settings, formal services must operate jointly with help from their carers, a point accorded high priority in *Caring for People* (1989).

CLOSING NOTE

The nature of dementia is such that the support of a range of services is required. These need to take account not only the consequences of cognitive deficits, the presence of noncognitive phenomena, such as behavioural problems or psychiatric symptoms, but also wider issues, such as personal preferences or how the service can fit in with help from other sources. People with dementia have been shown to be heavier users of services and service providers need to ensure that both specialist and generic services take this into account. Over time, the needs of a person with dementia will increase. Services felt to be unsuitable in the early stages may become useful, which is where providing information about services to families will prove its value. As dementia increases in its severity, so too does the likelihood of entry to long-term residential care. Therefore, services must seek to provide residential and community services in tandem. There is no doubt that many elderly people and their families neither wish for, nor feel the need to accept, services. There is equally no doubt that a growing body of research shows that, in the absence of help from formal services, some families are placed under unacceptable levels of strain and difficulty. It is not enough to examine services in terms of outcome for people with dementia if other factors, such as their well being, or that of their carers are ignored. Over the next few years, if the challenge for services lies in providing a 'seamless service' incorporating sources of help from the statutory, voluntary and private sector, it also requires a service which is seamless within itself, where rigid barriers between home-based care and care away from home are dismantled and the guiding principles are the needs of people with dementia and their carers.

REFERENCES

Allen, I. (1983). *Short Stay Residential Care for the Elderly*. Policy Studies Institute, London.

Askham, J. and Thompson, C. (1990). *Dementia and Home Care: A Research Report on a Home Support Scheme for Dementia Sufferers*. Age Concern, Mitcham.

Barer, B. and Johnson, C. (1990). A critique of the caregiving literature. *The Gerontologist*, **30**, 26–9.

Barton, A., Coles, O., Stone, M. *et al.* (1990). Home help and home care for the frail elderly: face to face in Darlington. *Research, Policy and Planning*, **8**, 7–13.

Bebbington, A. and Charnley, H. (1990). Community care for the elderly – rhetoric and reality. *British Journal of Social Work*, **20**, 409–32.

Brodaty, H. and Gresham, M. (1989). Effect of a training programme to reduce stress in carers of patients with dementia. *British Medical Journal*, **299**, 1375–9.

Brody, E. (1985). Parent care as a normative family stress. *The Gerontologist*, **25**, 19–29.

Brody, E., Saperstein, A. and Lawton, M. (1989). A multi-service respite program for caregivers of Alzheimer's patients. *Journal of Gerontological Social Work*, **14**, 41–74.

Burningham, S. (1991). Homeshare daycare. *Alzheimer's Disease Society Newsletter*, 10 October.

Cantor, M. (1985). Ageing and social care. In *Handbook of Ageing and the Social Sciences*, Binstock, R. and Shanas, E. (Eds), 2nd edition, pp. 745–81. Van Nostrand Reinhold Company, New York.

Challis, D., Chessum, R., Luckett, R. and Woods, R. (1988). Community care for the frail elderly: an urban experiment. *British Journal of Social Work*, **18** (Suppl.), 13–42.

Challis, D., Darton, R., Johnson, L. *et al.* (1989). *Supporting Frail Elderly People at Home: The Darlington Community Care Scheme*. Personal Social Services Research Unit, University of Kent, Canterbury.

Challis, D. and Davies, B. (1986). *Case Management in Community Care*. Gower, Aldershot.

Chappell, N. and Blandford, A. (1991). Informal and formal care: exploring the complementarity. *Ageing and Society*, **11**, 299–317.

Clark, P. and Bowling, A. (1989). Observational study of quality of life in NHS nursing homes and a long stay ward for the elderly. *Ageing and Society*, **9**, 123–48.

Coyne, A. (1991). Information and referral service usage among caregivers for dementia patients. *The Gerontologist*, **31**, 384–8.

Coyne, A., Meade, H., Petrone, M. *et al.* (1990). The diagnosis of dementia: demographic characteristics. *The Gerontologist*, **30**, 339–44.

Department of Health (1989). *Caring for People: Community Care in the Next Decade and Beyond*, CM 849. HMSO, London.

Donaldson, C., Clark, K., Gregson, B. *et al.* (1988). *Evaluation of a Family Support Unit for Elderly Mentally Infirm People and their Carers*. Health Care Research Unit, Report 34, Newcastle.

Ehrlich, P. and White, J. (1991). TOPS: A consumer approach to Alzheimer's respite programs. *The Gerontologist*, **31**, 686–91.

Fisher, M. (1990/91). Defining the practice content of care management. *Social Work and Social Sciences Review*, **2**, 204–30.

Foster, P. (1991). Residential care of frail elderly people: a positive reassessment. *Social Policy and Administration*, **25**, 108–20.

George, L. (1987). Easing caregiver burden: the role of informal and formal supports. In *Health in Ageing: Sociological Issues and Policy Directions*, Ward, R. and Tobin, S. (Eds), pp. 133–58. Springer, New York.

Gilleard, C. (1992). Community care services for the elderly mentally ill. In

Care-giving in Dementia: Research and Applications, Jones, G. and Miesen, B. (Eds). Routledge, London.

Gurland, B., Golden, R., Teresi, J. and Challop, J. (1984). The Short-CARE: an efficient instrument for the assessment of depression, dementia and disability. *Journal of Gerontology*, **39**, 166–9.

Henrard, J. (1991). Care for elderly people in the European Community. *Social Policy and Administration*, **25**, 184–92.

Jack, R. (1991). Social services and the ageing population. *Social Policy and Administration,* **25**, 284–99.

Jones, G., Ely, S. and Miesen, B. (1992). The need for an interdisciplinary core curriculum for professionals working with dementia. In *Care-giving in Dementia: Research and Applications*, Jones, G. and Miesen, B. (Eds). Routledge, London.

Kay, D., Beamish, P. and Roth, M. (1964). Old age mental disorders in Newcastle upon Tyne. Part 1. A study of prevalence. *British Journal of Psychiatry*, **110**, 146–58.

Knopman, D., Kitto, J., Deinard, S. and Heiring, J. (1988). Longitudinal study of death and institutionalization in patients with primary degenerative dementia. *Journal of the American Geriatric Society*, **36**, 108–12.

Lawton, M., Brody, E. and Saperstein, A. (1989). A controlled study of respite service for caregivers of Alzheimer's patients. *The Gerontologist*, **29**, 8–16.

Levin, E., Moriarty, J. and Gorbach, P. (1992). *'I Couldn't Manage Without the Breaks': Respite Services for the Carers of Confused Elderly People*, draft report to the Department of Health. National Institute for Social Work, London.

Levin, E., Sinclair, I. and Gorbach, P. (1989). *Families, Services and Confusion in Old Age*. Gower, Aldershot.

Lieberman, M. and Kramer, J. (1991) Factors affecting decisions to institutionalize demented elderly. *The Gerontologist*, **31**, 371–4.

Lindesay, J., Briggs, K., Lawes, M. *et al.* (1991). The domus philosophy: a comparative evaluation of a new approach to residential care for the demented elderly. *International Journal of Geriatric Psychiatry*, **6**, 727–36.

Litwak, E. (1985). *Helping the Elderly: The Complementary Roles of Informal Networks and Formal Systems*. Guilford Press, New York.

Liu, K. and Manton, K. (1989). The effect of nursing home use on Medicaid eligibility. *The Gerontologist*, **29**, 59–66.

Livingston, G., Thomas, A., Graham, N. *et al.* (1990a). The Gospel Oak Project: the use of health and social services by dependent elderly people in the community. *Health Trends*, **22**, 70–3.

Livingston, G., Hawkins, A., Graham, N. *et al.* (1990b). The Gospel Oak study: prevalence rates of dementia, depression and activity limitation among elderly residents in inner London. *Psychological Medicine*, **20**, 137–46.

Lodge, B. and McReynolds, S. (1990). *The Use of Multidisciplinary Assessment by the Community Dementia Team*, 2nd edition. Scottish Action on Dementia, Edinburgh.

Lodge, B. and McReynolds, S. (1984). *Quadruple Support for Dementia*. Age Concern, Leicestershire.

Marshall, M. (1990). *Working with Dementia: Guidelines for Professionals*. Venture Press, Birmingham.

Micklewood, P. (1991). *Caring for Confusion*. Scutari Press, London.

Midre, G. and Synak, B. (1989). Between family and state: ageing in Poland and Norway. *Ageing and Society*, **9**, 241–59.

Montgomery, R. and Borgatta, E. (1989). The effects of alternative support strategies on family caregiving. *The Gerontologist*, **29**, 457–64.

National Health Service and Community Care Act 1990 (CP 19) HMSO, London.

Nies, H., Tester, S. and Nuijens, J. (1991). Day care in the United Kingdom and the Netherlands: a comparative study. *Ageing and Society*, **11**, 245–73.

O'Connor, D., Pollit, P., Roth, M. *et al.* (1990). Problems reported by relatives in a community study of dementia. *British Journal of Psychiatry*, **156**, 835–41.

Ogawa, N. (1989). Population ageing and its impact upon health resource requirements at government and familial levels in Japan. *Ageing and Society*, **9**, 383–405.

Oldman, C. (1991). *Paying for Care: Personal Sources of Funding Care*. Joseph Rowntree Foundation, York.

Pattie, A. and Gilleard, C. (1979). *Manual of the Clifton Assessment Procedures for the Elderly*. Hodder and Stoughton, Kent.

Pearson, C. (1992). Overnight Success. *Social Work Today*, **23**, 21.

Penning, M. and Chappell, N. (1990). Self-care in relation to formal and informal care. *Ageing and Society*, **10**, 41–59.

Pollitt, P., O'Connor, D. and Anderson, I. (1989). Mild dementia: perceptions and problems. *Ageing and Society*, **9**, 261–75.

Robinson, C. (1991). *Home and Away: Respite Care in the Community*. Venture Press, Birmingham.

Sinclair, I., Parker, R., Leat, D. and Williams, J. (1990). *The Kaleidoscope of Care*. HMSO, London.

Social Services Inspectorate/Scottish Office Social Work Service Group (1991). *Care Management and Assessment: Summary of Practice Guidance*. HMSO, London.

Tester, S. (1989). *Caring by Day: A Study of Day Care Services for Older People*. Centre for Policy on Ageing, London.

Thornton, P. (1989). *Creating a Break: A Home Care Relief Scheme for Elderly People and their Supporters*. Age Concern, Mitcham.

Twigg, J., Atkin, K. and Perring, C. (1990). *Carers and Services: A Review of Research*. HMSO, London.

Wimo, A., Wallin, J., Lungren, K. *et al.* (1990). Impact of day care on dementia patients – costs, wellbeing and relatives' views. *Family Practice*, **7**, 279–86.

Wyn Thomas, B. (1990). *Consulting Consumers in the NHS: A Guideline Study: Services for Elderly People with Dementia Living at Home*. National Consumer Council, London.

Robin G. Morris

and

Lorna W. Morris

Institute of Psychiatry
London

13 PSYCHOSOCIAL ASPECTS OF CARING FOR PEOPLE WITH DEMENTIA: CONCEPTUAL AND METHODOLOGICAL ISSUES

INTRODUCTION

The majority of people with dementia live in the community and are cared for by relatives or friends, some of whom are themselves elderly and suffer from physical disabilities (Morris *et al.*, 1993). For want of better terminology, the term 'carer' or 'informal carer' has been applied in this context to denote somcone who takes on the principal role of looking after the needs of a person with dementia in the community. These informal carers thus make up the bulk of people who come into contact with dementia sufferers and, although many people willingly take on this role, it has been recognized increasingly that the social impact of dementia operates at this level. Recognition of this fact has led to the setting up of formal and voluntary organizations, such as the Alzheimer's Disease Society, whose prime role is to support the work of informal carers.

The argument for professional people focussing on the carer has always had a pragmatic element as well as a philosophical one. Clinicians have reorientated their approaches to mobilize and maintain the effectiveness of informal support systems with the aim of maintaining a person with dementia at home. For example, there is evidence that maintenance of a person with dementia in the community is closely related to the degree of family support (Bergmann *et al.*, 1978; Poulshock and Deimling, 1984), and that facilities such as day care and formal training programmes for carers can reduce the immediate need for institutionalization (Gilleard *et al.*, 1984; Brodarty and Gresham, 1989). However, this approach is not without cost for the informal carer. Much of the research into the experiences of carers has rightly adopted the notion of *objective* and *subjective* burden after the seminal work of Grad and Sainsbury (1965) in following the desegregation of elderly psychiatric patients into the community in the 1960s. Although informal carers may not necessarily see it in these terms, the objective burden refers to the practical problems associated with caregiving such as continuous nursing care and interference with the carers everyday routine and freedom. In addition, a negative aspect of caregiving is the restriction of social activities and consequent social isolation (Poulshock and Deimling, 1984). In contrast subjective burden, which in some cases is the most acute, refers to the emotional reaction of the carer including reduced morale, anxiety and depression (R.G. Morris *et al.*, 1988). For example, an informal carer may simultaneously have to cope with the physical burden of

* The writing of the chapter was supported in part by a grant from the Alzheimer's Disease Society (UK) to Dr Robin G. Morris.

having constantly to supervise someone who is at risk of leaving the house and becoming lost and the grief associated with the mental deterioration of their relative. Both subjective and objective burden can in turn be related to the well being of the carer, expressed in terms of such factors as quality of life, physical health and emotional well being (Haley et al., 1987b; Pruchno and Resch, 1989).

The concept of 'role' in caregiving is an important one, and to some extent is defined by society and the expectations placed on the carer. Several studies report that the manner in which the caregiver responds to their situation depends largely on the familial relationship (Cantor, 1983). For example, the degree of depression and strain associated with caregiving has been found to be related to the 'distance' in the blood/role relationship; the less the familial distance, the worse the mental health of the carer (Cantor, 1983; Gilhooly, 1984; George and Gwyther, 1986). This finding can easily be explained in terms of the amount of emotional and practical involvement with caregiving, particularly in the spouse caregiver (Cantor, 1983). It has often been noted that the responsibility of caregiving falls on one person, even though there are several family members who could conceivably adopt the same role. Indeed, there appears to be a 'cascade' effect in which each family member will take responsibility in turn, but not collectively. Another factor, to be explored below, is that the proportion of women carers is much greater (approximately 70 to 80%; Charlesworth et al., 1984). This is not explained solely by the imbalance in the number of elderly men who are married, but rather the different life experiences and socialization patterns experienced by women and men (Finch and Groves, 1983).

Understanding such factors should lead to improvement in the counselling and support of informal carers and in decision making about the use of formal care. These factors operate at many levels, for example, in deciding whether to admit a patient with dementia into temporary hospital care, how best to set up day care facilities for dementia sufferers that take into account the psychological needs of carers, and how to maximize the effectiveness of support groups for informal carers. Thus this chapter focusses on studies which have explored the stresses and strains experienced by carers, the factors that may effect this and the different approaches to improving psychological well being.

THE BURDEN OF CARE

The concept of 'objective burden' applies to the practical problems of caregiving. Similarly, the term 'daily hassles' has been used by Gilleard (1984) to describe the day-to-day impact of caring such as the need to organize and coordinate the various means of meeting the needs of the person with dementia and coping with the often irritating and frustrating demands. Poulshock and Deimling (1984) have used the term 'caregiving impact' to denote the social impact of caregiving, such as the effects on family relationships, employment and health (Rabins et al., 1982).

The objective burden of caregiving stems directly from changes in the behaviour of the person with dementia. These are described elsewhere (Chapter 10), but the main salient changes and how they affect the carer have been elicited by research using checklists. An early study by Sanford (1975) required carers to list all the problems that they encountered at home which if dealt with would make life more tolerable. The main problems included nocturnal wandering, faecal incontinence, an inability to wash, dress or feed unaided, immobility and dangerous behaviour such as using the gas cooker or heating appliances inappropriately. These problems can broadly be categorized into those concerned with sleep disturbance, incontinence and danger.

A somewhat different clustering of difficulties has been established by other studies, again using the checklist approach. Here, a large list of problem behaviours is established by professionals working with carers which is then rationalized and shortened to construct the checklist. Using this method and factor analysis Greene et al. (1982) derived three factors, termed 'apathy and withdrawal', 'behavioural disturbance' and 'mood disturbance'. this classification underlines the fact that lack of behaviour can be just as disturbing to the carer as behavioural disturbance. Gilleard et al. (1982) derived five factors which they labelled 'dependency', 'disturbance', 'disability', 'demand' and 'wandering'. An extension of this approach, similar to the methodology used by Sanford (1975), is to require the carer to rate the severity of elicited problems on a semantic differential scale. Using a large sample ($n = 214$) of carers they found that the perceived major problems were the need for constant supervision, proneness to falls, incontinence, night-time wandering and the inability of the person with dementia to engage in independent or meaningful activities. A more recent study by Pruchno and Resch (1989) derived three main factors, namely, 'forgetful' (items to do with memory disturbance), 'asocial' (to do with a breakdown in communication or social appropriateness) and 'disorientated' (to do with spatial or temporal disorientation). These factors, however, appear to leave out some of the more distressing behaviours associated with severe dementia, such as incontinence.

Curiously, the relationship between the well being of the carer and the severity of impairment of the person with dementia is not straightforward. Some studies have shown no association between such variables (Zarit et al., 1980; Gilhooly, 1984, 1986; Pagel et al., 1985; Fitting et al., 1986; George and Gwyther, 1986; Haley et al., 1987b). Other studies have found significant associations, but these do not apply to all aspects. For example, Machin (1980) and Greene et al. (1982) found that the degree of strain in the carer was related only to levels of withdrawal and apathy in the dementia sufferer. Gilleard et al. (1982) reported the strongest associations between strain and demanding behaviours, including demanding attention, disrupting social life and interpersonal conflicts. This lack of clear association points towards the complex nature of the caregiving process. It is likely that the multifacetted changes in the dementia sufferer will have different effects on the carer, whose reaction may not be uniform. This aspect has been explored by R.G. Morris et al. (1988) who support the view that a range of mediating factors mitigate against or exacerbate stress in the carer. These include the caregiving relationship, coping style of the carer, and the degree of formal social support, explored more fully below.

The studies reviewed above are cross-sectional in nature and make certain assumptions about the process of caring that should be studied in more detail. Townsend et al. (1989) have put forward several hypotheses about the relationship between the severity of the person's dementia and the caregiver outcome, some of which are held implicitly. The first is the *wear-and-tear* hypothesis that assumes that the dementia sufferer and the carer should experience a progressive deterioration in functioning as the dementia progresses. Thus as the person's symptoms increase, the caregiver should be overwhelmed by additional symptoms and problems. A second hypothesis, *adaptation*, is that the caregiver learns to adapt with experience, despite the mounting deterioration of the dementia sufferer. In other words, the caregivers' well being will stabilize or even improve over time. A third hypothesis, termed *trait*,

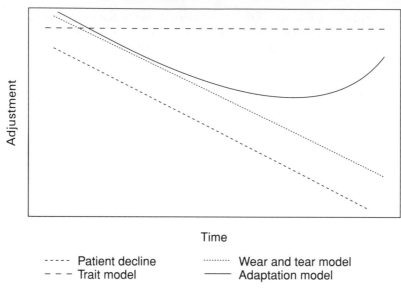

Fig. 13.1 Models of caregiver adjustment to patient decline. Reproduced with permission from Haley and Pardo (1989).

is that the carer maintains a constant level of adaptation over time. These three hypotheses are summarized in Fig. 13.1. Clearly, current knowledge is insufficient to distinguish between these three hypotheses and it may be that different groups of carers fit different models. For example, it is likely that some carers would show some of the characteristics of both the 'wear-and-tear' and 'adaptation' hypotheses.

Another equally important factor is that behaviour changes in dementia are not uniform over time. This is illustrated in Fig. 13.2. The higher level self-care

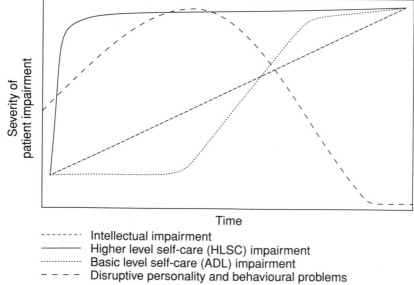

.... Intellectual impairment
———— Higher level self-care (HLSC) impairment
.... Basic level self-care (ADL) impairment
– – – – Disruptive personality and behavioural problems

Fig. 13.2 Severity of dementia and type of patient impairment. Adapted from Haley and Pardo (1989).

activities (HLSC), such as independence of managing finances, shopping, transportation and telephone use may deteriorate rapidly early on in the course of dementia. Problems concerned with basic self-care such as feeding and dressing, termed activities of daily living (ADL), occur much later on in the course of dementia. There is also evidence that disruptive behaviour problems, such as wandering, repeated questions and dangerous behaviour may peak in the middle phase of dementia and decrease at the final stage, although this is less well established (Haley and Pardo, 1989). This means that the objective burden of the carer will vary both in severity and character over time. For example, at the early stages the greatest burden may be having to adjust to taking over responsibility for the family finances, whilst in the middle phase it may be dealing with disruptive behaviour problems. Clearly this means that cross-sectional studies using a group of carers at different stages is unlikely to yield reliable associations between the severity of problems and carer well being.

LEVELS OF DEPRESSION AND STRAIN

The psychological well being of caregivers has been explored in several studies (cf. R.G. Morris et al., 1988), almost all of which report decreased morale and increased levels of depression and strain. For example, L.W. Morris et al. (1988) found that 14% of their sample of spouse carers had levels of depression on the Beck Depression Inventory (BDI) that were clinically significant. A range of other studies report similar findings (e.g. Fitting et al., 1986; George and Gwyther, 1986; Moritz et al., 1989; Pruchno and Resch, 1989). Very high levels of depression were found by Pagel et al. (1985) with 40% of their sample deemed to be depressed according to the Research and Diagnostic Criteria (RDC; Spitzer et al., 1978). Variations in levels of depression reported can be attributed in part to how the carers were recruited into the study. For example, carers who are contacted through a day centre may have more problems generally than those obtained through sampling people in the community. Morris et al. (1992) found low levels of depression in their sample of people applying to classes for carers of dementia sufferers.

Anxiety and stress is another negative outcome of caring and may be linked to the increased incidence of health problems in carers (Pruchno and Resch, 1989). Again levels of anxiety are higher than control samples of people who are not carers. A high number of stress symptoms and negative affect were reported by George and Gwyther (1986) using the Short Psychiatric Evaluation Schedule (Pfeiffer, 1979). Similarly, both Anthony-Bergstone et al. (1988) and Pruchno and Resch (1989) found high levels of anxiety in their studies of carers. Levels of probable 'caseness' of psychiatric disorder have also been investigated, measured using global ratings with varied results. The earlier study by Bergmann and Jacoby (1983) found that 33% of their sample had a psychiatric disorder based on the General Health Questionnaire (GCHQ). Gilleard et al. (1984) reported an even higher level with 68% of their carers exceeding the threshold value of 4/5 on the GHQ. This contrasts with the findings of a community study by Eagles et al. (1987) using the same scale where the number of cases were no more than expected in the community. Again, disparities in findings such as these point towards biases in the selection of carers. They may also, however, reflect the different levels of adaptation and impact of caring in people from different communities.

FACTORS MEDIATING THE IMPACT OF CAREGIVING

The caregiving relationship

As indicated above, a range of factors may mediate the impact of caregiving. This includes the caregiving relationship, partly because of the fact that the closer the blood/role relationship the more the carer is involved in the caregiving process (Cantor, 1983; George and Gwyther, 1986). Spouses are most likely to suffer from mental health problems, followed by siblings and other family members. The gender of the carer is also an important factor, to be explored on p. 000.

Another factor, explored in a preliminary fashion, is the premorbid quality of the relationship between the carer and dementia sufferer. A series of articles pointed towards the fact that if the relationship had been poor in the past, then this interfered significantly with a positive attitude to caregiving (Tobin and Kulys, 1981; Horowitz and Shindelman, 1983). Indeed, Gilleard et al. (1984) required carers to rate the quality of the past relationship on a single semantic differential scale and found that the lower the rating the higher the incidence of poor mental health. L.W. Morris et al. (1988) has since explored this issue using a version of the Waring et al. (1980) marital intimacy scale which investigated intimacy in terms of eight different facets, namely affection, cohesion, expressiveness, compatibility, conflict resolution, sexuality, autonomy and identity. Carers were required to fill in the scale according to their memory of the relationship prior to the onset of dementia, termed 'past intimacy'. It was found that levels of past intimacy were much lower in carers who reported greater strain and who scored more highly on the Beck Depression Inventory. To some extent, this result is predictable since a poor previous relationship would result in tensions, hostility and resentments in terms of fulfilling the caregiving role. It is also possible, however, that high levels of depression and strain would colour the persons perception of the past relationship in a negative fashion. Longitudinal studies of carers starting shortly after the onset of dementia would be of benefit in determining this issue more fully.

The decline in the level of intimacy has also been investigated in a similar fashion. L.W. Morris et al. (1988) also required their carers to rate the level of intimacy in the present. They found that there was a significant decline in intimacy comparing 'past' and 'present' levels (see Fig. 13.3) and also that the size of this difference significantly predicts the level of depression. There is very substantial evidence that depression is a common response to loss or bereavement. In the case of caregiving the person is not only losing the previously higher level of intimacy with the dementia sufferer but may be undergoing a process of 'premature' mourning or anticipatory grief. In addition, the social isolation associated with the breakdown of the relationship together with lack of time or opportunities to invest in new relationships may also make the person more vulnerable to depression (Brown et al., 1987).

Coping strategies

Professionals working with carers of people with dementia tend to focus on imparting knowledge and giving practical advice concerning how to manage the person, as well as providing support. As such the focus on training, knowledge and skills (e.g. Brodarty and Gresham, 1989) may ignore the fact that somebody caring for a person with dementia for any length of time may need to develop a repertoire of both cognitive and behavioural strategies that enables them to defend against despair and respond to the multitude of demands placed upon them (Pruchno and Resch, 1989). Coping strategies may

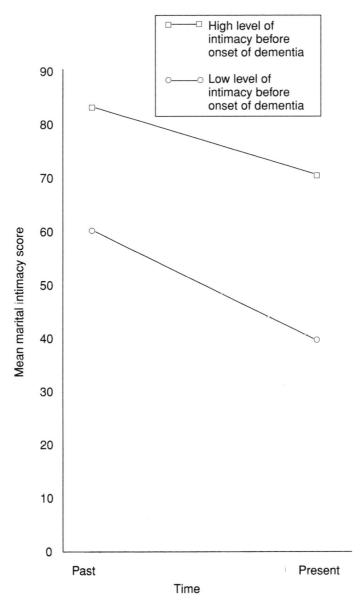

Fig. 13.3 Graph showing the loss of marital intimacy for subjects with high and low levels of intimacy before the onset of dementia in their spouse. Reproduced with permission from Morris (1986).

involve mastery of a situation, but can also mean minimizing, avoiding, tolerating and accepting it. In addition, as yet there is no clear consensus about which type of coping strategy is more effective for maintaining a positive level of mental health (Aldwin and Revenson, 1987). For this reason it should be an empirical question as to what coping strategies are most beneficial to carers of people with dementia.

A critical factor is that coping strategies tend to have different consequences when used in response to different types of stressors (Felton *et al.*, 1984). For example, it is generally accepted that emotion-focussed coping strategies, which are directed to regulating the individual's emotional response to a problem, are most effective in situations that are not amenable to individual control. Pruchno and Resch (1989) have pointed out that some of the uncontrollable stresses associated with dementia may be more successfully dealt with by focussing on the emotional distress aroused by the illness rather than attempts to alleviate the problem which are unlikely to succeed. On the other hand, the strategy of distancing oneself from the problem by wishful thinking or the use of fantasy has been found to be inversely associated with well being in carers (Quayhagen and Quayhagen, 1988). Possibly, although some of the problems associated with dementia are insoluble, mentally removing the caregiver from the realistic demands placed upon them may be antithetical to the needs of the situation (Pruchno and Resch, 1989).

A series of studies support the notion that problem-focussed coping strategies which concentrate on managing or altering the problem causing stress are associated with psychological well being in carers of people with dementia (Baruch and Spaid, 1989). Pratt et al. (1985) found that lower levels of subjective burden were experienced by carers who tended to be more confident in problem solving and reframing strategies, such as seeing a particular problem in a different light to arrive at a solution. In contrast, a passive approach was associated with higher levels of burden. Similarly, Wright et al. (1987) found that higher levels of life satisfaction were related to problem-focussed coping and reframing strategies whilst increased burden was specifically associated with avoidant-evasive and regressive coping styles. In their study of 54 carers Haley et al. (1987b) report that high levels of life satisfaction, better health and lower depression were all related to the greater use of problem-solving skills. In a very extensive study of 315 spouse caregivers of people with dementia Pruchno and Resch (1989) investigated the association between emotional well being and various types of coping strategies, including 'wishfulness', 'acceptance', 'intrapsychic' and 'instrumental' (see Table 13.1). Depression was measured with the Centre of Epidemiological Studies Depression Index (CES-D) (Radloff, 1977) and level of affect with the Bradburn Affect Scale (Positive Affect) derived from the Affect Balance Scale (Bradburn, 1969). Both the 'wishfulness' and 'intrapsychic' coping strategies were significantly associated with higher levels of depression, repeating the finding of Quayhagen and Quayhagen (1988). Use of instrumental coping strategies was related to more positive affect, again emphasizing the usefulness of a problem-solving approach. However, acceptance, unlike the two other emotion-focussed coping responses, was negatively related to all indexes of mental health used in the study. This latter finding has important implications since it suggests that a realistic appraisal and acceptance of a situation is an adaptive response.

Adaptation to the role of caregiving may depend to some extent on how the carer perceives the task of caregiving. Difficulties in adaptation can be attributed partly to the insidious nature of the illness, such that in the initial stages the caregiver may wrongly attribute the behaviour of the person with dementia (Morris et al., 1989a). For example, changes in behaviour or the personality of the person with dementia are attributed to something going wrong in the relationship. Such observations have led researchers to study the cognitions of carers in the context of attributional theory and to investigate whether certain attributional styles are more likely to be associated with poor emotional well being.

Early formulations of attributional theory conclude that internal, stable and global causal attributions for negative outcomes make people more prone to depression (Abramson et al., 1978). Although this is not accepted as a specific

Table 13.1 Coping strategies and their association with levels of depression measured using the Centre for Epidemiologic Studies Depression Index (CES-D) and levels of affect in spouse carers of people with dementia (Pruchno and Resch, 1989).

Coping strategy and questions	Outcome
1. *Wishfulness* Wished you were a stronger person to deal with it better Wished you could change what had happened ' Wished you could change the way you felt	Higher level of depression No association with affect
2. *Acceptance* Accepted the situation Refused to let it get to you Made the best of it You knew what had to be done, so you tried to make things work	Lower level of depression No association with affect
3. *Intrapsychic* Had fantasies about how things might turn out Told yourself things to help you feel better Hoped a miracle would happen Daydreamed/imagined a better time or place than the one you were in	Higher level of depression No association with affect
4. *Instrumental* Made a plan of action and followed it Felt inspired to be creative in solving the problem Came up with a couple of different solutions to the problem Changed something about yourself so you could deal with the situation better Did something totally new to solve the problem	Higher sense of positive affect No association with depression

cause of depression, there is evidence that people's concept of causality and control over their responses to specific negative *events* is related to the onset of depression (Brewin, 1984). The attributional style of carers has been studied initially by Pagel *et al.* (1985) and Coppel *et al.* (1985), and more recently by Morris *et al.* (1989a), the latter of which is considered here. Using the reformulated learned helplessness model of depression (Abramson *et al.*, 1978, 1988), Morris *et al.* (1989a) considered caregivers attributions of causality and control over their situation specifically in relation to caregiving. For example, to assess the internality dimension, carers were asked whether 'At present, despite all that your doctor has told you about your partner's illness, to what extent do you think his/her symptoms are due to something about yourself, or about your partner and circumstances?' To assess the stability dimension one of the questions was 'At present, when looking ahead to a year's time, do you expect that the strain and distress then will be greater or less than that which you are now experiencing?' An example of a globality dimension question was 'At present to what extent do you think that your partner's illness is affecting all the other areas of your life?' Only the stability and globality dimensions were significantly correlated with depression in their sample of spouse carers. Thus attributing the symptoms of the person with dementia to oneself was not predictive of depression, presumably because the carers tended not to blame themselves concerning their spouses illness. However, seeing their level of stress as stable and the impact of caregiving as affecting all aspects of their lives was predictive of depression. Perceived loss of control is also frequently seen as negative feature of the caregiving process (R.G. Morris et al., 1988). Following on from Coppel et al. (1985), Morris et al. (1989a) investigated the sense of control that the caregivers had over their spouses behaviour and their own emotional reactions. They report very high correlations, with an increased sense of control in the carer being associated with a low level of depression in both areas. In addition, these factors were also associated with low levels of strain.

To summarize, studies of coping strategies point towards instrumental or problem-solving approaches being the most adaptive, with the caveat that learning to accept and make the best of the situation also predicts good mental health (Pruchno and Resch, 1989). To some extent these findings are mirrored in the research on attributional style where it has been found that attributions of circumstances to do with caregiving that are seen as stable and global (i.e. unchangeable) are associated with higher levels of depression. The carers sense of control over the behaviour of the person with dementia and their own emotional reaction appear also to be important in mitigating against depression. This cluster of findings points towards the benefits of carers perceiving that they can take action to change certain things, whilst accepting and adapting to their overall circumstances. Conversely, carers who are unable to do this may be more at risk for psychiatric illness.

Gender differences in responding to the caregiving role
A consistent finding is that women carers experience a lower level of morale and higher levels of strain, anxiety and depression than men (Gilhooly et al., 1984; Gilleard et al., 1984; Fitting et al., 1986; Anthony-Bergstone et al., 1988; Moritz et al., 1989). Where studies have been conducted using comparisons with noncarers, the level of mental health problems have been found to be greater in women over and above the baseline levels in community samples. For example, Pruchno and Resch (1989) found that levels of depression on the CES-D rose more sharply in women carers and Anthony-Bergstone et al. (1988) found that symptoms of obsessive–compulsive neurosis, depression, hostility and psychoticism were relatively increased in women carers. The cause of this increase in mental health problems is likely to be multifaceted (Morris et al., 1991). One aspect possibly arises from the role expectations of women, although the explanation is more complicated, as will be shown below.

It has been argued that women carers, especially elderly spouses, were raised in a period when women were socialized to be more family orientated and take on nurturant roles; the role of carer in later life is an extension of the traditional responsibilities of wife and daughter (Treas, 1977). Support for this view is mixed, although there is consistent evidence that women are more involved in the process of caregiving than men and it is clear that the pattern of caregiving by men and women differs significantly. Horowitz's (1985) study of son and daughter caregivers of the frail elderly (including people with dementia) found that whilst women tend to aid in transportation, meal preparation, errands, shopping and personal care, men tend to help with decision making and personal assistance. In this study, women were more active in caregiving. Despite this, Miller (1987) found no difference between men and women in terms of help given with daily tasks. Another study of spouse carers by Pruchno and Resch (1989) reported that men and women give the same amount of help in activities of daily living, although the latter received more help from other people. In the Baruch and Spaid (1989) study men reported performing an average of 27 tasks within the month before the interview compared to 23 tasks reported by women. In this case, men reported more tasks concerned with communication, mobility, hygiene, dressing and feeding.

This lack of consistent findings has led some researchers to consider other factors to be important in the well being of the carer, in particular the persons perspective on the caregiving role which is in turn influenced by gender stereotypes. Miller (1987) proposed that taking on the role of caregiving may be at variance to a person's expectations or aspirations. For men, caregiving can be seen as an extension of the traditional role of an authority figure in the home or in work rather than an extension of the nurturing role. Thus male caregivers tend to be at ease in terms of taking responsibility for the instrumental aspects of caregiving. On the other hand, women find it harder to assume an authority position over an adult, particularly if they have been used to seeing their husband as an authority figure in the marriage. Miller's (1987) proposal may account for some situations, but not all partnerships appear to fit into this stereotype; for example, in many cases women assume responsibility for the family finances. Another factor, which is more relevant to daughter caregivers is reflected in changed demographic trends in which more women have entered the work place. In particular, middle-aged women may experience more 'role-conflict' with the competing demands of the immediate family, career aspirations and responsibilities and caring for a dependent parent. This conflict and the subsequent ambivalence about caregiving has led to the concept of the 'women-in-the-middle' where conflicting demands cannot be met.

A further factor, proposed by Gutmann (1987) and Eichorn et al. (1981) is the tendency for women to become more assertive and instrumental as they get older and less nurturing or expressive. Middle-aged women carers may be in the process of relinquishing child-rearing responsibilities and planning to take more control over their lives. Similarly, women spouse carers can be seen as viewing their later lives as a period for personal growth and fulfilment away from the responsibilities of a nurturing or caregiving role (Zarit et al., 1986). These factors would tend to mean that women would experience a greater role conflict, with a resulting increased experience of emotional distress (Gutmann, 1987). In line with both Gutmann (1987) and Eichorn et al.'s (1981) proposal there is evidence that male spouse carers are more likely to report an improvement in the marital relationship after the onset of dementia (Fitting et al., 1986). However, Fitting et al. (1986) suggest that male carers may derive a positive feeling from 'repaying' the wife for past nurturing, or from an atoning sense of guilt, in the case of a previously unhappy relationship.

In summary, there is consistent evidence for lower levels of emotional well being in women carers as a group. Various reasons have been proposed including the notion of higher 'role-conflict'. Nevertheless, the various explanations for increased incidence of strain and depression in women carers are likely to be broad generalizations and tend not to take into account the changing roles of women in society. Substantial overlap must exist between men and women in their responses to the caregiving role.

SUPPORTING THE CARER

Social support

The level of informal support is frequently considered as a factor that mitigates against high levels of strain in the caregiving relationship (Niederehe and Fruge, 1984; Morris *et al.*, 1989b). Indeed there is evidence that carers who have a larger network of social support from relatives and friends tend to feel in less need of professional help (Fitting *et al.*, 1986), and make less demands on community services (Caserta *et al.*, 1987). The dynamics of social support are clearly complex, since support can be given in a variety of different ways, which may or may not be helpful. For example, having a friend whom you can reliably call upon to help you out in a crisis, but who is not seen very frequently may be more useful than a close relation who provides frequent visits but is critical of the care being given.

This might explain why studies investigating the association between carer emotional well being and the quantity of social support have produced mixed results. For example, Zarit *et al.* (1980) found that carers who were receiving more family visits tended to have less feelings of burden. In contrast, both Gilleard *et al.* (1984) and Gilhooly (1984) found no association between well being and the degree of contact and help received from family friends. Measuring the quantity of activities associated with social support may not be a useful way of measuring the effectiveness of the support given. Thus Gilhooly (1984) reported that satisfaction with help from relatives is associated with carer well being.

More recently, Morris *et al.* (1989b) investigated the *quality* of social support using a scale derived from the Californian Human Population Laboratory Questionnaire (Berkman, 1983). This scale looks at the emotional, instrumental and financial help received by the carer and the network of social relations that surround them. Examples of the items in the questionnaire include 'If you can call on a relative or friend for help with a real problem, how often do you do so?' or 'When you need some extra help, can you count on anyone to help with daily tasks like shopping, cleaning, cooking and transport?' Morris *et al.* (1989b) found that caregivers were less depressed and experienced less strain when they received more social support. A study by Pearson *et al.* (1988) has also investigated the types of help that carers most appreciate. These include social visits and being able to leave the person with dementia with a relative so that the carer can go out of the house for social or recreational activities.

In recent years, professional carers have worked to improve the quality of social support. In cases where this is not an attempt to push the burden of care back on to the informal carer or create a language of activity to obscure the lack of priority given to people with dementia, this has been seen as a positive approach. For example, the community schemes pioneered by Challis and Davies (1986) are designed to coordinate professional and voluntary support to interweave with the carers' existing social support network, for example, by recruiting volunteers to provide practical help and decrease the social isolation of the carer.

Educational classes or support groups for carers

Different approaches

An alternative form of support for informal carers which is becoming increasingly popular is a series of meetings focussing on dementia and the caregiving process. These can take a variety of forms including formal classes for carers led by professional people, discussion groups focussing on the caregiving process, and support groups aimed at providing mutual emotional support. These classes or groups are most appropriate in a community setting such as a day hospital, where the informal carer is more likely to wish to communicate directly with individual care staff.

The most traditional mode is an educational class where informal carers attend a series of 'seminars' concerned with disseminating information about the illness, including the cause of dementia, understanding the person's behaviour and the types of help available for the informal carer (Zarit and Zarit, 1982). Another type of class focusses on improving caregiving skills. Although these tend to be facilitated by professionals, one of the aims of the classes is for carers to pass on management skills to each other in similar format to a 'workshop'. One method has been to use the problem-solving model (D'Zurilla and Goldfried, 1971) to structure this approach.

For example, approaches developed by Zarit and coworkers (Zarit and Zarit, 1982; Zarit et al., 1985) and by Morris and coworkers (Morris, 1992; Morris et al., 1993) involve encouraging the informal carer to identify and describe specific problems, generate and evaluate a plan of intervention and then implement and evaluate the plan. This approach is based on the finding that an instrumental or problem-solving focussed approach to caregiving is consistently associated with higher levels of carer well being (see p. 000). A specific course, developed by Morris and his coworkers is outlined in Table 13.2. The aim of the course is to apply problem-solving methods to the different aspects of caregiving, including managing the behaviour problems of the person with dementia and interacting with formal services. Specific techniques include getting the group to discuss the 'pros' and 'cons' of a particular course of action, and encouraging members to try out solutions at home and report back to the next session. This approach has been used more intensively in a 10-day residential programme by Brodarty and Gresham (1989). They admit up to four people with dementia and their respective principal carers into hospital. The person with dementia is given a range of occupational activities and therapy, including memory retraining, whilst the carer is involved in intensive education, group therapy and training in management skills.

An alternative to the 'skills' approach is a psychotherapeutic orientation (Barnes et al., 1981). Here the focus is on emotional adjustment stemming from the losses associated with dementia and changes in the life-style of the carer. The resulting emotions, including feelings of anger, frustration, guilt and despair are explored through the group which sees the caregiving process as an opportunity for personal growth. The strength of this approach appears to be that it focusses on emotional adaptation, which appears to be positively associated with carer well being (Quayhagen and Quayhagen, 1988). Despite this, focussing on negative emotions is not always beneficial to the members of carer's group as a whole. This may in part be due to the members of a group being at different stages of adjustment with some carers not yet ready to face up to the deep sense of loss and sadness experienced by others (Barnes et al., 1981; Schmidt and Keyes, 1985; Wasow, 1985). This highlights the need for groups that focus on the expression of emotions to have skilful leadership and screening of participants, with appropriate support outside the group (Morris, 1993).

Methodological issues in the evaluation of classes or groups
Attempts to evaluate the efficacy of classes or groups raises a number of methodological issues. Firstly, the different approaches should be considered in relation to what the class or group is aiming to achieve. For example, an

Table 13.2 Content of sessions used in the Morris *et al.* (1992) Carers Programme (Ways of Coping) (modified from Morris, 1993; supported by the Alzheimer's Disease Society, UK).

Session	Purpose
1. Individual interview of carer by a professional	To assess the level of dependency of the dementia sufferer, the degree of stress or strain experienced by the carer To explain the purpose of the group meetings
2. Group meeting Theme: 'understanding behaviour'	To introduce the carers to each other and enable them to explain their current situation To describe the different stages of dementia To introduce methods for observing the behaviour of the dementia sufferer

Material to take away: A record sheet for recording 'problem behaviours'

3. Group meeting Theme: 'generating solutions'	To discuss the use of the recording sheet, and share problems encountered To discuss ways of reframing problems To introduce ways of coping with behavioural problems (e.g. wandering, aggression) To introduce ways of generating and evaluating solutions (e.g. 'pros' and 'cons' method)

Material to take away: The carers are required to pick a particular problem and then to generate and evaluate different ways of tackling it

4. Group meeting Theme: 'coping with stress'	To review ways of tackling problem behaviours To introduce different ways in which carers may cope with stress and to evaluate positive and negative coping strategies

Material to take away: Participants would record a strategy that they had used to reduce stress and evaluate how successful it had been

5. Group meeting Theme: 'formal and informal support'	To review success of strategies for coping with stress To describe what is available in terms of local community services To discuss ways of identifying the need for and obtaining formal and informal support.

Material to take away: The participants would identify areas where they might benefit from help and decide on strategies they might use

6. Group meeting Theme: 'conclusion'	To discuss the outcome of the task assignment from session 5 To review the problem solving approach to improve coping strategies To provide feedback from the participants in terms of their evaluation of the course

7. Individual interview of carer by a professional	To assess the level of strain and stress of the carer To evaluate changes in coping strategies To obtain the individual's evaluation of the course To provide further information for the carer where necessary
8. Individual interview of carer by a professional	To repeat session 7 after a period of approximately 3 months

educationally focussed group might be expected to produce increases in knowledge, but no significant changes in terms of emotional adaptation. A problem-solving focussed group might produce increased management and instrumental care skills on the part of the carer, but this might only produce changes in levels of strain or depression after a longer term follow-up. Hence the choice of outcome measure should be considered carefully to avoid naive conclusions being made concerning efficacy. In addition, unless careful 'process' research is undertaken, it is not always clear that what occurs in a class or group reflects the title given to it. For example, a study by Morris et al. (1992) comparing educationally focussed classes with a problem-solving focussed group, found that 'problem solving' and skills training was occurring inadvertently in the 'education' classes due to the teaching methods of those leading these classes. An additional factor in longitudinal evaluation is the choice of a control group, which in some cases may be unethical or produce positive changes because the study has brought the carers into contact with the researchers.

Formal valuations studies have been conducted on time-limited clases or groups, as summarized in Table 13.3. These include a mixture of approaches or comparison of approaches which appear unsystematic as a whole, but give some indication of their efficacy. Two studies included groups that concentrated specifically on education *and* measured changes in knowledge (Chiverton and Caine, 1989; Morris et al., 1992). Both studies report a significant increase in knowledge about dementia, but Morris et al. (1993) found that this occurred in groups focussing on problem-solving focussed coping strategies. Kahan et al. (1985) also found a significant increase in knowledge in their groups which combined education and support. The no-specificity of the study by Morris et al. (1992) illustrates the difficulty of evaluating an approach since it is likely that the problem-solving groups would have also imparted knowledge to the carers.

Several studies have included groups focussing on problem solving. Out of these, four report positive changes in the emotional well being of carers (Kahan et al., 1985; Zarit et al., 1987; Brodarty and Gresham, 1989; Toseland et al., 1989), whilst two studies report no change (Haley et al., 1987a; Haley, 1989; Morris et al., 1992). However, in the studies producing positive changes only the intensive training package of Brodarty and Gresham (1989) produced differential increases in carer well being relative to an appropriate control group. It could be argued that the principal outcome measure for this approach is positive changes in coping strategies. The two studies that have measured coping strategies produced different results, with Haley et al. (1987a) finding no changes in coping responses but Morris et al. (1992) reporting an increase in

Table 13.3 Summary of the outcome of group intervention studies for carers of dementia sufferers (only studies using quantitative outcome measures included) (taken from Morris, 1993).

Reference	Approach	Length	Outcome
Brodaty and Gresham (1989)	Intensive training versus waiting list	Ten days, residential	Increase in carer well being dementia sufferer less likely to be institutionalized
Chiverton and Caine (1989)	Education	Three sessions weekly; 2 hours	Increase in knowledge about dementia
Gendron et al. (1986)	Stress management	Eight sessions weekly	Reduced anxiety; increased assertiveness
Glosser and Wexler (1985)	Education Support	Eight sessions weekly; 2 hours	Positive ratings for perceived helpfulness
Haley et al. (1987)	1. Support 2. Support and training 3. Waiting list control	Ten sessions weekly; 1.5 hours	Positive ratings for perceived helpfulness but no difference between groups in carer well being or coping strategies
Haley (1989)		Long-term follow-up	Confirmed outcome of previous study (above) after approximately 2 years
Kahan et al. (1985)	Education Support	Eight sessions weekly; 2 years	Decrease in level of depression and perceived burden; increase in knowledge about dementia
Lazarus (1981)	Support Therapy	Ten sessions weekly; 1 hour	No change in self esteem, but increase in sense of locus of control
Morris et al. (1992)	1. Education 2. Training focus to improve coping strategies	Five sessions weekly; 1.5 hours	Positive ratings of helpfulness in both groups but no change in emotional well being
Shibbal-Champagne and Lapinska-Stachow (1985–1986)	Education Support	Eight sessions weekly; 1.5 hours	Decrease in carer burden

Toseland et al. (1989)	1. Education and problem-solving focus 2. Peer-led support focus	Eight sessions weekly; 2 hours	Positive changes in psychological well being in both groups
Zarit et al. (1987)	1. Education and support 2. Individual and family counselling 3. Waiting list control group	Eight sessions weekly	Decrease in carer burden and frequency of emotional disorder, but equal change in all three groups

problem-solving skills. The study by Haley *et al.* used a different approach to that of Morris *et al* (1992). which involved using techniques derived from cognitive therapy. Nevertheless, the positive finding of Morris *et al* (1992). is not specific, being found in their 'education' comparison group.

To some extent all classes and groups include a 'support' element, but some groups are seen specifically as providing mutual support. Out of the six studies that include appropriate outcome measures to evaluate 'support' groups five indicate positive results, either in terms of a decrease in burden or an increase in emotional well being (Lazarus, 1981; Kahan *et al.*, 1985; Shibbal-Champagne and Lapinska-Stachow, 1985/1986; Zarit *et al.*, 1987; Toseland *et al.*, 1989). One study shows no positive change (Haley *et al.*, 1987a; Haley, 1989). Again, the specificity of the result is poor, with some studies showing no extra improvement above comparison or control groups.

Overall, these studies illustrate the methodological difficulties in evaluating the efficacy of different approaches, such that it is too early to say whether classes or groups are effective. Several factors, however, should be borne in mind in future evaluations. For example, all the groups evaluated were time-limited and relatively short. It is thus likely that only small changes in the carers would be observed, particularly as there are a huge range of other factors that might affect carer emotional well-being simultaneously. This is consistent with several studies showing high levels of consumer satisfaction in carers who have attended a group (Glosser and Wexler, 1985; Morris *et al.*, 1992), but small changes in terms of other outcome variables. A carer may quickly perceive the usefulness of a group without experiencing any substantial change in their emotional well being or behaviour. Longer and more intensive classes or groups might be expected to produce more powerful changes. In addition, very few studies refer to the fact that carers who attend classes or groups are highly selected. For example, in the study by Morris *et al.* (1992) it was decided to exclude carers with depression on the grounds that they would be likely to be undergoing concurrent treatment. However, levels of psychological disorder in carers attending groups tends to be much lower anyway. Thus the purpose of running a class or group might, for example, be to improve the quality of life of the carer through improving coping skills, rather than increase emotional well being which is relatively normal. Finally, with the exception of Haley (1989), none of the studies achieved a long-term follow-up. Problems of attrition, noted by Haley (1989) present obvious difficulties, but it is possible that the differential efficacy of the approached reviewed above will only be apparent over a longer period.

Formal support

The prevailing view, at least in the UK, is that as a whole informal carers of dementia sufferers continue to give support to their dependants at a great cost to themselves and with inadequate support from community services (Jones and Vetter, 1985). Nevertheless, more attention is being paid to the provision of community care and a range of services has been implemented, including home helps, meals on wheels, laundry services and the provision of day care and respite care.

Such services are often vital to carers, enabling them to continue functioning as well as improving the quality of life of the person with dementia. Key worker schemes for promoting the carer have been experimented with by Challis and Davies (1986) who found that the use of local volunteers and flexibly allocated funds successfully maintained approximately 50% of people with dementia is the community compared to 23% of a control population. There is also evidence that increased formal support reduces the amount of strain experienced by the carer. Levin *et al.* (1986) found that the build up of strain was less in carers who were receiving a high level of local authority services. This was despite the fact that they tended to be dissatisfied with services. Similarly, Gilhooly (1984) found a significant correlation between morale in the caregiver and the degree of home help services or visits from a community nurse. Despite this, it is often found that support services respond to strain and breakdown in the carer rather than prevent it occurring. Thus, some studies report that carers who have higher levels of strain or depression are receiving higher levels of formal support (Morris *et al.*, 1989b). Interestingly, it has been found that carers who have a good quality of social support tend to be more satisfied with the formal support they receive (Morris *et al.*, 1989b).

Another important form of formal support is day or respite care. A positive feature of day care is that it releases time for the carer to concentrate on other activities and reduce the level of social isolation (Gilleard, 1987). However, in some cases, attendance at a day hospital or day centre may precipitate institutionalization by bringing the carer into closer contact with formal services (Greene and Timbury, 1979; Bergmann and Jacoby, 1983). Respite care also provides relief for the carer and formal evaluations have shown improvements in the physical and mental health of the carer and increased confidence to continue caring (Scharlach and Frenzel, 1986; Burdz *et al.*, 1988). Future research in this area, however, may be directed to establishing which types of carers benefit most from this service. For example, some carers appear to be reluctant to relinquish care and become more distressed after leaving their relative in another place if they are not satisfied with the individual care and attention received.

DISCUSSION

Research into informal carers during the last decade has clarified the factors affecting their psychological well being, and what aspects can reduce the degree of objective and subjective burden that they experience. These show that the relationship with the person with dementia, the role and coping strategies adopted by the carer and the different forms of social and formal support are important interlocking factors. These had been summarized in a review by R.G. Morris *et al.* (1988), but since this review there has been burgeoning of the literature in this field, reflecting the continued interest. It was indicated then that the dominant research strategy has been to correlate different measures and thus establish associated links between different factors through the use of multivariate analyses. This is still the dominant research study, but more investigators are concentrating on longitudinal investigations that have greater predictive power (Levin *et al.*, 1986; Haley, 1989). In addition, creative approaches to the management of dementia which incorporate the carer are being developed, for example, the intensive training programme developed by Brodarty and Gresham (1989).

These approaches are likely to yield further knowledge in the future. Nevertheless, methodological difficulties are substantial, such as developing longitudinal measures that can follow carers in different stages of fulfilling their role and coping with the differential rates of changes associated with varying severities of dementia. For example, how does the adaptation of a carer whose spouse deteriorates and dies in 3 years in their sixties compare with a slow deterioration in old age? One approach, which mirrors recent developments in investigating the time course of dementia, is to explore the 'natural history' of caregiving by following emotional development of individual carers in detail.

In conclusion, the psychosocial factors that surround the process of caregiving are varied and generate interest in their own right, but also provide an opportunity for basic research into how people cope with chronic, unpredictable and long-term stressors and how these can be ameliorated. The practical value of knowing more about the carer is substantial, and is unlikely to diminish as community-based approaches become more established and carers themselves become more recognized in an ageing population.

REFERENCES

Abramson, L.Y., Alloy, L.B. and Metalsky, G.I. (1988). The cognitive diathesis-stress theories of depression: Toward an adequate test of the theories validities. In *Cognitive Processes in Depression*, Alloy, L.B. (Ed.). Guilford Press, New York.

Abramson, L.Y., Seligman, M.E.P. and Teasdale, J. (1978). Learned helplessness in humans: critique and reformulation. *Journal of Abnormal Psychology*, **87**, 49–79.

Aldwin, C.M. and Revenson, T.A. (1987). Does coping help? A re-examination of the relation between coping and mental health. *Journal of Personality and Social Psychology*, **53**, 337–48.

Anthony-Bergstone, C., Zarit, S.H. and Gatz, M. (1988). Symptoms of psychological distress among caregivers of dementia patients. *Psychology and Aging*, **3**, 245–8.

Barnes, R.F., Raskind, M.A., Scott, M. and Murphy, C. (1981). Problems of families caring for Alzheimer patients: The use of a support group. *Journal of the American Geriatrics Association*, **14**, 355–60.

Barusch, A.S. and Spaid, W.M. (1989). Gender differences in caregiving: Why do wives report greater burden? *The Gerontologist*, **29**, 667–76.

Bergmann, K. and Jacoby, R. (1983). The limitation and possibilities of community care for the elderly demented. *Elderly People in the Community: Their Service Needs*. HMSO, London.

Bergmann *et al.* (1978).

Berkman, L.F. (1983). The assessment of social networks and social support in the elderly. *Journal of the American Geriatrics Society*, **31**, 743–9.

Bradburn, N. (1969). *The Structures of Psychological Wellbeing*. Aldine, Chicago.

Brewin, C.R. (1984). Attributions for industrial accidents: Their relationship to rehabilitation outcome. *Journal of Social and Clinical Psychology*, **2**, 156–64.

Brodarty, H. and Gresham, M. (1989). Effects of a training programme to reduce stress in carers of patients with dementia. *British Medical Journal*, **299**, 1375–9.

Brown, G.W., Bifulco, A. and Harris, T.O. (1987). Life events, vulnerability and the onset of depression: some refinements. *British Journal of Psychiatry*, **150**, 30–42.

Burdz, M.P., Eaton, W.O. and Bond, J.B. (1988). Effect of respite care on dementia and nondementia patients and their caregivers. *Psychology and Aging*, **3**, 38–42.

Cantor, M.H. (1983). Strain among caregivers: a study of experience in the United States. *The Gerontologist*, **23**, 597–604.

Caserta, M.S., Lund, D.A., Wright, S.D. and Redburn, D.E. (1987). Caregivers of dementia patients: the utilisation of community services. *Gerontologist*, **27**, 209–14.

Challis, D. and Davies, B. (1986). *Case Management in Community Care: An Evaluated Experiment in the Home Care of the Elderly*. Gower, Aldershot.

Charlesworth, A., Wilkin, D. and Durie, A. (1984). *Carers and Services: A Comparison of Men and Women Caring for Dependent Elderly People*. Equal Opportunities Commission, Manchester.

Chiverton, P. and Caine, E.D. (1989). Education to assist spouses in coping with Alzheimer's disease: a controlled trial. *Journal of the American Geriatrics Association*, **37**, 593–8.

Coppel, D.B., Burton, C., Becker, J. and Fiore, J. (1985). Relationships of cognition associated with coping reactions to depression in spousal caregivers of Alzheimer's disease patients. *Cognitive Therapy and Research*, **9**, 253–66.

D'Zurilla, T.J. and Goldfried, M.R. (1971). Problem solving and behaviour modification. *Journal of Abnormal Psychology*, **78**, 107–26.

Eagles, J.M., Beattie, J.A.G., Blackwood, G.W. *et al.* (1987). The mental health of elderly couples – I: The effects of the cognitively impaired spouse. *British Journal of Psychiatry*, **150**, 293–8.

Eichorn, D.H., Clausen, J.A., Hann, N. *et al.* (1981). *Present and Past Middle Life*. Seadonic Press, New York.

Felton, B.J., Revenson, T.A. and Hinrichsen, G.A. (1984). Stress and coping in the explanation of psychological adjustment among chronically ill adults. *Social Science and Medicine*, **18**, 889–98.

Finch, J. and Groves, D. (1983). *Labour of Love: Women, Work and Caring*. Routledge & Kegan Paul, London.

Fitting, ?., Rabins, P., Lucas, M.J. and Eastham, J. (1986). Caregivers for demented patients: A comparison of husbands and wives. *The Gerontologist*, **26**, 48–252.

Gendron, C.E., Poitras, L.R. and Engels, M.L. (1986). Skills training with supporters of the demented. *Journal of the American Geriatrics Society*, **34**, 875–80.

George, L.K. and Gwyther, L.P. (1986). Caregiver well-being: a multidimensional examination of family caregivers of demented adults. *The Gerontologist*, **26**, 253–9.

Gilhooly, M.L.M. (1984). The impact of caregiving on caregivers: factors associated with the psychological well-being of people supporting a dementing relative in the community. *British Journal of Medical Psychology*, **57**, 35–44.

Gilhooly, M.L.M. (1986). Senile dementia: factors associated with caregiver's preference for institutional care. *British Journal of Medical Psychology*, **59**, 165–71.

Gilleard, C.J. (1984). *Living with Dementia: Community Care of the Elderly Mentally Infirm*. Croom Helm, London.

Gilleard, C.J. (1987). Influence of emotional distress among supporters on the outcome of psychogeriatric day care. *British Journal of Psychiatry*, **150**, 219–23.

Gilleard, C.J., Boyd, W.D. and Watt, G. (1982). Problems in caring for the elderly mentally infirm at home. *Archives of Gerontology and Geriatrics*, **1**, 151–8.

Gilleard, C.J., Belford, H., Gilleard, E. *et al.* (1984). Emotional distress among the supporters of the elderly mentally infirm. *British Journal of Psychiatry*, **145**, 172–7.

Glosser, G. and Wexler, D. (1985). Participants' evaluation of educational/

support groups for families of patients with Alzheimer's disease and other dementias. *Gerontologist*, **25**, 232–6.

Grad, J. and Sainsbury, P. (1965). An evaluation of the effects of caring for the aged at home. In *Psychiatric Disorders in the Aged*. WPA symposium. Geigy, Manchester.

Greene, J.G. and Timbury, G.C. (1979). A geriatric psychiatry day hospital service: a five year review. *Age and Ageing*, **8**, 49–53.

Greene, J.G., Smith, R., Gardiner, M. and Timbury, G.C. (1982). Measuring behavioural disturbance of elderly demented patients in the community and its effects on relatives: A factor analytic study. *Age and Ageing*, **11**, 121–6.

Gutmann, D.L. (1987). *Reclaimed Powers: Towards a New Psychology of Men and Women in Later Life*. Basic Books, New York.

Haley, W.E. (1989). Group intervention for dementia family caregivers: A longitudinal perspective. *The Gerontologist*, **29**, 478–80.

Haley, W.E., Brown, S.L. and Levine, E.G. (1987a). Experimental evaluation of the effectiveness of group intervention for dementia caregivers. *The Gerontologist*, **27**, 376–82.

Haley, W.E., Levine, E.G., Brown, S.L. and Bartolucci, A.A. (1987b). Stress, appraisal, coping and social support as predictors of adaptational outcome among dementia caregivers. *Psychology and Aging*, **2**, 232–330.

Haley, W.E. and Pardo, K.M. (1989). Relationship of severity of dementia to caregiver stressors. *Psychology and Aging*, **4**, 389–92.

Horowitz, A. (1985). Sons and daughters as caregivers to older parents: differences in role performance and consequences. *The Gerontologist*, **25**, 612–17.

Horowitz, A. and Shindelman, L.W. (1983). Reciprocity and affection: past influences on current caregiving. *Journal of Gerontological Social Work*, **5**, 5–20.

Jones, D.A. and Vetter, N.J. (1985). Formal and informal support received by carers of elderly dependents. *British Medical Journal*, **291**, 643–5.

Kahan, J., Kemp, B., Staples, F.R. and Brummel-Smith, K. (1985). Decreasing the burden in families caring for a relative with a dementing illness: a controlled study. *Journal of the American Geriatrics Society*, **33**, 664–70.

Lazarus, R.S. (1981). The stress and coping paradigm. In *Models of Clinical Psychopathology*, Eisdorfer, C. (Ed.), pp. 177–214. Spectrum, New York.

Levin, E., Sinclair, I. and Gorbach, P. (1986). *The Supporters of Confused Elderly Persons at Home*. National Institute of Social Work, London.

Machin, E. (1980). A survey of the behaviour of the elderly and their supporters at home. Unpublished MSc thesis, University of Birmingham.

Miller, B. (1987). Gender and control among spouses of the cognitively impaired: a research note. *The Gerontologist*, **27**, 447–53.

Moritz, D.J., Kasl, S.V. and Berkman, L.F. (1989). The health impact of living with a cognitively impaired elderly spouse: depressive symptoms and social functioning. *Journal of Gerontology*, **14**, 517–27.

Morris, L.W. (1986). The psychological factors affecting emotional wellbeing of the spouse caregivers of dementia sufferers. Unpublished MSc thesis, University of Newcastle upon Tyne.

Morris, L.W., Morris, R.G. and Britton, P.G. (1988). The relationship between marital intimacy, perceived strain and depression in spouse carers of dementia sufferers. *British Journal of Medical Psychology*, **61**, 231–6.

Morris, L.W., Morris, R.G. and Britton, P.G. (1989a). Cognitive style and perceived control in spouse carers of dementia sufferers. *British Journal of Medical Psychology*, **62**, 173–9.

Morris, L.W., Morris, R.G. and Britton, P.G. (1989b). Social support networks and formal support as factors influencing the psychological adjustment of spouse caregivers of dementia sufferers. *International Journal of Geriatric Psychiatry*, **4**, 47–51.

Morris, R.G. (1993). Psychological aspects of dementia. In *The Psychology of Dementia*, Miller, E. and Morris, R.G. J. Wiley Press, Chichester, New York.

Morris, R.G., Morris, L.W. and Britton, P.G. (1988). Factors affecting the emotional wellbeing of caregivers of dementia sufferers. *British Journal of Psychiatry*, **153**, 147–56.

Morris, R.G., Woods, R.T., Davies, K.S. *et al.* (1992). The use of a coping strategy focused support group for carers of dementia sufferers. *Counselling Psychology Quarterly*, **5** (4), 337–48

Morris, R.G., Woods, R.T., Davies, K.S. and Morris, L.W. (1991). Gender differences in carers of dementia sufferers. *British Journal of Psychiatry*, **158** (Suppl. 10): 69–74.

Niederehe, G. and Fruge, E. (1984). Dementia and family dynamics: clinical research issues. *Journal of Geriatric Psychiatry*, **17**, 21–56.

Pagel, M.D., Becker, J. and Coppel, D.B. (1985). Loss of control, self-blame and depression: an investigation of spouse caregivers of Alzheimer's disease patients. *Journal of Abnormal Psychology*, **94**, 169–82.

Pearlin and Schooler (1978).

Pearson, J., Verma, S. and Nellet, C. (1988). Elderly psychiatric patient status and caregiver perceptions as predictors of caregiver burden. *The Gerontologist*, **28**, 79–83.

Pfeiffer, E. (1979). A short psychiatric evaluation schedule: a new 15 item monotonic scale indicative of functional psychiatric disorder. In *Brain Function in Old Age*. Proceedings of Bayer Symposium VII. Springer, New York.

Poulshock, S.W. and Deimling, G.T. (1984). Families caring for elders in residence: issues in the measurement of burden. *Journal of Gerontology*, **39**, 230–9.

Pratt, C., Schmall, V., Wright, S. and Cleland, M. (1985). Burden and coping strategies of caregivers to Alzheimer's patients. *Family Relations*, **34**, 27–33.

Pruchno, R.A. and Resch, N.L. (1989). Aberrant behaviors and Alzheimer's disease: Mental health effects on spouse caregivers. *Journal of Gerontology*, **44**, 177–82.

Quayhagen, M.P. and Quayhagen, M. (1988). Alzheimer's stress: Coping with the caregiving role. *The Gerontologist*, **28**, 391–6.

Rabins, P.V., Mace, H.L. and Lucas, M.J. (1982). The impact of dementia on the family. *Journal of the American Medical Association*, **248**, 333–5.

Radloff, L. (1977). The CES-D scale: A self-report depression scale for research in the general population. *Applied Psychological Measurement*, **1**, 385–401.

Sanford, J.R.A. (1975). Tolerance of debility in elderly dependants by supporters at home: its significance for hospital practice. *British Medical Journal*, **iii**, 471–5.

Scharlach, A. and Frenzel, C. (1986). An evaluation of institution-based respite care. *The Gerontologist*, **26**, 77–82.

Schmidt, G.L. and Keyes, B. (1985). Group psychotherapy with family caregivers of dementia patients. *The Gerontologist*, **25**, 347–50.

Shibal-Champagne, S. and Lapinksa-Stachow, D.M. (1985/1986). Alzheimer's educational/support group: considerations for success – awareness of family tasks, pre-planning, and active professional facilitation. *Journal of Gerontological Social Work*, **9**, 41–8.

Spitzer, R., Endicott, J. and Robins, E. (1978). *Research Diagnostic Criteria for a Selected Group of Functional Disorders*. New York Psychiatric Institute.

Tobin, S. and Kulys, R. (1981). The family in the institutionalisation of the elderly. *Journal of Social Issues*, **37**, 145–57.

Toseland, T.W., Rossiter, C.M. and Labrecque, M.S. (1989). The effectiveness of peer-led groups to support family caregivers. *The Gerontologist*, **29**, 465–71.

Townsend, A., Noelker, L., Deimling, G. and Bass, D. (1989). Longitudinal impact of interhousehold caregiving on adult children's mental health. *Psychology and Aging*, **4**, 393–401.

Treas, J. (1977). Family support systems for the aged: Some social and demographic considerations. *The Gerontologist*, **17**, 486–91.

Waring, E.M., Tillman, M.P., Frelick, L. *et al.* (1980). Concepts of intimacy in the general population. *Journal of Nervous and Mental Diseases*, **168**, 471–4.

Wasow, M. (1985). Support groups for family caregivers of patients with Alzheimer's disease. *Social Work*, **31**, 93–7.

Wright, S.D., Lund, D.A., Pratt, C. and Caserta, M.S. (1987). *Coping and Caregiver Wellbeing: The Impact of Maladaptive Strategies or How Not to Make a Situation Worse*. Paper presented at the meeting of the Gerontological Society, Washington DC.

Zarit, S.H., Anthony, C.R. and Boutselis, M. (1987). Interventions with caregivers of dementia patients: Comparison of two approaches. *Psychology and Aging*, **2**, 225–32.

Zarit, S.H., Orr, N.K. and Zarit, J.M. (1985). *The Hidden Victims of Alzheimer's Disease: Families under Stress*. New York University Press, New York.

Zarit, S.H., Todd, P.A. and Zarit, J.M. (1986). Subjective burden of husbands and wives as caregivers: A longitudinal study. *The Gerontologist*, **20**, 260–6.

Zarit, S.H. and Zarit, J.M. (1982). Families under stress: interventions for caregivers of senile dementia patients. *Psychotherapy: Theory Research and Practice*, **19**, 461–71.

Zarit, S.H., Reever, K.E. and Bach-Peterson, J. (1980). Relatives of impaired elderly: correlates of feeling of burden. *The Gerontologist*, **20**, 649–55.

Hans Förstl

and

Walter Hewer

Central Institute of Mental Health
Mannheim

14 MEDICAL MORBIDITY IN ALZHEIMER'S DISEASE

MORTALITY AND MORBIDITY IN DEMENTIA: A REVIEW

Numerous studies have documented increased mortality in demented patients compared to nondemented controls (e.g. Christie, 1985; Martin *et al.*, 1987; Häfner and Bickel, 1989; van Dijk *et al.*, 1991). The life expectancy of demented patients admitted for inpatient treatment is reduced to 10% of nondemented controls (Go *et al.*, 1978). Patients may die from a variety of coexistent or coincidental diseases, for example, pneumonia or stroke, but they rarely seem to die as a 'direct' consequence of dementia in Alzheimer's disease, the most frequent form of dementia (Cummings and Benson, 1992).

Polymorbidity has been called the essential feature of geriatric medicine (Wertheimer, 1989), but this feature has attracted little attention in patients with senile or presenile dementia of the Alzheimer type. The term 'primary degenerative' dementia seems to imply that the disease is not related to other medical illnesses which exert a relevant influence on its development. A review of current literature about Alzheimer's disease seems to confirm this impression. Epidemiology, differential diagnosis, the development of new therapeutic strategies and molecular biology are in the focus of current interest. Potentially important pre-existing, concurrent or associated medical disease has only received marginal interest in a small number of recent publications. Previously healthy patients who develop an illness in late adulthood or old age could be part of a survival elite with a lower risk for internal medical illness. One recent US paper asked 'Are Alzheimer patients healthier?' and the answer was 'yes' (Wolf-Klein *et al.*, 1988). This question will be reconsidered in this contribution.

Pre-existing medical illness as a risk factor
It has been shown that mild cognitive impairment in the elderly is frequently associated with evidence of past 'biological life events', for example, present or past treatment for diseases with possible brain impact such as renal dysfunction or hypertension (Houx *et al.*, 1991). But, as stated by Larson *et al.* (1963), there is insufficient cause to assume that internal medical illness would exert any influence on the development of Alzheimer's disease. Epidemiological studies on risk factors for dementia have examined the importance of a large number of medical illnesses. The results are inconclusive and sometimes in disagreement (e.g. Table 14.1).

Infections and allergies
Tuberculosis or pyelonephritis have been discussed as risk factors for senile dementia of the Alzheimer type (Soininen and Heinonen, 1982) and were

Table 14.1 Odds ratios for frequently investigated medical disorders in patients with Alzheimer's disease and controls (case-control studies).

References	Number of cases	Odds ratios			
		Thyroid disease	Diabetes	Hayfever; allergies	Herpes zoster
Heyman et al. (1984)	40	3.5*	0.8		
French et al. (1985)	78	1.7	0.8	2.8; 0.8	
Amaducci et al. (1986)	116	0.2*–2.3†	0.7–1.0†	0.8–2.2†	0.6–1.3†
Chandra et al. (1987)	64	0.3			1.3
Shalat et al. (1987)	98	5.2	1.6	1.1 (all)	
Kokmen et al. (1991)	415	0.9	1.2		
Mendez et al. (1992)	407	1.8	0.7		
Breteler et al. (1991)‡		1.0		0.8; 0.9	0.9

* $P < 0.05$.
† Range between hospital-based and community samples.
‡ Meta-analysis of eight case-control studies.

rejected (Heyman et al., 1983; French et al., 1985; Dewey et al., 1988). Herpes zoster was reported to be significantly more frequent in a sample of patients developing Alzheimer's disease, but this result has not been reproduced (Heyman et al., 1983; Chandra et al., 1987). Genital herpes and allergic dermatitis were considered to be slightly more frequent in the history of patients with Alzheimer's disease, but not asthma or allergic rhinitis (Heyman et al. 1983; Amaducci et al., 1986). Also, the allegedly more frequent exposure to pets, particularly dogs (Amaducci et al., 1986), could not be confirmed (Dewey et al., 1988).

Endocrinology and nutrition
Compared to a control group, thyroid disease was significantly more frequent in patients with Alzheimer's disease (Heyman et al., 1983; Mendez et al., 1992), equally frequent (Thal et al., 1988) or less frequent (Amaducci et al., 1986). It was suggested that there was an inverse relationship between the occurrence of diabetes mellitus and Alzheimer's disease (Bucht et al., 1988), that the risk for diabetes in Alzheimer's disease was only slightly lower (Shalat et al., 1987; Mendez et al., 1992), unchanged (Soininen and Heinonen, 1982) or increased (Henderson, 1988).

It was claimed that smoking would increase the risk of developing Alzheimer's disease (Shalat et al., 1987), but the majority of reports could not find evidence to this effect (Heyman et al., 1983; French et al., 1985; Amaducci et al., 1986; Dewey et al., 1988). A recent meta-analysis has demonstrated an inverse relationship between smoking and the development of dementia (Graves et al., 1991). A large number of further nutritive toxic factors are currently under discussion (Henderson, 1988).

Cardio- and cerebrovascular disease
Most studies could not find any evidence for an increased frequency of hypertension in patients prior to developing Alzheimer's disease (Heyman et al., 1983; French et al., 1985; Dewey et al., 1988; Henderson, 1988). Henderson (1988) suggested that vascular brain changes, in particular vascular dementia, would increase the risk for Alzheimer-type changes. This hypothesis was based on the observation that the coincidence of reported vascular and Alzheimer-type changes in demented patients was significantly higher than would be

expected by chance (Tomlinson *et al.*, 1970; Kokmen *et al.*, 1987; Wade *et al.*, 1987; Boller *et al.*, 1989). A potential relationship between vascular disease and Alzheimer-type changes is suggested further by the observation that 75% of the nondemented patients dying from critical coronary artery disease had abundant cortical senile plaques compared to only 15% of patients dying of other illnesses (Sparks *et al.*, 1990).

The resumé of these epidemiological studies appears modest. Only seemingly trivial results stood the test of time: age and familial disposition were largely confirmed as risk factors (Heyman *et al.*, 1983; Henderson, 1988). Marginal and probably chance findings proved highly significant in individual investigations: headache and vertigo decreased the risk of developing dementia (Dewey *et al.*, 1988), prostatectomy would be more frequent in men with Alzheimer's disease (Wolf-Klein *et al.*, 1988) etc. The question whether there was a plausible pathogenic role for internal medical illnesses in the development of Alzheimer's disease has been examined in numerous studies but none of the hypotheses raised has been generally confirmed. A meta-analysis of eight case-control studies yielded odds ratios near to 1 for frequently examined potential risk factors (Breteler *et al.*, 1991; Table 14.1). This does not indicate meaningful interactions between individual medical diseases and the development of dementia.

Coexisting medical disease and causes of death
The notion of better health in patients with Alzheimer's disease was based on a retrospective study (Wolf-Klein *et al.*, 1988): in comparison with another patient sample seen in an outpatient clinic, patients with Alzheimer's disease had a smaller number of diagnoses (three compared to five) and received a smaller number of prescribed drugs (on average less than 2 compared to 2.8). These results have to be questioned in view of the methodological drawbacks of the study (retrospective examination, unspecified control group).

Infection and inflammation
Case control studies have shown that Alzheimer patients had a significantly higher rate of pneumonia and other infections of the upper airways, septicaemia, cystitis and kidney infection. The use of indwelling urinary catheters in incontinent patients is one cause for these infections. The increased rate of wounds of the head, trunk, shoulders and arms is caused by more frequent falls, and these are related to sensory and motor disturbances (Spanó and Förstl, 1992). A significantly increased rate of trophic ulcers was found consistently (Chandra *et al.*, 1986b; Henderson, 1988; Mölsä *et al.*, 1986).

Nutrition and metabolism
Compared to patients with other diagnoses, patients with Alzheimer's disease have a lower body weight and lose a greater percentage of their weight after admission to a hospital or nursing home (Fisman *et al.*, 1988; Singh *et al.*, 1988; Thal *et al.*, 1988; Burns *et al.*, 1989a). On clinical examination, they show thin, light hair, cheilosis, atrophic tongue or skin wounds with a poor healing tendency (Chandra *et al.*, 1986b; Burns *et al.*, 1989a). It has been shown in a controlled study that these changes are not related to obvious disturbances of vitamin, electrolyte or energy metabolism. They occurred in spite of the patients' improved dietary intake with improved amounts of calories, protein, vitamins and minerals and may be due to gastrointestinal malabsorption (Abalan, 1984; Bucht *et al.*, 1988; Burns *et al.*, 1989a). Vice versa, the alteration of a glucose/insulin interaction could be the consequence of rather than the

cause of the weight loss in Alzheimer's disease (Fisman *et al.*, 1988). Moreover, diabetes mellitus has been described in up to 20% of patients with Alzheimer's disease (Heyman *et al.*, 1983; French *et al.*, 1985; Shalat *et al.*, 1987). There are no consistent results regarding a higher (Small *et al.*, 1985) or lower rate of thyroid illness in Alzheimer's disease (Thal *et al.*, 1988; Wolf-Klein *et al.*, 1988; Table 14.1).

Neurosensory and vegetative disturbances
Hearing impairment, cataract and glaucoma are more frequent in Alzheimer's disease than in nondemented controls (Kay, 1962; Chandra *et al.*, 1986b). The visual field becomes increasingly limited in patients with advance Alzheimer's disease (Steffes and Thralow, 1987). The processing of accoustic stimuli is disturbed at the peripheral (Peters *et al.*, 1988) and central levels (Rapcsak *et al.*, 1989). It has been shown that hearing impairment is a predictor of more severe cognitive decline (e.g. Peters *et al.*, 1988).

Impaired vision and hearing can contribute to the 'sundowning' phenomenon, i.e. increased confusion and agitation in the evening hours and at night. Neurovegetative dysregulation represents another cause for this disturbance. Patients with Alzheimer's disease show an increased apnoea index. These disturbances were directly related to the development of nocturnal confusional states (Hoch *et al.*, 1989).

Cause of death
The term 'cause of death' has been subject to different interpretations. Some authors have considered Alzheimer's disease in itself as a cause of death (Mölsä *et al.*, 1986), whereas others have only taken the immediate causes of death into consideration, i.e. the acute events, for example, of acute pneumonia or septicaemia (Chandra *et al.*, 1986b). According to Kay and Roth (1955), cerebral degeneration is the primary cause of death in dementia and leads to death from 'nonspecific' causes (i.e. bronchopneumonia, circulatory disorders other than myocardial infarcation and dementia *per se*) as opposed to 'specific' causes of death (e.g. myocardial infarction, malignancy and others). Certain psychiatric phenomena may determine increased mortality in Alzheimer's disease (Förstl *et al.*, 1993).

Airway infections have been reported consistently as the most frequent cause of death in Alzheimer's disease accounting for up to 70% of the cases (Sulkava *et al.*, 1983; Chandra *et al.*, 1986b; Mölsä *et al.*, 1986; Burns *et al.*, 1990). Disturbances of swallowing, altered eating habits and an impaired immunological status have been considered as the most likely causes of these frequent and fatal airway infections (Sulkava *et al.*, 1983; Mölsä *et al.*, 1983). Pulmonary artery embolism from deep venous thrombosis, acute cerebral or cardiovascular events or consequences of peripheral arterial illness have been identified as causes of death in 5% or more of the patients (Kay, 1962; Sulkava *et al.*, 1983; Chandra *et al.*, 1986b; Mölsä *et al.*, 1986; Hewer *et al.*, 1991). Malignant disorders account for less than 10% of the deaths in patients with Alzheimer's disease and this is less than in the general population. This does not indicate a 'protective' effect of Alzheimer's disease against malignant disorders, as life expectancy in patients with Alzheimer's disease is significantly reduced (Sulkava *et al.*, 1983; Chandra *et al.*, 1986a, b; Mölsä *et al.*, 1986). There is agreement between different studies regarding the pattern of mortality in dementia (Alstrom, 1942; Kay, 1962; Ryan, 1992): 'nonspecific' causes of death are consistently more frequent in dementia, whereas 'specific' causes of death are less common than in the general population.

MEDICAL ILLNESS IN NEUROPATHOLOGICALLY VERIFIED ALZHEIMER'S DISEASE, VASCULAR DEMENTIA AND OTHER FORMS OF DEMENTIA

Patients and methods

We have recently assessed the medical histories and *post-mortems* of 60 demented patients. Alzheimer's disease was verified neuropathologically in 30 patients (8 male; 22 female; mean age 80.1 years; mean duration of illness 7.9 years). Twenty patients suffered from vascular dementia (5 male; 15 female; age 82.9 years; duration of illness 5.5 years) and a group of 10 patients had other forms of dementia (Lewy body dementia, progressive supranuclear palsy; 5 male; 5 female; 71.8 years; duration of illness 5.1 years). A full hospital *post-mortem* examination was performed in every case. The brains were examined extensively according to current practice in the Medical Research Council's Alzheimer's Disease Brain Bank at the Institute of Psychiatry in London, UK (Förstl *et al.*, 1991; 1992). Statistical differences between the diagnostic groups were examined using the Kruskal-Wallis Test.

Results

Alzheimer patients received treatment for an average of 2.0 medical diseases [standard deviation (S.D.) 1.1] and patients with vascular dementia for 2.1 diseases (S.D. 1.1). The most frequent medical diseases diagnosed during life are listed in Table 14.2. No significant differences were found between the different diagnostic groups.

The most frequent *post-mortem* findings are given in Table 14.3. The numbers of clinically and pathologically diagnosed chronic medical diseases were similar in neuropathologically proven Alzheimer's disease, in vascular dementia and in the group with other forms of dementia.

Pneumonia was the most frequent cause of death in all dementia groups, followed by myocardial infarction and septicaemia (Table 14.4). No significant differences were found between the groups.

Discussion

The finding of a higher proportion of occlusive peripheral arterial disease in vascular dementia is in keeping with earlier results (Tresch *et al.*, 1985; Erkinjuntti, 1987; Thal *et al.*, 1988). Several investigations have shown that

Table 14.2 Frequently diagnosed medical diseases in samples of patients with neuropathologically verified Alzheimer's disease, vascular dementia and other forms of dementia: no significant differences were found between the different groups of dementia.

	Alzheimer's disease	Vascular dementia	Other forms of dementia
n	30	20	10
Cardiovascular disease			
Hypertension	3	3	2
Cardiac disease	7	6	2
Metabolic disease			
Diabetes	4	3	—
Hypothyroidism	2	2	—
Upper respiratory infection	14	6	5
Malignant disease	3	3	1

Table 14.3 Most frequent *post-mortem* findings.

	Alzheimer's disease	Vascular dementia	Other dementias	P
Cardiovascular disease				
Coronary artery disease	14	10	2	*
Peripheral arterial occlusive disease	11	13	3	†
Myocardial infarction	7	3	—	n.s.
Myocardial dilatation	4	3	1	n.s.
Myocardial hypertrophy	3	4	1	n.s.
Bronchopneumonia	6	5	1	n.s.
Kidney disease	9	4	2	n.s.
Thyroid enlargement	4	2	2	n.s.

*$P < 0.05$ for the comparison of vascular dementia versus the other dementias.
†$P < 0.10$ for the comparison of Alzheimer's disease versus vascular dementia.
n.s. = not significant.

cardiovascular disorders can also occur in a signficiant number of Alzheimer patients (Tresch *et al.*, 1985; Thal *et al.*, 1988). However, other clinical investigations claim that Alzheimer's disease, in contrast to vascular dementia, would be characterized by the absence of cardiovascular disorders (Erkinjuntti, 1987).

The discrepancy between our results and some of the earlier clinical and epidemiological studies, which relied on strict clinical criteria for the intravital diagnosis of probable dementia of the Alzheimer type (McKhann *et al.*, 1984), can be explained by a selection artefact: in clinical studies, demented patients who show additional evidence of cardiovascular disorders or other conditions which might cause cognitive impairment, cannot be classified as suffering from probable Alzheimer's disease. In practice, this approach may lead to an underestimation of relevant general medical disorders in patients with a specialist diagnosis of probable Alzheimer's disease.

Our results regarding the causes of death (Table 14.4) are in agreement with previous data (Sulkava *et al.*, 1983; Mölsä *et al.*, 1986). Pneumonia represented the most frequent cause of death accounting for 50% or more of the cases in the three groups investigated. Irrespective of the underlying diagnosis of dementia, this was followed by acute myocardial infarction and septicaemia.

CONCLUSIONS

The *literature review* has shown consistent evidence for an increased mortality in patients with dementia compared to nondemented controls. The most frequent diseases leading to death are 'nonspecific', for example, broncho-

Table 14.4 The most frequent causes of death: no significant differences were found between the different dementia groups.

	Alzheimer's disease	Vascular dementia	Other dementias	P
Pneumonia	17 (57%)	10 (50%)	6 (60%)	n.s.
Myocardial infarction	4 (13%)	3 (15%)	1 (10%)	n.s.
Septicaemia	1 (3%)	1 (5%)	—	n.s.

n.s. = not significant.

pneumonia or other complications of dementia, which have been considered the primary cause of death. There is no agreement about certain medical disorders acting as risk factors for the development of Alzheimer's disease or about the relative risk of specific internal medical diseases occurring together with Alzheimer's disease. An increased prevalence of neurosensory or vegetative disturbances in Alzheimer's disease has been demonstrated by several authors.

The total numbers of clinically or pathologically diagnosed medical disorders in our *clinicopathologic study* did not show significant differences between the different forms of dementia. Metabolic, infectious, degenerative and malignant disorders were found with similar frequency in all groups investigated. Cardiovascular diseases were only slightly more common in patients with vascular dementia than in patients suffering from Alzheimer's disease or other forms of dementia. In contrast to several earlier clinical or epidemiological studies, it has to be concluded that patients with Alzheimer's dementia cannot be considered physically healthier than patients with other forms of dementia. They need more medical attention than other elderly patients because they are less able to report their symptoms. We suggest that the erroneous concept of a relatively well-preserved medical condition in Alzheimer's disease results from a selection artefact which is due to strict diagnostic criteria developed for scientific studies.

REFERENCES

Abalan, F. (1984). Alzheimer's disease and malnutrition: a new aetiological hypothesis. *Medical Hypothesis*, **15**, 385.

Alstrom, C.H. (1942). Mortality in mental hospitals with a special regard to tuberculosis. *Acta Psychiatrica Scandinavica* (Suppl. 24).

Amaducci, L.A., Fratiglioni, L., Rocca, W.A. *et al.* (1986). Risk factors for clinically diagnosed alzheimer's dementia: a case-control study of an Italian population. *Neurology (Minneap.)*, **36**, 922–31.

Boller, F., Lopez, O.L. and Moossy, J. (1989). Diagnosis of dementia: clinico-pathologic correlations. *Neurology (Minneap.)*, **39**, 76–9.

Breteler, M.M.B., van Duijn, C.M., Chandra, V. *et al.* (1991). Medical history and the risk of Alzheimer's disease: a collaborative re-analysis of case-control studies. *International Journal Epidemiology*, **20**, S36–S42.

Bucht, G., Adolfsson, R., Lithner, F. and Winblad, B. (1988). Changes in blood glucose and insulin secretion in patients with senile dementia of the Alzheimer type. *Acta Medica Scandinavica*, **213**, 387–92.

Burns, A., Jacoby, R., Luthert, P. and Levy, R. (1990). Cause of death in Alzheimer's disease. *Age and Ageing*, **19**, 341–4.

Burns, A., Marsh, A. and Bender, D.A. (1989a). Dietary intake and clinical, anthropometric and biochemical indices of malnutrition in elderly demented patients and non-demented subjects. *Psychological Medicine*, **19**, 383–91.

Burns, A., Marsh, A. and Bender, D.A. (1989b). A trial of vitamin supplementation in senile dementia. *International Journal of Geriatric Psychiatry*, **4**, 383–91.

Chandra, V., Bharucha, N.E. and Schoenberg, B.S. (1986a). Patterns of mortality from types of dementia in the United States, 1971 and 1973–1978. *Neurology (Minneap.)*, **36**, 204–8.

Chandra, V., Bharucha, N.E. and Schoenberg, B.S. (1986b). Conditions associated with Alzheimer's disease at death: case control study. *Neurology (Minneap.)*, **36**, 204–8.

Chandra, V., Philipose, V., Bell, P.A. *et al.* (1987). Case-control study of late onset probable Alzheimer's disease. *Neurology,* **37,** 1295–1300.

Christie, A.B. (1985). Survival in dementia: a review. In *Recent Advances in Psychogeriatrics,* Arie, T. (Ed.). Churchill Livingstone, Edinburgh.

Cummings, J.L. and Benson, D.F. (1992). *Dementia, A Clinical Approach.* Butterworth–Heinemmann, Oxford, Stoneham MA.

van Dijk, P.T.M., Dippel, D.W.J. and Habbema, J.D.F. (1991). Survival of patients with dementia. *Journal of the American Geriatrics Society,* **39,** 603–10.

Dewey, M.E., Davidson, I.A. and Copeland, J.R.M. (1988). Risk factors for dementia: evidence from the Liverpool study of continuing health in the community. *International Journal of Geriatric Psychiatry,* **3,** 245–9.

Erkinjuntti, T. (1987). Differential diagnosis between Alzheimer's disease and vascular dementia: evaluation of common clinical methods. *Acta Neurologica Scandinavica,* **76,** 433–42.

Fisman, M., Gordon, B., Feleki, V. *et al.* (1988). Metabolic changes in Alzheimer's dementia. *Journal of the American Geriatrics Society,* **36,** 298–300.

Förstl, H., Burns, A., Luthert, P. and Cairns, N. (1991). Dementia and internal medical illness: a comparison of Alzheimer's disease, vascular dementia and other dementing disorders. *Zeitschrift Gerontologie,* **24,** 91–3.

Förstl, H., Burns, A., Levy, R. *et al,* (1992). Neurologic signs in Alzheimer's disease: results of a prospective clinical and neuropathologic study. *Archives of Neurology,* **49,** 1038–42.

Förstl, H., Besthorn, C., Geiger-Kabisch C. *et al.* (1993). Psychotic feature and the course of Alzheimer's disease: relationship to cognitive electroencephalographic and computerized tomography findings. *Acta Psychiatrica Scandinavica* (in press).

French, L.R., Schuman, L.M., Mortimer, J.A. *et al.* (1985). A case-control study of dementia of the Alzheimer type. *American Journal of Epidemiology,* **121,** 414–21.

Go, R.C.P., Todorov, A.B., Elston, R.C. and Constantinidis, J. (1978). The malignancy of dementias. *Annals of Neurology,* **3,** 559–61.

Graves, A.B., van Duijn, C.M. and Chandra, V. (1991). Alcohol and tobacco consumption as risk factors for Alzheimer's disease: a collaborative re-analysis of case-control studies. *International Journal of Epidemiology,* **20** (Suppl. 1), 548–57.

Häfner, H. and Bickel, H. (1988). Physical morbidity and mortality in psychiatric patients. In *Interaction between Mental and Physical Illness,* Öhman, R. (Ed.), pp. 29–47, Springer, New York.

Henderson, A. (1988). The risk factors for Alzheimer's disease; a review and a hypothesis. *Acta Psychiatrica Scandinavica,* **78,** 257–75.

Hewer, W., Rössler, W., Fätkenheuer, B. and Jung, E. (1991). Mortalität von Patienten mit organisch bedingten psychischen Störungen während des Zeitraums stationärer Behandlung. *Nervenarzt,* **62,** 170–6.

Heyman, A., Wilkinson, W.E. and Hurwitz, B.J. (1983). Alzheimer's disease: genetic aspects and associated clinical disorders. *Annals of Neurology,* **14,** 507–15.

Heyman, A., Wilkinson, W.E., Stafford, J.A. *et al.* (1984). Alzheimer's disease: a study of epidemiologic aspects. *Annals of Neurology,* **15,** 335–41.

Hoch, C.C., Reynolds, C.F., Nebes, R.D. *et al.* (1989). Clinical significance of sleep disordered breathing in Alzheimer's disease: preliminary data. *Journal of the American Geriatrics Society,* **37,** 139–44.

Houx, P.J., Vreeling, F.W. and Jolles, J. (1991). Age-associated cognitive decline is related to biological life events. In *Alzheimer's Disease: Basic Mechanisms, Diagnosis and Therapeutic Strategies*, Iqbal, K., McLaghlan, D.R.C., Winblad, B. and Wisnewski, H.M. Eds). John Wiley & Sons Ltd, Chichester.

Kay, D.W.K. (1962). Outcome and cause of death in mental disorders of old age: a long-term follow-up of functional and organic psychoses. *Acta Psychiatrica Scandinavica*, **38**, 249–76.

Kay, D.W.K. and Roth, M. (1955). Physical accompaniments of mental disorder in old age. *Lancet*, **ii**, 740–5.

Kokmen, E., Offord, K.P. and Okazaki, H. (1987). A clinical and autopsy study of dementia in Olmsted County, Minnesota, 1980–81. *Neurology (Minneap.)*, **37**, 426–30.

Kokmen, E., Beard, C.M., Chandra, V. *et al.* (1991). Clinical risk factor's for Alzheimer's disease: a case control study. *Neurology*, **41**, 1393–7.

Larson, T., Sjögren, T. and Jacobson, G. (1963). Senile dementia: a clinical, sociomedical and genetic study. *Acta Psychiatrica Scandinavica*, **167** (Suppl.), 1–259.

Martin, D.C., Miller, J.K., Kapoor, W. *et al.* (1987). A controlled study of survival with dementia. *Archives of Neurology*, **44**, 1122–6.

McKhann, G., Drachman, D., Folstein, M. *et al.* (1984). Clinical diagnosis of Alzheimer's disease: report of the NINCDS–ADRDA work group under the auspices of Department of Health and Human Services Task Force on Alzheimer's disease. *Neurology (Minneap.)*, **34**, 939–44.

Mendez, M.F., Underwood, K.L., Zander, B.A. *et al.* (1992). Risk factors in Alzheimer's disease: a clinicopathologic study. *Neurology*, **42**, 770–5.

Mölsä, P.K., Marttila, R.J. and Rinne, U.K. (1986). Survival and cause of death in Alzheimer's disease and multi-infarct dementia. *Acta Neurologica Scandinavica*, **69** (Suppl. 98), 103–7.

Peters, C.A., Potter, J.F. and Scholer, S.G. (1988). Hearing impairment as a predictor of cognitive decline in dementia. *Journal of the American Geriatrics Society*, **36**, 981–6.

Rapcsak, S.Z., Kentros, M. and Rubens, A.B. (1989). Impaired recognition of meaningful sounds in Alzheimer's disease. *Archives of Neurology*, **46**, 1298–300.

Ryan, D.H. (1992). Death in dementia: a study of causes of death in dementia patients and their spouses. *International Journal of Geriatrica Psychiatrica*, **7**, 465–72.

Shalat, S.L., Seltzer, B., Pidcock, C. and Baker, E.L. (1987). Risk factors for Alzheimer's disease: a case control study. *Neurology (Minneap.)*, **37**, 1630–3.

Singh, S., Mulley, G.P. and Losowsky, M.S. (1988). Why are Alzheimer patients thin? *Age and Aging*, **17**, 21–18.

Small, G.W., Matsuyama, S.S. and Komanduri, R. (1985). Thyroid disease in patients with dementia of the Alzheimer type. *American Journal of Geriatrics Society*, **33**, 538–9.

Soininen, H. and Heinonen, O.P. (1982). Clinical and etiological aspects of senile dementia. *European Neurology*, **21**, 401–10.

Spanó, A. and Förstl, H. (1992). Falling and the fear of it. *International Journal of Geriatric Psychiatry*, **7**, 149–51.

Sparks, D.L., Hunsaker III, J.C., Scheff, S.W. *et al.* (1990). Cortical senile plaques in coronary artery disease, aging and Alzheimer's disease. *Neurobiology of Aging*, **11**, 601–7.

Steffes, R. and Thralow, J. (1987). Visual field limitation in the patient with dementia of the Alzheimer's type. *Journal of the American Geriatrics Society*, **35**, 198–204.

Sulkava, R., Haltia, M., Paetau, A. *et al.* (1983). Accuracy of clinical diagnosis in primary degenerative dementia: correlation with neuropathological findings. *Journal of Neurology, Neurosurgery and Psychiatry*, **46**, 9–13.

Thal, L.J., Grundman, M. and Klauber, M.R. (1988). Dementia: characteristics of referral population and factors associated with progression. *Neurology (Minneap.)*, **38**, 1083–90.

Tomlinson, B., Blessed, G. and Roth, M. (1970). Observations on the brains of demented old people. *Journal of Neurological Science*, **11**, 205–42.

Tresch, D.D., Folstein, M.F., Rabins, P.V. and Hazzard, W.R. (1985). Prevalence and significance of cardiovascular diseases and hypertension in elderly patients with dementia and depression. *Journal of the American Geriatrics Society*, **33**, 530–7.

Wade, J.P.H., Mirsen, T.R., Hachinski, V.C. *et al.* (1987). The clinical diagnosis of Alzheimer's disease. *Archives of Neurology*, **44**, 24–9.

Wertheimer, J. (1988). Polymorbidity. In *Psychiatrie der Gegenwart*, Vol. 8, Kisker, K.P. *et al.* (Eds). Springer, Berlin.

Wolf-Klein, G.P., Silverstone, F.A., Brod, M.S. *et al.* (1988). Are Alzheimer patients healthier? *Journal of the American Geriatrics Society*, **36**, 219–44.

INDEX

effect on memory 203
Gegenhalten 152, 153, 156
  as function of global deterioration
    scale 163
  examination 156
Genes
  longevity assurance 21, 33
Genetics of dementia 51
Geriatric Mental Status Schedule 1, 6,
  44, 45, 225
Gerontogenes 33
Glabellar blink reflex 151, 152, 153, 155
  examination of 159
Glaucoma 278
Glial fibrillary acidic protein 186
Global Deterioration Scale (GDS) 67, 104,
  160, 168, 169
  reflexes as function of 162, 163, 164,
    165, 166
Glucose metabolism 117
Glutamate in Alzheimer's disease 194,
  209
Glycation
  metabolic effects of 29
Grasp reflex 149, 153, 155, 167
Growth factors 184, 185

Hand grasp reflex 151, 152, et seq 158
Head injury
  Alzheimer's disease and 51
Hearing impairment 76, 278
Heart disease 52
Heat-shock response 31
Hepatitis 206
Herpes zoster 276
Hippocampal atrophy
  as Alzheimer's disease marker 121
  cognitive impairment and 118, 121
  in normal ageing 103, 107
  in normal pressure hydrocephalus 118
  symmetry of in Alzheimer's disease
    110
Hippocampus
  cross-sectional studies 106
  GABA in 195
  glutamate in 195
  in Huntington's disease 177
  MRI in 107, 109, 110, 114–6
  neuroimaging in 104
  noradrenaline in 194
  positron emission tomography 116–8
  post-mortem studies 119
  reflexes in 145
  role in memory 118
  transverse fissure 105, 114, 115
History and Aetiology Schedule 45
Home care 241
Hughes Hall Project for Later Life 240
Hydrocephalus
  hippocampal atrophy in 118
5-Hydroxytryptamine
  aggression and 232
Hypertension 275
Hypothyroidism 13, 52

Incontinence 137
  in Alzheimer's disease 77
Infections 278
  as risk factors 275, 277
Informant Questionnaire on Cognitive
    Decline in the Elderly 44
Information Memory Concentration Test
  71
Information processing
  loss of 65
Isopeptides 26

Kendrick Object Learning Test 89
Kent Community Care Scheme 239
Korsakoff syndrome 94, 198, 208

Language
  in Alzheimer's disease 73, 76, 105
Lecithin in Alzheimer's disease 205
Lectins 188
Lewisham Case Management Scheme
  240
Lewy bodies 179
Lewy body dementia 4, 5
  compared with other dementias 6
  ubiquitinated proteins in 35, 36
Life-span 21
Lipofuscin 25, 179
Longevity assurance genes 21, 34
Lorazepam 204

Magnetic resonance imaging 107, 109,
  110, 114–6, 232
Maillard reaction 29
Memory
  acetylcholine and 197
  age-associated impairment 160
  in Alzheimer's disease 73, 105
  benzodiazepine affecting 203
  catecholamines and 203–4
  cholinergic blockade affecting 198,
    199, 200, 201
  effect of drugs on 193–220
  GABA affecting 203
  5HT and 209
  relation to attention deficits 201
  role of hippocampus 118
  role of neurotransmitters in 197
  scopolamine affecting 197, 201
  vasopressin affecting 203
Memory and Behaviour Problems
    Checklist 228
Memory impairment 93, 162
Meningitis 52
Meta-analysis 12
Metabolism
  Alzheimer's disease and 277
Methylphenidate 209
Microglia 188
Mini Mental State Examinations (MMSE)
  11, 42, 43, 65, 71, 73, 89, 104, 109,
    135, 206
Mitochondria
  DNA in 23
  role in ageing process 25, 27